Student Success in the Prescribing Safety Assessment (PSA)

VILIUS SAVICKAS
MPharm, MRPharmS, CertGPP
Senior Clinical Pharmacist
Surrey and Sussex Healthcare NHS Trust

and

REEM KAYYALI
PhD, MSc, BPharm, MRPharmS
Principal Lecturer, School of Pharmacy and Chemistry
Kingston University

Edited by

DR NEEL SHARMA
BSc (Hons), MBChB, MSc, MRCP (UK)
National University Hospital
Singapore

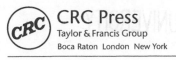

CRC Press
Taylor & Francis Group
Boca Raton London New York

CRC Press is an imprint of the
Taylor & Francis Group, an **informa** business

Radcliffe Publishing Ltd
St Mark's House
Shepherdess Walk
London N1 7BQ
United Kingdom

www.radcliffehealth.com

British Library Cataloguing in Publication Data

A catalogue record for this book is available from the British Library.

ISBN-13: 978 184619 978 3

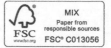

Typeset by Darkriver Design, Auckland, New Zealand

Contents

Contents

About the Authors

Vilius Savickas, MPharm, MRPharmS, CertGPP

Vilius is a Senior Clinical Pharmacist at Surrey and Sussex Healthcare NHS Trust. He is a former Future Pharmacist Editor, Educational Development Officer and Honorary Life Member of the British Pharmaceutical Students' Association (BPSA). Vilius continues to support BPSA by coordinating the Facebook Group 'Professional Development Matters!' for students and pre-registration trainees. He has also recently initiated the 'Buddy Scheme' and the Foundation Pharmacist Forum for postgraduate pharmacists in Kent, Surrey and Sussex regions.

Dr Reem Kayyali, PhD, MSc, BPharm, MRPharmS

Reem graduated from Nottingham University with a bachelor degree in pharmacy. She then undertook a Master of Science in Biopharmacy at King's College London and then a PhD related to the use of iron chelators in the management of thalassaemia. She was then awarded the Mapplethorpe Fellowship for 2 years at King's College London to conduct research related to redox activity and apoptosis by iron chelators. After that, she worked as a research fellow at University College London Medical School. The reforms that the pharmacy profession has witnessed in the last decade were the driver for her to make a career transition from pure scientific research to an academic post focusing on pharmacy practice and clinical pharmacy. In 2006, she joined the School of Pharmacy and Chemistry at Kingston University as a senior lecturer working within the clinical and pharmacy practice team. In 2010, she was promoted to Principal Lecturer, acting as part of her role as the pharmacy practice/clinical pharmacy subject area lead. She is a registered pharmacist with the General Pharmaceutical Council and is a member of the Royal Pharmaceutical Society.

Neel Sharma (Editor)

Neel Sharma graduated from The University of Manchester with bachelor degrees in pharmacology and medicine. He also holds a Master of

Science in Gastroenterology from Barts and The London School of Medicine and Dentistry. Neel undertook his foundation and core medical training in London and maintains a strong interest in medical education. He was appointed Clinical Lecturer at the Centre for Medical Education at Barts in 2011, and he previously held the position of Tutor at the Institute of Medical and Health Sciences Education, Li Ka Shing Faculty of Medicine, The University of Hong Kong, from 2012 to 2013. He is also a member of the Curriculum Development Team for the newly established Lee Kong Chian School of Medicine in Singapore.

I would like to dedicate this book to all my colleagues at East Surrey Hospital, particularly those within the pharmacy department. Thank you very much for all your help and support over the last two years. I feel honoured having been a part of such an incredible team.

VS

I would like to dedicate this book to my lovely children; Hala and Sammy, my mum, Samira and my husband, Khaled. Thank you for your continuous love and support all through the years.

RK

I would like to dedicate this book to my parents, Ravi and Anita, and my sister Ravnita. Without their continued support and encouragement none of this would have truly been possible.

NS

Introduction

THE PRESCRIBING SAFETY ASSESSMENT

Medical students are subject to robust training in a variety of disciplines ranging from anatomy and pathophysiology to law and psychology. However, it is widely recognised that current medical degrees in the UK incorporate a limited amount of training in clinical pharmacy/pharmacology and prescribing,[1] yet junior doctors are often responsible for the majority of routine prescribing practice.

Junior house officers' prescribing has been associated with more than half of all the prescribing errors among the medical practitioners of different grades in hospitals, as opposed to only 2% by medical consultants.[2] Furthermore, the EQUIP study, 'An in depth investigation into causes of prescribing errors by foundation trainees in relation to their medical education' carried out by the General Medical Council (GMC) in 2009, demonstrated that prescribing errors were twice as common among the Foundation Year 1 (FY1) and Foundation Year 2 (FY2) doctors as compared to consultants. It was obvious that junior doctors may not have been capable of meeting the prescribing-related expectations fully from day one of their independent practice.

The GMC responded with *Tomorrow's Doctors* (2009), outlining a number of competencies for medical graduates that should be achieved before they qualify.[3] The document included eight competencies relating to good practice in prescribing, to ensure that graduates are able to prescribe drugs 'safely, effectively and economically'.[3] There is no formal prescribing assessment across the UK to ensure that all graduates are at the same level of competence required to enter their prescribing practice. As a result, the Prescribing Safety Assessment (PSA) was proposed by the Medical Schools Council (MSC) and the British Pharmacological Society (BPS) to help medical graduates achieve these learning outcomes before they are released into the real world.[4]

The PSA has been defined as the 'pass/fail, summative examination of the skills, judgment and supporting knowledge related to prescribing medicines in the NHS'.[4] The content of the assessment maps into prescribing competencies indicated by the GMC and is intended to test knowledge in the following areas:

- prescribing
- prescription review
- planning management
- communicating information
- calculation skills
- adverse drug reactions
- drug monitoring
- data interpretation.[3,4]

Candidates will have to demonstrate their ability to meet these competencies across a range of clinical domains, including:

- medicine
- surgery
- elderly care
- paediatrics
- psychiatry
- obstetrics and gynaecology
- general practice.[3,4]

The PSA is a two-hour open-book online examination which comprises eight sections based on eight main types of peer-reviewed questions (as indicated by the areas of knowledge already mentioned). Students are allowed to use the *British National Formulary* (BNF) and a calculator (provided as part of PSA interface). Questions are structured around certain clinical case-based scenarios and require the candidate to employ a holistic approach to analysing information provided before identifying suitable answers.[5]

Despite the development of this assessment being almost in its final stages, there are currently limited resources and support for students who are expected to sit the actual assessment in 2013–14. At the moment such resources include Prescribe, an online e-learning platform developed by the BPS and MSC,[6] and any additional individual support students may receive within their medical school.

AIMS AND STRUCTURE OF THIS BOOK

Student Success in the Prescribing Safety Assessment is designed specifically to meet the professional development needs of the PSA candidates as well as the prescribing competencies outlined by the GMC. This book provides a bank of 150 open-book case-based scenarios. The questions are based on the clinical domains and areas of knowledge to be tested in the PSA. Although specifically designed for final year medical students, this book is also likely to benefit other students and healthcare professionals who wish to improve their prescribing skills and clinical pharmacy knowledge, such as pharmacy students, pharmacists undertaking a postgraduate qualification, or healthcare professionals training to become supplementary or independent prescribers.

Working through this bank of questions should enable PSA candidates and other students or healthcare professionals to:
- understand and learn the questioning techniques used during the assessment
- appreciate the principles used in clinical pharmacy and pharmaceutical care
- develop the skills and knowledge required to conduct an effective clinical review of a patient's pharmaceutical care
- enhance their knowledge of clinical pharmacology and pharmacokinetics of commonly used medicines
- improve their prescribing clinical decision-making skills
- enhance their ability to extract correct clinical information from the BNF in a timely fashion
- become familiar with the main evidence-based prescribing guidelines and prescribing information – e.g. National Institute for Health and Care Excellence (NICE), British Thoracic Society, European Society of Cardiology, numerous peer-reviewed articles, Medusa Injectable Medicines Guide and primary care databases (e.g. NICE Clinical Knowledge Summaries)
- overall, improve their ability to prescribe safely, effectively and cost-effectively.

Student Success in the Prescribing Safety Assessment is divided into eight chapters according to the eight prescribing competencies to be assessed as part of the PSA (*see* Table 1). The proportions of these chapters have been designed to match the outline of the assessment. For instance, since the prescribing section of the PSA is worth as much as 80 out of the total 200 marks, Chapter 1 is by far the largest and contains 48 prescribing questions, which are based on four templates proposed by the MSC and the BPS.

Each scenario also relates to one or more of the seven clinical domains indicated above (i.e. medicine, surgery, etc.). Considering the spectrum of activities faced by FY1 doctors, the main clinical domains covered in this book are medicine, surgery and elderly care. However, other clinical domains, such as paediatrics and psychiatry, are also integrated in adequate proportions (*see* Table 1). The answers to each question are provided in the Answers section near the back of the book and are grouped by chapter.

This publication adopts the structure of questions used during the PSA pilot and available on the website. At the time of publication of this volume, there was a slight alteration to the question style for Chapters 3, 4, 6 and 7. These now only require you to choose the single most appropriate option. From the exam perspective this makes the process of question answering much easier. We have, however, maintained the inclusion of choosing the two most appropriate answers. This will benefit you in terms of revision and will help mimic the real-life situation whereby prescribers are often required to develop a strategy of more than one action in order to achieve a favourable outcome for the patient. It is of course not possible to emulate the exam in its entirety and we wanted to ensure that a prescribing relevant resource was available in sufficient time to help ease the strain of revision during what is already a compact year.

In addition to the main eight chapters, the publication also contains four appendices. Appendix 1 includes the templates of prescriptions that are to be used when answering the questions presented in Chapter 1. The candidates may photocopy these templates and use them as a practice and/or revision tool. Appendix 2 contains a list of common abbreviations used in the publication. Appendix 3 is an introduction to the principles of prescribing and pharmaceutical care. Appendix 4, or 'The Guide to Using and Revising the BNF', provides a list of the most important sections and revision points in the BNF, which the candidate should be aware of when revising for the PSA and in everyday practice.

The primary source of information to be used by all PSA candidates is the BNF and therefore the majority of questions included in this book can be answered by solely using this reference source (note that the questions are based on *BNF 65*, the latest edition of the BNF available during the production of this volume). However, a number of questions, particularly those

TABLE 1 Estimated Proportions of Clinical Contexts in Questions Appearing in Different Chapters of this Book

Chapter	Question Type (Number of Questions)	Medicine	Surgery	Elderly Care	Paediatrics	Psychiatry	Obstetrics and Gynaecology	General Practice
1	Prescribing (48)	12	7	7	7	3	4	8
2	Prescription Review (24)	5	5	3	2	3	3	3
3	Planning Management (13)	3	2	2	2	1	2	1
4	Communicating Information (13)	3	1	1	3	1	2	2
5	Calculation Skills (13)	2	2	2	2	1	2	2
6	Adverse Drug Reactions (13)	3	2	3	2	1	1	1
7	Drug Monitoring (13)	3	3	1	2	1	1	2
8	Data Interpretation (13)	2	2	4	1	2	1	1
	Total of 150 questions	33	24	23	21	13	16	20

relating to intravenous (IV) fluid regimens, will require practitioners to use some common knowledge, to exercise professional judgement, and to at times refer to other sources of information, such as Medusa Injectable Medicines Guide[7] or the *Handbook on Injectable Drugs* by LA Trissel.[8]

Candidates are advised to choose their own preferred method of using this book. As an example, they may wish to work through all of the questions in one of the chapters before moving to the next chapter. Alternatively, they may select one question from each chapter. It may also be reasonable for candidates to time themselves once they become familiar with the templates of questions used in the examination. The PSA is a 2-hour examination and therefore the candidates are expected to spend as little as 2 minutes solving some of the question items. On the other hand, some types of questions, particularly those in Chapters 1 and 2, may take up more of the candidate's time than others.

Student Success in the Prescribing Safety Assessment is a collaboration between a doctor, an academic pharmacist and a clinical pharmacist. The emphasis of the publication is placed on clinical pharmacy and pharmaceutical care, and therefore the majority of candidates will find forming a diagnosis straightforward in most of the questions, except perhaps the cases where a rare adverse drug reaction is suspected. Nevertheless, it is important that candidates use their medical knowledge in conjunction with pharmaceutical knowledge to appreciate the links between the two and to understand how they are used together in practice to ensure the most appropriate pharmaceutical care is provided to the patient.

The authors of this book hope that you will enjoy solving the problems presented by each case scenario while at the same time developing your skills and knowledge to help you become a competent prescriber. We would like to wish all candidates the best of luck, both during the revision process and in the assessment itself. We are also more than happy to answer any further queries you may have through direct contact with Radcliffe Publishing www.radcliffehealth.com/contact-us-0.

REFERENCES

1. Dornan T, Ashcroft D, Heathfield H, *et al*. *An In Depth Investigation into Causes of Prescribing Errors by Foundation Trainees in Relation to Their Medical Education. EQUIP study*. London: General Medical Council; 2009.
2. Dean B, Schachter M, Vincent C, *et al*. Prescribing errors in hospital inpatients: their incidence and clinical significance. *Qual Saf Health Care*. 2002; **11**(4): 340–4.

3. *Tomorrow's Doctors: outcomes and standards for undergraduate medical education*. London: General Medical Council; 2009.
4. *Prescribing Safety Assessment* [Online]. Medical Schools Council; British Pharmacological Society [cited 2 October 2011]. Available at: www.prescribe. ac.uk/psa/
5. *Prescribing Safety Assessment: Assessment Structure* [Online]. Medical Schools Council; British Pharmacological Society [cited 2 October 2011]. Available at: www.prescribe.ac.uk/psa/?page_id=23
6. www.prescribe.ac.uk
7. www.injguide.nhs.uk
8. Trissel LA. *Handbook on Injectable Drugs* [Online]. London: Pharmaceutical Press; 2013. Available at: www.medicinescomplete.com

Chapter 1
Prescribing

READ BEFORE YOU START

- There are eight 'Prescribing' question items in the PSA worth 10 marks each (80 marks in total).
- You will be marked in two main areas of 'Drug Choice' and 'Dose and Route' (each worth 4 marks). You will be eligible for all 4 marks if you provide an optimal answer that cannot be improved and 3 marks if you provide an answer that is good but is suboptimal on some grounds (e.g. cost-effectiveness, likely adherence). You shall be eligible for 2 marks if you provide an answer that is likely to provide benefit but which is clearly suboptimal for more than one reason, and 1 mark for an answer that has some justification and deserves some credit. The correct date (timing) on the prescription and prescriber's signature are worth 1 mark each.

NB the authors of this publication appreciate the fact that a variety of answers (in a decreasing order of appropriateness for the patient) may be accepted for the purpose of the examination. However, the inclusion of clinically inappropriate or less-appropriate options or any option that may be unethical or which may breach any legislation has been avoided whenever possible. Therefore, while in some cases as many as four or more answer options may be acceptable, the majority of questions include one or a maximum of two correct answers.

- There are four types of prescribing questions in the PSA assessment and in this chapter (hospital once-only medicines, hospital regular medicines, hospital fluid prescription charts and FP10 prescriptions). *See* the templates for each prescription type presented in Appendix 1 together with the examples of correctly written prescriptions – use these templates when answering the questions. The templates may be photocopied if necessary.

- Each question will ask you to prescribe one medicine that is most appropriate for the management of an acute condition, a chronic condition or the patient's symptoms (e.g. pain).
- The questions may include high-risk medicines (e.g. anticoagulants, opioids, insulin), medicines that are in common use (e.g. antibiotics) and intravenous (IV) fluids.
- Note that to answer some of the questions, which involve IV infusions (particularly IV fluids), you may need to refer to additional reference sources, such as Medusa Injectable Medicines Guide[1] or the *Handbook on Injectable Drugs* by LA Trissel.[2]

QUESTION 1

A 66-year-old Caucasian gentleman attends your primary care diabetes clinic for a routine check-up.

PMH: T2DM, hypertension, angina, atrial fibrillation
DH: metformin 1 g OM, 500 mg at noon and 500 mg in the evening, ramipril 5 mg OM, atenolol 50 mg OD, glyceryl trinitrate sublingual spray 400 micrograms PRN, simvastatin 40 mg ON and aspirin 75 mg OM
SH: smokes 21 cigarettes a day

On Examination

Temperature 36.7°C, HR 87/min and irregular, BP 132/80 mmHg, RR 15/min, O_2 sat 98% on air

Investigations

Na^+ 136 mmol/L (135–146), K^+ 4.7 mmol/L (3.5–5.0), Cr 95 µmol/L (79–118), eGFR 73 mL/min/1.73 m^2, glucose 13.2 mmol/L (4–9), HbA_{1c} 62 mmol/mol (48–59); weight: 110 kg; height: 1.82 m

On questioning, the gentleman admits that he is very reluctant to take more tablets but would rather take another oral medication than use an injectable one, as he has a terrible fear of needles.

Write a prescription for ONE drug that will help to improve the long-term control of this patient's T2DM.

(Use the general practice prescription form provided in Appendix 1)[3]

QUESTION 2

A 67-year-old woman presents to the A&E department with a 7-day history of shortness of breath, chest tightness, productive cough and fever.

PMH: iron deficiency anaemia
DH: ferrous sulphate 200 mg BD
SH: glass of wine every other day, non-smoker

On Examination

Temperature 39.2°C, HR 120/min and regular, BP 89/55 mmHg, RR 25/min, O_2 sat 95% on air
Patient appears to be confused (GCS 9/15)
Weight: 62 kg

Investigations

WBC 17.4×10^9/L (4–11), Neut 12.5×10^9/L (2.0–7.5), Plt 378×10^9/L (150–400), Hb 9.2 g/dL (11.5–16.5), D-dimer 140 nanograms/mL (<500 nanograms/mL), PT 13 seconds (12–16)
Na^+ 153 mmol/L (135–146), K^+ 4.8 mmol/L (3.5–5.0), Cr 98 μmol/L (79–118), U 14.3 mmol/L (2.5–6.7), CRP 219 mg/L (<10)
CXR: right basal consolidation

Following an initial assessment your colleague writes a prescription for benzylpenicillin IV 1.2 g QDS. However, after checking your local antibiotic guidelines and the BNF, you realise that benzylpenicillin monotherapy may be inadequate for the severity of this patient's condition.

Write a prescription for ONE medicine that would be appropriate to add to the current treatment regimen for this patient.

(Use the hospital 'regular medicines' prescription chart provided in Appendix 1)

QUESTION 3

You are a house officer on the Acute Stroke Unit. A 45-year-old man has suffered an ischaemic stroke and has been nil by mouth for about a week. He was recommenced on oral nutritional feeds 3 days ago. While undertaking routine blood test result analysis, your SpR points out some electrolyte disturbances and suspects this patient might be developing re-feeding syndrome.

PMH: asthma, generalised anxiety disorder, insomnia

DH: salbutamol 100 micrograms pressurised-metered dose inhaler one to two puffs PRN, beclomethasone (Clenil Modulite®) 100 micrograms pressurised-metered dose inhaler two puffs BD, lorazepam 1 mg BD PRN and 1 mg at bedtime

SH: smokes 25 cigarettes a day (for 26 years); alcohol, 10–14 units/week

On Examination

Temperature 36.3°C, HR 85/min and regular, BP 134/78 mmHg, RR 18/min, O_2 sat 97% on air

Investigations

Na^+ 142 mmol/L (135–146), K^+ 3.0 mmol/L (3.5–5.0), PO_4^{3-} 0.3 mmol/L (0.8–1.5), Mg^{2+} 0.9 mmol/L (0.7–1.1), corrected Ca^{2+} 2.3 mmol/L (2.20–2.67), U 3.4 mmol/L (2.5–6.7), Cr 67 μmol/L (79–118)

Weight: 43 kg; height: 1.64 m

Write a prescription for ONE intravenous fluid that would correct the electrolyte disturbances encountered by this patient.

(Use the hospital fluid prescription chart provided in Appendix 1)

QUESTION 4

A 25-year-old woman is admitted to the A&E department at 10 a.m. with persistent nausea and vomiting that started around 11 p.m. last night. Her sister who lives in the same flat found an empty box of paracetamol (16 × 500 mg tablets) at home and suspects the patient might have taken an overdose.

PMH: major depression and epilepsy
DH: fluoxetine 20 mg daily and phenytoin 300 mg daily
SH: 16 units of alcohol/week

On Examination

Temperature 36.5°C, HR 101/min and regular, BP 143/85 mmHg, RR 25/min, O_2 sat 98% on air

Investigations

Na$^+$ 148 mmol/L (135–146), K$^+$ 3.1 mmol/L (3.5–5.0), U 3.2 mmol/L (2.5–6.7), Cr 75 μmol/L (79–118), albumin 42 g/L (35–50), ALP 67 U/L (39–117), ALT 101 U/L (5–40), total bilirubin 45 μmol/L (<17), phenytoin 12 mg/L (10–20 mg/L), paracetamol 40 mg/L
Weight: 58 kg

Write a prescription for ONE medicine in an infusion fluid that will help to treat the acute problem suffered by this patient.

(Use the hospital 'once-only medicines' prescription chart provided in Appendix 1)

QUESTION 5

A 30-year-old woman who is 32 weeks pregnant presents to her GP practice complaining of persistent constipation. She has had trouble opening her bowels on at least 4–5 days each week for the last 4 months despite an increase in her dietary intake of fruits, vegetables and fluids. The patient is worried that this straining together with her asthma might have an impact on her pregnancy.

PMH: stable asthmatic
DH: salbutamol 100 micrograms inhaler PRN
SH: non-smoker, non-drinker

On Examination

Temperature 36.3°C, HR 75/min and regular, BP 125/78 mmHg, RR 13/min, O_2 sat 99% on air

Investigations

Na^+ 140 mmol/L (135–146), K^+ 4.0 mmol/L (3.5–5.0)
PEFR: >400 L/min and <20% diurnal variation

Write a prescription for ONE medicine that will help to relieve the symptoms of constipation experienced by this patient.

(Use the general practice prescription form provided in Appendix 1)

QUESTION 6

You are house officer on a paediatric ward. A 6-year-old boy is brought to hospital after having his hand bitten by a dog in the playground about 2 hours ago.

PMH: nil
DH: nil; penicillin allergy
SH: lives locally with his mum and dad

On Examination

Temperature 36.5°C, HR 105/min and regular, BP 108/82 mmHg, RR 19/min, O_2 sat 100% on air; the child is otherwise well

Investigations

WBC 5.4×10^9/L (4–11), Neut 2.5×10^9/L (2.0–7.5), Plt 210×10^9/L (150–400), Na$^+$ 138 mmol/L (135–146), K$^+$ 4.1 mmol/L (3.5–5.0), Cr 81 μmol/L (79–118), U 2.7 mmol/L (2.5–6.7), CRP 2 mg/L (<10)

The boy has all of his childhood immunisations up to date, including the primary immunisation for tetanus (at 2, 3 and 4 months). However, he has not had a booster dose of tetanus vaccine, which is recommended before the age of 5.

You have prescribed a prophylactic antibiotic regimen and a tetanus immunoglobulin for the prevention of infection from animal bites for this child. Your SpR now asks you to prescribe a booster dose of tetanus vaccine as appropriate.

(Use the hospital 'once-only medicines' prescription chart provided in Appendix 1)

QUESTION 7

A 68-year-old man comes for a routine GP appointment complaining of persistent wheezing and breathlessness despite using his medicines as prescribed. He finds it increasingly more difficult to undertake normal activities of daily living.

PMH: hypertension (diagnosed 10 years ago), COPD (diagnosed 6 months ago)
DH: amlodipine 10 mg OD, indapamide 2.5 mg OM, salbutamol pressurised metered-dose inhaler 100 micrograms two puffs PRN up to QDS
SH: smoker (32 pack-years)

On Examination

Temperature 35.4°C, HR 110/min and regular, BP 125/80 mmHg, JVP not elevated, RR 25/min, O_2 sat 95% on air; no peripheral oedema noted

Investigations

Hb 17.4 g/dL (13.5–17.7), Na^+ 133 mmol/L (135–146), K^+ 4.0 mmol/L (3.5–5.0), U 4.3 mmol/L (2.5–6.7), Cr 58 μmol/L (79–118), FEV_1 60%
Weight: 52 kg; height: 1.76 m
ECG: sinus tachycardia

Write a prescription for ONE medicine that will help to improve this patient's breathlessness and his quality of life.

(Use the general practice prescription form provided in Appendix 1)[4]

QUESTION 8

A 56-year-old woman has been admitted to hospital with new-onset (<48 hours' duration) atrial fibrillation.

PMH: surgically treated breast cancer (6 years ago), deep vein thrombosis (2 years ago)
DH: letrozole 2.5 mg OD; she also buys aspirin 75 mg over the counter and takes it OM
SH: lives with her husband and two children; non-smoker, nil alcohol

On Examination

Temperature 36.2°C, HR 140/min, irregular, BP 96/67 mmHg, RR 26/min, O_2 sat 97% on air

Investigations

WBC 9.6×10^9/L (4–11), Neut 6.7×10^9/L (2.0–7.5), Plt 260×10^9/L (150–400), D-dimer 55 nanograms/mL (<500 ng/mL), PT 14 seconds (12–16), INR <1
Na^+ 138 mmol/L (135–146), K^+ 4.2 mmol/L (3.5–5.0), Cr 85 μmol/L (79–118), U 3.6 mmol/L (2.5–6.7), CRP 4 mg/L (<10), albumin 38 g/L (35–50), ALP 24 U/L (39–117), ALT 6 U/L (5–40), total bilirubin 2 μmol/L (<17), TSH 2.5 mU/L (0.3–3.5), free T_4 15 pmol/L (10–25)
ECG: absent P waves, irregular
CXR: no significant abnormalities detected
Weight: 63 kg; height: 1.62 cm

The patient is prescribed adequate thromboprophylaxis and, while investigating the underlying pathophysiology of the patient's AF, the consultant cardiologist decides to try some pharmacological interventions. He asks you to write a prescription for an appropriate anti-arrhythmic given by intravenous infusion that could help restore the sinus rhythm for this patient.

(Use the hospital fluid prescription chart provided in Appendix 1)

QUESTION 9

You are a house officer in the orthogeriatric team. An 83-year-old woman is admitted to your ward with a tibial fracture following a fall in the snow. She is due for external fixation.

PMH: recurrent falls, hypertension, anaemia, dementia

DH: nifedipine MR (Adalat® Retard) 20 mg BD, ferrous sulphate 200 mg BD and donepezil 10 mg OD

SH: widower, twice-a-day care package at home; non-smoker, non-drinker

On Examination

Temperature 36.6°C, HR 85/min and regular, BP 135/80 mmHg, RR 13/min, O_2 sat 98% on air

Investigations

WBC 3.2×10^9/L (4–11), Neut 2.4×10^9/L (2.0–7.5), Hb 11.2 g/dL (13.5–17.7), Plt 320×10^9/L (150–400), Na^+ 136 mmol/L (135–146), K^+ 4.3 mmol/L (3.5–5.0), U 3.4 mmol/L (2.5–6.7), Cr 63 μmol/L (79–118); weight: 55 kg; height: 1.64 m

Your registrar asks you to prescribe some thromboprophylaxis for this lady to be continued while she is in hospital.

Write a prescription for ONE injectable thromboprophylactic medicine that is appropriate for this patient.

(Use the hospital 'regular medicines' prescription chart provided in Appendix 1)

QUESTION 10

A 5-year-old is brought to A&E following a history of severe, rapid-onset headache, vomiting, neck stiffness, general malaise and fever.

PMH: nil; childhood immunisations up to date
DH: nil; penicillin allergy
SH: lives with his parents

On Examination

Temperature 39.4°C, HR 105/min and regular, BP 93/65 mmHg, RR 21/min, O_2 sat 95% on air
Kernig's sign positive and a non-blanching purple rash notable on the trunk

Investigations

WBC 14.3 × 10^9/L (4–11), Neut 11.4 × 10^9/L (2.0–7.5). Na^+ 147 mmol/L (135–146), K^+ 3.2 mmol/L (3.5–5.0), U 6.8 mmol/L (2.5–6.7), Cr 54 μmol/L (79–118), CRP 134 mg/L (<10)
Weight: 18 kg, height: 1.10 m
Head CT: no significant abnormalities
CSF on lumbar puncture: turbid and purulent, polymorphs 1600/mm³, protein 18 g/L, glucose (% blood glucose) <50

Bacterial meningococcal disease is strongly suspected, and your SHO asks you to initiate empirical antibiotic treatment for this child until microbiological culture and sensitivity data is available.

Follow BNF recommendations to write a prescription for a STAT dose of an injectable antibiotic to treat bacterial meningococcal meningitis, which is then to be continued on a regular hospital prescription chart.

(Use the hospital 'once-only medicines' prescription chart provided in Appendix 1)

QUESTION 11

Mr Y, a 58-year-old male, is brought into hospital by ambulance after his wife noticed him behaving in a way that she described as 'weird and unusual'. His symptoms involved slurred, incoherent speech, right-sided weakness and hemianopia.

PMH: T2DM, hypertension, osteoarthritis
DH: metformin MR tablets 1 g OM, glimepiride 4 mg OM, simvastatin 40 mg ON, lisinopril 20 mg OM, paracetamol 1 g QDS
SH: lives with his wife; smokes 19 cigarettes/day; alcohol, 5–8 units/day

On Examination

Temperature 36.5°C, HR 98/min and regular, BP 155/93 mmHg, RR 24/min, O_2 sat 94% on air

Investigations

Hb 13.4 g/dL (11.5–16.5), WBC 7.6×10^9/L (4–11), Na^+ 141 mmol/L (135–146), K^+ 4.4 mmol/L (3.5–5.0), Mg^{2+} 1.0 mmol/L (0.7–1.1), corrected Ca^{2+} 2.44 mmol/L (2.20–2.67) U 4.6 mmol/L (2.5–6.7), Cr 126 μmol/L (79–118), glucose 9.6 mmol/L (4–9), recent HbA_{1c} 54 mmol/mol (48–59), CRP 5 mg/L (<10), ESR 8 (<20 mm in 1 hour)
Weight: 124 kg; height: 1.83 m
Head CT: occlusion of the main trunk of the middle cerebral artery (MCA)

Mr Y is thrombolysed, and the consultant asks you to initiate antiplatelet therapy 24 hours later.

Write a prescription for ONE antiplatelet medicine that should be initiated for this patient following an MCA stroke.

(Use the hospital 'regular medicines' prescription chart provided in Appendix 1)

QUESTION 12

Tom is a 19-year-old who has recently moved out of his parents' house in Leeds to Nottingham to start a degree in economics. After one of the many university parties, his friends found him severely confused, sweating and shaking in the morning which did not resemble his normal hangover. They decided to bring him to A&E.

PMH: T1DM
DH: NovoMix® 30 (biphasic insulin aspart) FlexPen® 10 units OM, 16 units in the evening
SH: non-smoker; alcohol: up to 20 units/week

On Examination

Temperature 36.8°C, HR 125/min and regular, BP 84/60 mmHg, JVP not elevated, RR 26/min, O_2 sat 94% on air, chest clear

Investigations

WBC 8.4×10^9/L (4–11), Neut 5.6×10^9/L (2.0–7.5), Na⁺ 154 mmol/L (135–146), K⁺ 4.8 mmol/L (3.5–5.0), U 8.9 mmol/L (2.5–6.7), Cr 135 μmol/L (79–118), CRP 15 mg/L (<10), glucose 2.8 mmol/L (4–9)
Weight: 68 kg; height: 1.79 m
Head CT: no significant abnormalities

An inadvertent insulin overdose is suspected, and Tom is given 20 g of GlucoGel®, but 10 minutes later he loses consciousness. Your SHO asks you to initiate treatment of hypoglycaemia immediately.

Prescribe ONE drug that would help this patient recover from a hypogly-caemic crisis.

(Use the hospital 'once-only medicines' prescription chart provided in Appendix 1)

QUESTION 13

A 10-year-old boy is brought in by ambulance following a bee sting in his left arm. Soon after the event he started developing widespread swelling, itchiness, wheezing and became drowsy.

PMH: nil; childhood immunisations up to date
DH: nil
SH: lives with his mother

On Examination

Temperature 35.4°C, HR 154/min and regular, BP 65/48 mmHg, RR 28/min, O_2 sat 94% on air
Facial erythema, progressive oedema, wheezing

Investigations

WBC 8.6×10^9/L (4–11), Neut 6.5×10^9/L (2.0–7.5), Na$^+$ 137 mmol/L (135–146), K$^+$ 3.6 mmol/L (3.5–5.0), U 2.8 mmol/L (2.5–6.7), Cr 75 μmol/L (79–118), CRP 9 mg/L (<10), glucose 4.6 mmol/L (4–9)
Weight: 33 kg; height: 1.40 m

Prescribe ONE medicine that should initially be used to reverse the signs and symptoms experienced by this boy.

(Use the hospital 'once-only medicines' prescription chart provided in Appendix 1)

QUESTION 14

Mrs JM is an 85-year-old lady who is admitted to the Care of the Elderly ward with an increasing acopia, with agitation and worsening memory. Her daughter explains to you that her mum has started to behave progressively 'more indifferent' over the last year or so. Mrs JM is very confused and is unable to recognise her relatives.

PMH: hypothyroidism, Parkinson's disease
DH: levothyroxine 125 micrograms OM, co-beneldopa (Madopar®) 62.5 mg at 8 a.m., 2 p.m. and 9 p.m., ropinirole 500 micrograms TDS
FH: nil
SH: lives alone, looked after by her daughter who comes to see her daily; non-smoker, non-drinker

On Examination

Temperature 35.8°C, HR 75/min and regular, BP 110/70 mmHg, RR 12/min, O_2 sat 97% on air
MMSE 16

Investigations

Na^+ 134 mmol/L (135–146), K^+ 3.8 mmol/L (3.5–5.0), corrected Ca^{2+} 2.5 mmol/L (2.20–2.67), U 5.6 mmol/L (2.5–6.7), Cr 74 μmol/L (79–118), serum B_{12} 154 nanograms/L (150–925), serum folate 2.7 micrograms/L (2.9–18), free T_4 22 pmol/L (10–25), TSH 2.5 mU/L (0.3–3.5).
Weight: 63 kg; height: 1.60 m
Urine dip: nil blood, nitrites, protein 1+
MRI head: frontal lobe atrophy

Mrs JM is offered a course of cognitive behavioural therapy, but your consultant also wishes to commence an acetylcholinesterase inhibitor therapy for suspected new onset Alzheimer's disease.

Write a prescription for ONE acetylcholinesterase inhibitor that would be the most appropriate option for Mrs JM.

(Use the hospital 'regular medicines' prescription chart provided in Appendix 1)

QUESTION 15

A 72-year-old gentleman is brought in by ambulance with a month-long history of increasing breathlessness, fatigue and severe oedema in both ankles.

PMH: STEMI, hypertension, AF (failed cardioversion)
DH: aspirin 75 mg OM, bisoprolol 5 mg OM, ramipril 10 mg OM, atorvastatin 80 mg ON
SH: retired builder, lives with his wife in London Bridge; alcohol: ≈18 units/week; smoker: 20/day (25 years)

On Examination

Temperature 36.5°C, HR 160/min and irregular, BP 180/110 mmHg, RR 25/min, O_2 sat 95% on air
Pitting oedema over the ankles, jugular venous distension, bilateral basal crepitations on chest auscultation, third heart sound audible

Investigations

WBC 4.3 × 10^9/L (4–11), Neut 3.5 × 10^9/L (2.0–7.5), Plt 320 × 10^9/L (150–400), Na$^+$ 145 mmol/L (135–146), K$^+$ 4.6 mmol/L (3.5–5.0), Cr 143 μmol/L (79–118), U 5.8 mmol/L (2.5–6.7), CRP 2 mg/L (<10), BNP 630 pg/mL (<400), D-dimer 120 nanograms/mL (<500 nanograms/mL), PT 12 seconds (12–16), albumin 43 g/L (35–50), ALP 27 U/L (39–117), ALT 12 U/L (5–40), total bilirubin 7 μmol/L (<17), glucose 7.6 mmol/L (4–9)
ECG: AF
CXR: pulmonary congestion, cardiomegaly
Weight: 95 kg; height: 1.78 cm

Your consultant suspects this patient might be suffering from an acute exacerbation of previously undiagnosed heart failure and asks you to prescribe a diuretic infusion that would help to reduce his fluid overload.

(Use the hospital fluid prescription chart provided in Appendix 1)[1,5–7]

QUESTION 16

Michael is a 52-year-old former rugby player who is known to suffer from osteoarthritis of both knees. Despite losing some weight, undertaking regular exercise and using current pharmacological treatments, Michael still feels significant pain and stiffness in his joints.

PMH: previous gastric ulcer, osteoarthritis
DH: omeprazole 20 mg OM, paracetamol 1 g QDS, OTC Voltarol® (diclofenac 1%) gel
SH: non-smoker, occasional alcohol (2–4 units/week)

On Examination

Temperature 36.5°C, HR 85/min and regular, BP 120/75 mmHg, JVP not elevated, RR 14/min; no peripheral oedema

Investigations

Baseline (6 months ago): Na$^+$ 137 mmol/L (135–146), K$^+$ 4.1 mmol/L (3.5–5.0), corrected Ca^{2+} 2.6 mmol/L (2.20–2.67), U 3.5 mmol/L (2.5–6.7), Cr 81 μmol/L (79–118)
Previous knee arthroscopy (6 months ago): early fissuring and surface erosion of the cartilage of both joints
Weight: 102 kg; height: 1.95 m

Michael does not feel that paracetamol or Voltarol® gel are 'doing any good' and would like to give another painkiller a go. However, he is quite reluctant to take any opioid-based analgesics, as the last time he took co-codamol he became constipated.

Write a prescription for ONE medicine that will help to relieve his osteoarthritis-related pain.

(Use the general practice prescription form provided in Appendix 1)[8,9]

QUESTION 17

You are a house officer on an orthopaedic ward. Mrs TY is an 82-year-old who has fallen down the staircase at home and fractured her left neck of femur.

PMH: breast cancer
DH: letrozole 2.5 mg OD
SH: widower, ex-smoker (15 pack-years, gave up 10 years ago)

On Examination

Temperature 36.2°C, HR 76/min and regular, BP 134/87 mmHg, RR 14/min, O_2 sat 97% on air

Investigations

Na^+ 138 mmol/L (135–146), K^+ 3.8 mmol/L (3.5–5.0), Mg^{2+} 0.9 mmol/L (0.7–1), corrected Ca^{2+} 2.51 mmol/L (2.20–2.67), PO_4^{3-} 1.1 mmol/L (0.8–1.5), U 3.4 mmol/L (2.5–6.7), Cr 65 μmol/L (79–118)
Weight: 48 kg; height: 1.59 m
DXA scan: T-score –4.0

The registrar asks you to prescribe a bone-protective therapy for this lady. On discussion Mrs TY admits that she sometimes finds it difficult to swallow her letrozole and would rather not take any more tablets as such. Taking this into consideration you therefore prescribe some effervescent Adcal-D3® and decide to initiate a prophylactic treatment against osteoporotic fractures.

Write a prescription for ONE medicine that would be a preferred therapy to prevent further osteoporotic fractures for this patient.[10,11]

(Use the hospital 'regular medicines' prescription chart provided in Appendix 1)[10,11]

QUESTION 18

Peter is a 52-year-old taxi driver who is brought to A&E with sudden-onset left-sided chest pain while at work.

PMH: GORD
DH: lansoprazole 30 mg OM
SH: alcohol: one to two cans of lager a day; smokes 20 cigarettes a day

On Examination

Temperature 36.6°C, HR 165/min and regular, BP 143/95 mmHg, JVP elevated, RR 32/min, O_2 sat 95% on air

Investigations

WBC 7.3×10^9/L (4–11), Neut 4.6×10^9/L (2.0–7.5), Hb 15.4 g/dL (13.5–17.7), Plt 354×10^9/L (150–400)

Na^+ 147 mmol/L (135–146), K^+ 4.9 mmol/L (3.5–5.0), U 6.5 mmol/L (2.5–6.7), Cr 92 μmol/L (79–118), CRP 12 mg/L (<10), troponin I 20.5 ng/mL (<1.5),[12] glucose 13.2 mmol/L (4–9)

Weight: 112 kg; height: 1.79 m

ECG: pending

Peter is given a few sublingual sprays of glyceryl trinitrate (GTN) 400 micrograms; however, that does not relieve his chest pain. The senior A&E nurse asks you to prescribe ONE stronger painkiller that would provide Peter with temporary relief of his pain.

(Use the hospital 'once-only medicines' prescription chart provided in Appendix 1)

QUESTION 19

Mrs LK, a 92-year-old lady, is admitted to hospital with left-sided weakness. Following an MRI she is diagnosed as suffering from a large ischaemic stroke. Five days later her inflammatory markers rise and she starts to feel feverish. This is accompanied by severe shortness of breath and a cough. She is subsequently treated empirically for an aspiration pneumonia with co-amoxiclav 1.2 g IV TDS and metronidazole 500 mg IV TDS. Unfortunately, such a regimen is ineffective, and co-amoxiclav is switched to piperacillin/tazobactam 4.5 g IV TDS. Three days into this treatment, Mrs LK's clinical condition deteriorates further. On discussion with her relatives, the decision is made to put Mrs LK on the Liverpool Care Pathway. She is prescribed glycopyrronium 1.2 mg to reduce excessive respiratory secretions and haloperidol 10 mg to combat her restlessness – both for administration in a continuous subcutaneous infusion pump over a 24-hour period. Mrs LK is also prescribed morphine sulphate 10 mg IV/SC every 2–4 hours PRN as breakthrough pain relief.

On Examination

Temperature 37.7°C, HR 110/min and regular, BP 155/93 mmHg, RR 19/min, O_2 sat 94% on air

Despite haloperidol, Mrs LK still appears very restless and profoundly confused. Some twitching in her legs and trunk is noted. The sister in charge asks you to review this lady and to prescribe a medicine to help relieve these symptoms.

Write a prescription for ONE parenteral medicine that would help relieve the symptoms experienced by Mrs LK.

NB the typical volumes used for continuous subcutaneous infusion syringe drivers are between 10 and 30 mL.

(Use the hospital fluid prescription chart provided in Appendix 1)[2,13]

QUESTION 20

Mr Richards, an 85-year-old gentleman, undergoes shoulder arthroscopy for acromioclavicular joint osteoarthritis.

PMH: Parkinson's disease, glaucoma, benign prostatic hyperplasia, osteoarthritis
DH: Stalevo® 75 mg/18.75 mg/200 mg tablets T at 8 a.m., noon, 4 p.m. and 10 p.m.; rasa-
giline 1 mg at 8 a.m.; travoprost 40 micrograms/mL eye drops T to both eyes at night;
finasteride 5 mg OM, co-dydramol 10/500 T-TT PRN QDS
SH: ex-smoker, occasional whisky

On Examination

Temperature 36.7°C, HR 81/min and regular, BP 134/85 mmHg, RR 13/min, O_2 sat 98% on
air; weight: 68 kg

Mr Richards is prescribed tramadol 50–100 mg PO QDS and Oramorph® liquid 5–10 mg PRN PO QDS to complement his co-dydramol after the procedure. This exacerbates his post-operative nausea, and your SHO asks you to write-up an anti-emetic prescription for this gentleman.

Write a prescription for ONE medicine that would be the most appropriate option in the treatment of nausea experienced by Mr Richards.

(Use the hospital 'regular medicines' prescription chart provided in Appendix 1)[14]

QUESTION 21

Mrs da Silva, an 88-year-old, is discovered to have a liver abscess and is treated using IV teicoplanin, PO ciprofloxacin and PO metronidazole.

PMH: T2DM, hypertension, polymyalgia rheumatica, depression
DH: gliclazide 180 mg OM, 60 mg in the evening, sitagliptin 100 mg OM, enalapril 20 mg OM, prednisolone 7 mg OM, naproxen 250 mg BD, mirtazapine 45 mg OM; allergies: penicillin (anaphylaxis)
SH: lives alone, twice daily social care package

Over the next 2 weeks Mrs da Silva's condition markedly improves. The antibiotic regimen is switched to PO doxycycline 100 mg BD, ciprofloxacin 500 mg BD and metronidazole 400 mg TDS. However, a few days later she suddenly develops severe diarrhoea with spiking temperatures.

On Examination

Temperature 38.6°C, HR 120/min and regular, BP 101/95 mmHg, RR 16/min, O$_2$ sat 96% on air

Investigations

Stool cultures – *Clostridium difficile* toxins A and B: positive

After Completing Antibiotics	Today
U 4.2 mmol/L (2.5–6.7)	U 9.4 mmol/L (2.5–6.7)
Cr 89 µmol/L (79–118)	Cr 167 µmol/L (79–118)
CRP 4 mg/L (<10)	CRP 101 mg/L (<10)
WBC 7.4 × 10^9/L (4–11)	WBC 15.3 × 10^9/L (4–11)

You stop Mrs da Silva's current antibiotic therapy.

Write a prescription for ONE medicine that would help to treat the infection causing the signs and symptoms experienced by Mrs da Silva.[15,16]

(Use the hospital 'regular medicines' prescription chart provided in Appendix 1)[15,16]

QUESTION 22

Miss JH, a 42-year-old, is brought into hospital A&E with a swollen right calf.

PMH: T2DM (right foot ulcer 3 months ago), trisomy 21, swallowing dysfunction (PEG tube in place), constipation, generalised anxiety, conduct disorder
DH: metformin sachets 500 mg TDS, senna liquid 15 mg ON, Laxido® sachets T BD, risperidone liquid 1 mg/mL 0.5 mL OM, diazepam oral solution 2 mg/5 mL 5 mL TDS
SH: lives in a nursing home, poorly mobile

On Examination

Temperature 36.5°C, HR 78/min and regular, BP 131/76 mmHg, RR 14/min, O$_2$ sat 97% on air
You suspect a possible DVT

Investigations

WBC 8.4 × 10^9/L (4–11), Neut 6.7 × 10^9/L (2.0–7.5), Plt 265 × 10^9/L (150–400), Hb 12.3 g/dL (11.5–16.5), APTT 22 seconds (23–31), INR 1.1, D-dimer 1136 nanograms/mL (<500 nanograms/mL)
Na$^+$ 148 mmol/L (135–146), K$^+$ 3.8 mmol/L (3.5–5.0), Cr 86 μmol/L (79–118), U 8.2 mmol/L (2.5–6.7), CRP 23 mg/L (<10), glucose 14.3 mmol/L (4–9), HbA$_{1c}$ 52 mmol/mol (48–59)
Weight: 76 kg; height: 157 cm

Write a prescription for ONE medicine that would help to treat the underlying cause of Miss JH's leg problem.[17,18]

(Use the hospital 'regular medicines' prescription chart provided in Appendix 1)[17,18]

QUESTION 23

Mr Bush is a 56-year-old gentleman who suffers from metastatic gastric cancer. He comes in to hospital with intractable pain and stomach upset.

PMH: gastric cancer, BPH

DH: tamsulosin MR 400 micrograms OM, paracetamol 1 g PRN QDS, Oramorph® 10 mg/5 mL solution 15 mL PRN every 6 hours, MST Continus® 70 mg BD, cyclizine 50 mg TDS PRN, metoclopramide 10 mg TDS PRN

SH: lives with his wife at home; visited by hospice nurses on a daily basis

On Examination

Temperature 36.6°C, HR 64/min and regular, BP 124/86 mmHg, RR 13/min, O_2 sat 98% on air

Mr Bush is reviewed by the Palliative Care Team who increase his dose of MST Continus® from 70 mg BD to 90 mg BD and recommend initiating omeprazole 40 mg OD. After 5 days at this dose of MST Continus® with (on average) additional three daily doses of Oramorph® (10 mg/mL) 20 mL PRN, his pain settles down. However, his 'tummy' upset is persistent despite omeprazole treatment.

Your consultant thinks that high doses of oral morphine may be causing this problem and asks you to review Mr Bush's pain management for alternative options.

Write a prescription for ONE medicine that could be used as an alternative option to oral morphine for Mr Bush.

(Use the hospital 'regular medicines' prescription chart provided in Appendix 1)

QUESTION 24

Mr Stratford, a 47-year-old music producer, is taken to hospital by his wife who reports him as being 'terribly sick' over the past few weeks. He is often nauseous and 'brings stuff up'. According to her, Mr Stratford has also lost over 2 stone in the last 6 months and has been feeling persistently depressed, particularly in the last week or so. His diabetes has been under control, so she's quite worried this may be something new and serious.

PMH: TIA (2 years ago), hypertension, T1DM

DH: aspirin 75 mg OM, dipyridamole 200 mg MR BD, simvastatin 20 mg ON, ramipril 5 mg OM, NovoMix® 30 Flexpen® 26 units OM, 18 units ON

SH: cocaine-dependence (allegedly gave up 3 years ago), four to five cans of beer a week, smokes 15 cigarettes a day

On Examination

Temperature 35.4°C, HR 112/min and regular, BP 89/57 mmHg (taken while standing), JVP not elevated, RR 19/min, O_2 sat 96% on air

GCS 13/15, lethargic, hyperpigmentation of buccal mucosa present, sunken eyes, dry skin

Investigations

Na^+ 125 mmol/L (135–146), K^+ 5.3 mmol/L (3.5–5.0), U 8.7 mmol/L (2.5–6.7), Cr 124 μmol/L (79–118), corrected Ca^{2+} 2.84 mmol/L (2.20–2.67), glucose 3.3 mmol/L (4–9), CRP 5 mg/L (<10), WBC 12.4 × 10^9/L (4–11), Neut 9.8 × 10^9/L (2.0–7.5)

Mr Stratford is prescribed 0.9% saline and IV hydrocortisone. The registrar asks you to order ONE diagnostic test for this gentleman.

(Use the hospital 'once-only medicines' prescription chart provided in Appendix 1)[19]

QUESTION 25

Emily is a 78-year-old retired post office executive who is referred to hospital by her GP with shortness of breath, dizziness and palpitations. She is diagnosed with fast atrial fibrillation (AF) and is digitalised and warfarinised as appropriate.

PMH: NSTEMI and PCI to right coronary artery (2 years ago)
DH: aspirin 75 mg OM, bisoprolol 5 mg OM, atorvastatin 40 mg ON, ramipril 2.5 mg OM, amoxicillin 500 mg TDS for 7/7 (2 weeks ago for a chest infection)
SH: lives on her own, fully independent

No precipitant of Emily's AF is identified on further investigations, and she is being prepared for discharge. However, about 4 days later, Emily starts developing a chesty cough accompanied by high temperature, confusion and difficulty in breathing. You are asked to see the patient.

On Examination

Temperature 38.9°C, HR 101/min irregular, BP 121/72 mmHg, RR 25/min, O_2 sat 95% on air
Chest examination: crepitations left base

Investigations 2 Days Ago

WBC 15 × 10^9/L (4–11), Neut 9 × 10^9/L (2.0–7.5), Plt 450 × 10^9/L (150–400), Hb 12.4 g/dL (11.5–16.5), D-dimer 97 nanograms/mL (<500 nanograms/mL), INR 1.5, PT 14 seconds (12–16)
Na^+ 141 mmol/L (135–146), K^+ 4.2 mmol/L (3.5–5.0), Cr 94 μmol/L (79–118), U 5.7 mmol/L (2.5–6.7), CRP 37 mg/L (<10)

You prescribe O_2 and give an extra dose of bisoprolol 2.5 mg.

Write a prescription for ONE other medicine that should be used for an immediate treatment of Emily's condition.[20,21]

(Use the hospital 'regular medicines' prescription chart provided in Appendix 1)[20,21]

QUESTION 26

Daniel, a 3-year-old, is taken to hospital by his mother following a 3-day history of high fever, wheeze and severe cough, which she describes as 'seal-like barking'. These symptoms have been particularly bad at night.

PMH: nil
DH: nil
SH: lives with mum and dad in Twickenham

On Examination

Temperature 39.7°C, HR 142/min and regular, BP 101/75 mmHg, RR 35/min, O$_2$ sat 94% on air
Chest: marked chest wall retraction with decreased air entry

Investigations

WBC 19.5 × 10^9/L (4–11), Neut 13.4 × 10^9/L (2.0–7.5), Plt 246 × 10^9/L (150–400), Hb 13.2 g/dL (11.5–16.5)
Na$^+$ 148 mmol/L (135–146), K$^+$ 3.7 mmol/L (3.5–5.0), Cr 68 μmol/L (79–118), U 9.3 mmol/L (2.5–6.7), CRP 114 mg/L (<10)
Weight: 14 kg; height: 95 cm

Daniel is prescribed O$_2$, a STAT dose of 700 mg IV ceftriaxone, 300 mL of IV sodium chloride 0.9%, 200 mg of PO paracetamol and 2 mg of PO dexamethasone. Despite a repeated dose of dexamethasone 12 hours later, he is still deteriorating and starts to become less responsive.

Prescribe ONE medicine that is most appropriate for the treatment of Daniel's condition at this stage.

(Use the hospital 'once-only medicines' prescription chart provided in Appendix 1)[22–24]

QUESTION 27

Mr Tomlin, a 59-year-old, undergoes a successful drug-eluting stent place-ment in the left circumflex coronary artery following confirmed evidence of stenosis on elective coronary angiography.

PMH: unstable angina (6 years ago), diabetes mellitus
DH: aspirin 75 mg OM, bisoprolol 5 mg OM, atorvastatin 40 mg ON, ramipril 10 mg OM, GTN 400 micrograms sublingual spray T-TT PRN, gliclazide MR 60 mg OM
SH: gave up smoking 6 years ago; one to two cans of beer a week

The patient is given the loading doses of relevant medications as part of the procedure.

Weight: 90 kg; height: 178 cm

Write a prescription for ONE medicine that should be added to Mr Tomlin's regular prescription for a defined period of time (assuming that the patient had been pre-medicated before PCI).

(Use the hospital 'regular medicines' prescription chart provided in Appendix 1)[25,26]

QUESTION 28

Miss MN, a 28-year-old, has recently been diagnosed with HIV and comes to your contraception clinic for a review.

PMH: migraine with aura

DH: rizatriptan (Maxalt® Melt Wafers) 10 mg PRN, repeated after 2 hours if migraine recurs, Migraleve® PRN two pink tablets at onset of attack, followed by two yellow tablets every 4 hours if necessary (up to two pink and six yellow in 24 hours), Cerazette® 75 micrograms OD; allergies: copper allergy (skin rash)

SH: smokes 35–40 cigarettes a day

On Examination

Temperature 36.6°C, HR 68/min and regular, BP 115/68 mmHg, RR 12/min, O$_2$ sat 98% on air

Weight: 59 kg; height: 1.57 m

Miss MN has recently been prescribed Combivir® tablets T BD and Viramune® 'immediate-release' tablets 200 mg OD for the first 14 days, then 200 mg BD.

You consult the GP and decide to adjust her pharmaceutical contraceptive measures accordingly. Miss MN understands this necessity but also admits that she is 'terribly scared of needles' and would like to avoid them if possible. She also has a fairly erratic lifestyle and has forgotten to take her pill on several occasions.

Assuming that an immediate switch to adjusted contraceptive measures is possible, write a prescription for ONE pharmaceutical contraceptive option that will be suitable for Miss MN.

(Use the general practice prescription form provided in Appendix 1)[27]

QUESTION 29

You are bleeped by the Neonatal Intensive Care Unit sister who asks you to come to see newborn baby Stevens that needs a medication prescribing. The sister thinks that the SpR may have forgotten to prescribe it before she left the unit. Baby Stevens had an endotracheal tube inserted (verified by colorimetric CO_2 detection) for mechanical ventilation soon after birth. He is to be transferred onto continuous positive airway pressure as soon as reasonably possible.

PMH: 27 weeks' gestation (born 25 minutes ago)
DH: mother received two 6 mg doses of dexamethasone IM 12 hours apart prior to delivery
Weight: 740 g

Baby Stevens has already been given a bolus of normal saline, which helped restore his BP. He is also due for some IV caffeine to facilitate weaning from the mechanical ventilation.

On Examination

Temperature 36.7°C, HR 131/min and regular, BP 61/35 mmHg, RR 36/min, O_2 sat 86% on air
Mild grunting, intermittent apnoea, no cyanosis

Prescribe a STAT dose of one medicine that is most essential for baby Stevens at this stage.

(Use the hospital 'once-only medicines' prescription chart provided in Appendix 1)[28–32]

QUESTION 30

Kevin, a 64-year-old retired mechanical engineer, is referred to hospital by the walk-in centre with progressive shortness of breath. He finds it difficult to undertake any normal activities, and his sleep has become increasingly worse.

PMH: STEMI (2 years ago), angina, five × coronary stents, diabetes, CHF, AF
DH: warfarin 5.5 mg daily, atorvastatin 80 mg ON, bisoprolol 10 mg OM, lisinopril 20 mg OM, GTN 400 micrograms sublingual spray PRN, nicorandil 20 mg BD, furosemide 80 mg at 8 a.m. and 80 mg at noon, metformin 1 g OM, 500 mg at noon, 500 mg in the evening, Victoza® 1.8 mg by SC injection OM; NKDA
SH: non-smoker, occasional drinker; weight: 127 kg; height: 183 cm

Kevin is placed on 1 L/24 hours' fluid restriction and is switched to IV furosemide. He recovers over a few days, and you decide to review his current pharmaceutical management.

On Examination

Temperature 36.4°C, HR 62/min and irregular, BP 110/74 mmHg, RR 21/min, JVP 5 cm elevated, O_2 sat 96% on air
Peripheral oedema noted, crepitations audible at lung bases; third heart sound present

Investigations

Na^+ 141 mmol/L (135–146), K^+ 3.3 mmol/L (3.5–5.0), Cr 91 μmol/L (79–118), eGFR 77 mL/min/1.73 m^2, glucose 8.3 mmol/L (4–9), HbA_{1c} 46 mmol/mol (48–59)
Echo: LVEF 35%; CXR: cardiomegaly, pulmonary congestion seen

Write a prescription for ONE medicine that should be added to Kevin's regular prescription to improve his clinical condition.

(Use the hospital 'regular medicines' prescription chart provided in Appendix 1)[6,7,33,34]

QUESTION 31

Mrs VB, a 49-year-old, is brought into hospital by her concerned partner. He thinks this time she is 'honestly sick'. Mrs VB has exceeded her credit card limit, has been 'driving like crazy', and he often cannot understand what she is talking about. He describes how his wife has been having 'some ridiculous thoughts'.

PMH: bipolar disorder
DH: Camcolit® 400 tablets TT OM, valproic acid 1 g BD, fluoxetine 20 mg OM
Weight: 51 kg; height: 1.53 m

Her fluoxetine is stopped, and she is prescribed some diazepam IM. However, that only calms her down for a few minutes. She refuses to take any medicines by mouth.

On Examination

Temperature 35.9°C, HR 145/min and regular, BP 159/97 mmHg, RR 27/min, O_2 sat 97% on air

During your examination you note Mrs VB is agitated and restless with rapid speech and an illogical thought process. You observe her flamboyant clothing and excessive make-up.

Investigations

WBC 4.1×10^9/L (4–11), Neut 2.4×10^9/L (2.0–7.5), Plt 235×10^9/L (150–400)
Na$^+$ 137 mmol/L (135–146), K$^+$ 4.1 mmol/L (3.5–5.0), Cr 77 μmol/L (79–118), U 2.7 mmol/L (2.5–6.7), CRP 3 mg/L (<10), ALP 41 U/L (39–117), ALT 8 U/L (5–40), total bilirubin 7 μmol/L (<17), TSH 2.8 mU/L (0.3–3.5), free T_4 17 pmol/L (10–25), lithium 1 mmol/L (0.4–1.0)
ECG: sinus tachycardia

Prescribe a STAT dose of one medicine that is most suitable for Mrs VB in order to relieve her symptoms.

(Use the hospital 'once-only medicines' prescription chart provided in Appendix 1)[35,36]

QUESTION 32

Miss TY, a 24-year-old art student, is referred to the sexual health clinic. She complains of non-menstrual bleeding and pain during sexual intercourse. She has also been suffering from some unusual, foul-smelling vaginal discharge.

PMH: myasthenia gravis (well controlled)

DH: pyridostigmine 120 mg at 8 a.m., 60 mg at 2 p.m. and 60 mg at 8 p.m.; metronidazole 400 mg PO TDS for 7/7 (8 days ago); vaccinations up to date; NKDA

SH: smokes up to 20 cigarettes/day, occasional alcohol, more than two sexual partners in the last 12 months

On Examination

Temperature 36.5°C, HR 73/min and regular, BP 123/84 mmHg, RR 13/min
Weight: 59 kg; height: 1.63 m
The cervix is inflamed, malodorous vaginal discharge present

Investigations

HIV test: negative
Hepatitis B test: pending
Endocervical swabs for chlamydia/gonorrhoea: pending
Urine: negative for nitrites, leucocytes and protein

You give her a STAT dose of IM ceftriaxone and decide to prescribe one other medicine just to be on the safe side.

Write a prescription for ONE other medicine that will be most suitable for Miss TY while awaiting confirmation of the diagnosis.

(Use the general practice prescription form provided in Appendix 1)[37–43]

QUESTION 33

Mrs Williams, a 39-year-old journalist, will be travelling to Brazil (Maranhão state) in a week's time. Up until recently, she did not realise that she needed to take some antimalarial prophylaxis during the trip. Today she comes into your travel health clinic for some advice and an antimalarial prescription.

PMH: epilepsy, acute porphyria; NKDA
DH: gabapentin 300 mg TDS, clonazepam 4 mg ON
SH: social drinker, non-smoker

On Examination

Temperature 36.7°C, HR 76/min and regular, BP 131/80 mmHg, RR 12/min; weight: 67 kg; height: 1.66 m.

Write a prescription for ONE antimalarial medicine that will be most suitable for Mrs Williams' trip to Brazil.

(Use the general practice prescription form provided in Appendix 1)

QUESTION 34

Mr LK, a 54-year-old Jamaican gentleman, attends your hypertension clinic. He routinely monitors his BP at home and has recently noticed it is persistently elevated (often >160/100 mmHg).

PMH: NSTEMI (2 years ago), heart failure
DH: aspirin 75 mg OM, carvedilol 25 mg BD, furosemide 80 mg OM and 40 mg midday, candesartan 32 mg OM (increased from 16 mg OM about 8 weeks ago), eplerenone 50 mg OM, atorvastatin 40 mg ON, GTN 300 microgram sublingual tablets one to two tablets PRN; allergies: ramipril – dry cough
SH: gave up smoking (20 pack year history) and drinking 2 years ago

On Examination

Temperature 36.5°C, HR 62/min and regular, BP 163/102 mmHg, RR 14/min; weight: 93 kg; height: 1.77 m

Investigations

Na⁺ 145 mmol/L (135–146), K⁺ 4.5 mmol/L (3.5–5.0), Cr 86 μmol/L (79–118), U 3.1 mmol/L (2.5–6.7), eGFR 103 mL/min/1.73 m², glucose 6.2 mmol/L (<11.1)
6 months ago: echo – LVEF 40% and LVH; ECG: sinus rhythm

Write a prescription for ONE medicine that may help optimise the BP control for Mr LK.

(Use the general practice prescription form provided in Appendix 1)[44–46]

QUESTION 35

Mrs Brown, a 29-year-old lady, is 38 weeks pregnant. She is admitted for elective Caesarean section.

PMH: deep vein thrombosis (6 months ago), gastric ulcer (12 months ago), first pregnancy complicated by spina bifida
DH: dalteparin 8000 units BD, omeprazole 20 mg OM
Weight: 83 kg; height: 1.69 m

The procedure is successful and a healthy baby is born. The consultant asks you to prescribe a STAT dose of one prophylactic medicine for this neonate at birth.

Prescribe a STAT dose of one prophylactic medicine that is most suitable for baby Brown at birth.

(Use the hospital 'once-only medicines' prescription chart provided in Appendix 1)[47,48]

QUESTION 36

Mrs VM, a 67-year-old ex-ambassador, comes to see you complaining of increasing pain in the big toe of her left foot. The pain started one day prior and has been getting worse. She finds it hard to put on her shoes and is suffering from extreme discomfort.

PMH: COPD, unstable angina (2 years ago), duodenal ulcer (10 years ago)
DH: ipratropium bromide pressurised metered-dose inhaler 20–40 micrograms up to QDS PRN, Seretide® 500 Accuhaler® T BD, aspirin 75 mg OM, ramipril 10 mg OM, carvedilol 12.5 mg BD, ezetimibe 10 mg ON, isosorbide mononitrate MR 30 mg OM, esomeprazole 20 mg OM, co-codamol 8/500 T-TT QDS PRN; allergies/sensitivities: simvastatin (myopathy)
SH: alcohol: one to two glasses of red wine a day, diet includes a significant amount of seafood

On Examination

Temperature 36.4°C, HR 65/min and regular, BP 124/85 mmHg, RR 17/min; weight: 82 kg; height: 1.67 m
Swelling, erythema and exquisite tenderness of the first metatarsophalangeal joint of her left foot; no other joints are affected in the feet, knees, ankles, shoulders, wrists; no rash or stiffness noted

Investigations

Na$^+$ 138 mmol/L (135–146), K$^+$ 3.9 mmol/L (3.5–5.0), Cr 89 μmol/L (79–118), U 3.5 mmol/L (2.5–6.7), eGFR 58 mL/min/1.73 m^2, urate 0.9 mmol/L (0.18–0.42)

Write a prescription for ONE medicine that may help to relieve the symptoms experienced by Mrs VM.

(Use the general practice prescription form provided in Appendix 1)[49–51]

QUESTION 37

Christine, a 19-year-old lady, is 8 weeks pregnant. She has been continuously vomiting over the last couple of days, and came into hospital after starting to feel weak and dizzy. It is so bad that she is unable to 'keep anything down'. Christine has tried Buccastem®, which she normally uses for her migraines, but that 'has not been of any good'.

PMH: migraine
DH: Buccastem® tablets 3 mg T-TT BD, paracetamol 500 mg–1 g PRN QDS, folic acid 400 micrograms OM; NKDA
SH: lives with her partner in a shared-house; non-drinker; smokes 10 cigarettes/day
Weight: 52 kg; height: 153 cm

On Examination

Temperature 36.6°C, HR 83/min and regular, BP 93/67 mmHg, RR 19/min, O_2 sat 99% on air; GCS 14/15

Investigations

Na^+ 157 mmol/L (135–146), K^+ 2.6 mmol/L (3.5–5.0), U 2.7 mmol/L (2.5–6.7), Cr 76 μmol/L (79–118), eGFR 90 mL/min/1.73 m², glucose 3.8 mmol/L (<11.1)

Christine is provided fluid/electrolyte support and is prescribed some oral thiamine.

Write a prescription for ONE medicine that would be most suitable for management of the signs and symptoms exhibited by Christine at this stage.

(Use the hospital 'regular medicines' prescription chart provided in Appendix 1)[52–54]

QUESTION 38

Mr FG, a 35-year-old history teacher, presents to your clinic complaining of some itchiness and burning sensation in the eyelids that started a few weeks ago. Both of his eyes are affected. The symptoms are worse in the mornings, and he often wakes up with his eyelids stuck together. He has tried applying warm compresses, massaging and cleaning the eyelids as advised by his local chemist, however that has been of little help.

PMH: dry eye syndrome (does not wear contact lenses)
DH: Systane Ultra® multiple-use eye drops T PRN to both eyes
FH: mother had methotrexate-induced bone marrow aplasia
SH: non-smoker, non-drinker

On Examination

Temperature 36.7°C, HR 78/min and regular, BP 115/68 mmHg, RR 14/min; weight: 69 kg; height: 1.69 m
Red, inflamed, swollen anterior margins of the eyelids of both eyes; mildly blurred vision; pronounced telangiectasia, trichiasis and madarosis present; collarettes around the lashes noted

Write a prescription for ONE medicine that is most suitable for Mr FG at this stage.

(Use the general practice prescription form provided in Appendix 1)[55,56]

QUESTION 39

Victoria, a 21-year-old student from Ghana, is admitted to hospital with unbearable body pain, blood-tinged sputum and breathlessness.

PMH: sickle-cell disease, anorexia nervosa
DH: folic acid 5 mg OM, hydroxycarbamide 500 mg OM, olanzapine 5 mg ON, cyclizine 50 mg TDS PRN, co-codamol 50/300 T-TT PRN QDS, tramadol 50–100 mg PRN QDS, senna 7.5 mg T-TT PRN ON; vaccinations up to date; allergies: penicillin (reaction unknown)
FH: mother suffers from sickle-cell disease
SH: unknown

On Examination

Temperature 38.4°C, HR 110/min and regular, BP 102/67 mmHg, RR 27/min, O_2 sat 95% on air; weight: 52 kg; height: 1.63 m
GCS 13/15; sharp pain and swelling of the legs; splenomegaly noted; chest auscultation: crepitations bibasally; heart sounds normal

Investigations

WBC 14.6×10^9/L (4–11), Neut 11.9×10^9/L (2.0–7.5), Plt 155×10^9/L (150–400), Hb 7.6 g/dL (11.5–16.5), reticulocyte count 18%
Na^+ 162 mmol/L (135–146), K^+ 2.5 mmol/L (3.5–5.0), Cr 152 μmol/L (79–118), U 12.2 mmol/L (2.5–6.7), CRP 89 mg/L (<10); CXR: bilateral pulmonary infiltrates; urine culture: negative; blood cultures: pending

Victoria is prescribed cefuroxime 1.5 g IV TDS together with adequate analgesia, O_2 and fluid support. Four days later she recovers and is restarted on her regular medicines. The haematologist thinks that the pre-admission drug history is incomplete and asks you to reinitiate one more essential medicine.

Write a prescription for ONE medicine that is most needed for Victoria at this stage.

(Use the hospital 'regular medicines' prescription chart provided in Appendix 1)[57–61]

QUESTION 40

Mr Barnett, a 65-year-old writer, is brought in to hospital by his wife after not being able to swallow any food or drink for several days. Mr Barnett's appetite has significantly declined over the past few weeks and he has lost as much as 2 stone in weight over the last month or so. He has also developed a painful cough.

PMH: squamous cell carcinoma of the oesophagus, hiatus hernia, IBS
DH: 5-fluorouracil 1000 mg/m^2/24 hours IV and cisplatin 75 mg/m^2 IV; completed four cycles (12 months ago), Oramorph® 10 mg/5 mL 5–10 mL PRN QDS, MST Continus® 30 mg BD, metoclopramide 10–20 mg PRN TDS, lansoprazole 30 mg OM, Mintec® capsules T TDS
SH: lives with his wife in a private mansion in Horsham

On Examination

Temperature 35.9°C, HR 67/min and regular, BP 110/78 mmHg, RR 14/min, O$_2$ sat 97% on air. Weight: 49 kg; height: 1.69 m. Respiratory examination: minimal crepitations right upper lobe.

Investigations

WBC 4.2×10^9/L (4–11), Neut 2.9×10^9/L (2.0–7.5), Plt 236×10^9/L (150–400), Hb 9.6 g/dL (11.5–16.5)
Na$^+$ 154 mmol/L (135–146), K$^+$ 5.2 mmol/L (3.5–5.0), Cr 134 μmol/L (79–118), U 8.3 mmol/L (2.5–6.7), CRP 6 mg/L (<10)
CXR: multiple cavitating lesions in the right upper lobe; CT of chest/liver/adrenals: pending

Mr Barnett is prescribed adequate pain relief and fluid support.

Write a prescription for ONE medicine that is most necessary for Mr Barnett at this stage.

(Use the hospital 'regular medicines' prescription chart provided in Appendix 1)[62–66]

QUESTION 41

Kelly is a 22-year-old lady who is 41 weeks pregnant. This is her first pregnancy. Today Kelly is admitted to the labour ward for elective membrane sweeping and labour induction. She is not planned for caesarean section.

PMH: nil
DH: nil
Weight: 72 kg; height: 1.66 m

On Examination

Temperature 36.3°C, HR 71/min and regular, BP 119/83 mmHg, RR 11/min, O_2 sat 99% on air; Bishop score 5/13
No evidence of uterine hyperstimulation or uterine rupture

Investigations

WBC 5.3×10^9/L (4–11), Neut 3.2×10^9/L (2.0–7.5), Plt 351×10^9/L (150–400), Na$^+$ 141 mmol/L (135–146), K$^+$ 4.0 mmol/L (3.5–5.0), Cr 88 μmol/L (79–118), U 4.1 mmol/L (2.5–6.7)
Electronic foetal monitoring (cardiotocography): HR 152/min, normal uterine contractions
Ultrasound: no abnormalities detected

Adequate pain relief is prescribed, and Kelly is prepared for induction of labour. The obstetrician asks you to prescribe one medicine that is most suitable to induce labour for this lady.

Prescribe a STAT dose of one medicine that is most suitable to help induce labour for Kelly.

(Use the hospital 'once-only medicines' prescription chart provided in Appendix 1)[67–70]

QUESTION 42

Mrs Bedford, a 74-year-old retired nurse, is brought into hospital after not being able to cope at home. Ever since her husband died of cancer 2 months ago, Mrs Bedford has been feeling very low and hopeless. To make it worse, she has been getting these 'horrible water problems'. Her GP has recently prescribed her some antibiotics but those didn't really work. She doesn't have much urgency but gets some leakage without noticing, primarily when she tries to do some gardening.

PMH: iron-deficiency anaemia, ulcerative colitis (in remission)
DH: ferrous fumarate 305 mg T BD, Salazopyrin EN-Tabs® 500 mg T QDS, Forceval® capsules T OM, nitrofurantoin 50 mg QDS for 3/7 (3 weeks ago)
SH: lives on her own in a house; daughter visits her twice a week

On Examination

Temperature 36.4°C, HR 73/min and regular, BP 129/83 mmHg, RR 14/min, O_2 sat 98% on air
Weight: 54 kg; height: 1.59 m
Some urine leakage on intentional coughing

Investigations

WBC 3.2×10^9/L (4–11), Neut 2.1×10^9/L (2.0–7.5), Plt 192×10^9/L (150–400), Hb 11.3 g/dL (11.5–16.5)
Na^+ 143 mmol/L (135–146), K^+ 3.6 mmol/L (3.5–5.0), Cr 69 μmol/L (79–118), U 2.6 mmol/L (2.5–6.7)

The consultant asks you to prescribe one medicine that will help to tackle both of Mrs Bedford's problems.

Write a prescription for ONE medicine that is most suitable for Mrs Bedford at this stage.

(Use the hospital 'regular medicines' prescription chart provided in Appendix 1)[69,71]

QUESTION 43

Mrs Khan, an 81-year-old lady, is admitted to hospital with a 2-week history of increased urinary frequency and urgency. She also complains of severe discomfort on urination.

PMH: GORD, hypertension
DH: lansoprazole dispersible tablets 30 mg OM, Gaviscon® 10 mL TDS + 10 mL ON PRN, amlodipine 10 mg OM, bendroflumethiazide 2.5 mg OM, trimethoprim 200 mg PO BD for 3/7 (7 days before admission); allergies: flucloxacillin (rash + swelling)
SH: lives in a nursing home

On Examination

Temperature 37.5°C, HR 82/min and regular, BP 129/83 mmHg, RR 14/min, O_2 sat 98% on air
Weight: 78 kg; height: 5'3"
A degree of suprapubic tenderness is present

Investigations

WBC 13×10^9/L (4–11), Neut 9×10^9/L (2.0–7.5), CRP 50 mg/L (<10), Plt 184×10^9/L (150–400), Hb 12.4 g/dL (11.5–16.5), Na^+ 152 mmol/L (135–146), K^+ 3.1 mmol/L (3.5–5.0), Cr 101 μmol/L (79–118), eGFR 48 mL/min/1.73 m^2, U 5.8 mmol/L (2.5–6.7), urine dipstick: positive for nitrites (+++) and leukocytes (++)

Mrs Khan is prescribed adequate fluid and electrolyte replacement as well as ciprofloxacin 750 mg PO BD. The next day the following urine culture sensitivity data is obtained: *Klebsiella* species resistant to trimethoprim and ciprofloxacin, sensitive to nitrofurantoin, co-amoxiclav and gentamicin.

Write a prescription for ONE antibacterial that is most suitable for Mrs Khan at this stage.

(Use the hospital 'regular medicines' prescription chart provided in Appendix 1)[15,72,73]

QUESTION 44

Mr Robinson, a 55-year-old policeman, experiences an attack of fulminant colitis and undergoes a panproctocolectomy with ileostomy.

PMH: ulcerative colitis, hiatus hernia, asthma

DH: mesalazine MR (Pentasa®) 2 g OM, mesalazine rectal foam 2 g ON, azathioprine 150 mg OM, omeprazole 40 mg OM, salbutamol 100 microgram Evohaler® T-TT PRN QDS, Symbicort Turbohaler® 200/6 TT BD

SH: smokes 14 cigarettes/day; occasional pint of beer

Post-operatively, Mr Robinson's ulcerative colitis medicines are stopped. He recovers well with adequate fluid, electrolyte and nutritional support. A few days into his recovery period, the sister in charge asks you to see him. His daily stoma output has been consistently around 1300 mL (normal output 400–800 mL/day).[74] Ever since patient-controlled analgesia was stopped, Mr Robinson has also been in pain despite paracetamol 1 g PO QDS and Oramorph® liquid 5–10 mg PRN QDS.

On Examination

Temperature 36.5°C, HR 105/min and regular, BP 95/76 mmHg, RR 16/min, O_2 sat 99% on air

Weight: 89 kg; height: 1.88 m

Investigations

WBC 4.3×10^9/L (4–11), Neut 2.8×10^9/L (2.0–7.5), CRP 8 mg/L (<10), Plt 239×10^9/L (150–400), Hb 11.7 g/dL (11.5–16.5), Na+ 139 mmol/L (135–146), K+ 4.2 mmol/L (3.5–5.0), Cr 130 μmol/L (79–118), U 9.5 mmol/L (2.5–6.7)

Write a prescription for ONE medicine that is most suitable for Mr Robinson at this stage.

(Use the hospital 'regular medicines' prescription chart provided in Appendix 1)[74–77]

QUESTION 45

Mr BW, a 60-year-old gentleman, undergoes coronary artery bypass graft (CABG) surgery. Unfortunately, he loses a significant amount of blood during the operation ($\approx$1 100 mL) and starts developing signs of hypovolaemic shock.

PMH: CKD, T2DM, sciatica

DH: gliclazide 80 mg BD, ramipril 2.5 mg OM, simvastatin 40 mg ON, co-codamol 30/500 T-TT PRN QDS

SH: vegan, nil alcohol, non-smoker

On Examination

Temperature 35.3°C, HR 138/min and regular, BP 90/86 mmHg, JVP not elevated, RR 29/min, O_2 sat 96% on air

Cool, clammy skin; capillary refill time 5 seconds; confused and restless

Weight: 89 kg; height: 1.92 m

Investigations (Pre-surgical)

WBC 4.9×10^9/L (4–11), Neut 3.2×10^9/L (2.0–7.5), Plt 398×10^9/L (150–400), Hb 12.8 g/dL (11.5–16.5)

Na^+ 149 mmol/L (135–146), K^+ 3.7 mmol/L (3.5–5.0), Cr 164 μmol/L (79–118), U 7.6 mmol/L (2.5–6.7), albumin 38 g/L (35–50), ALP 52 U/L (39–117), ALT 17 U/L (5–40), total bilirubin 7 μmol/L (<17), CRP 12 mg/L (<10)

Urine output: 21 mL/hr

The consultant asks you to prescribe some fluids to provide adequate volume expansion until whole blood becomes available for transfusion.

Write a prescription for ONE fluid that is most suitable for Mr BW prior to blood transfusion.

(Use the hospital fluid prescription chart provided in Appendix 1)[1,78–83]

QUESTION 46

Mrs ME, a 56-year-old administrator, undergoes elective total hip replacement surgery. The operation is successful and she is recovering well.

PMH: angina, hypertension, non-valvular atrial fibrillation (AF), CKD, osteoarthritis, asthma, needle phobia

DH: Securon SR® 240 mg OM, amiodarone 200 mg and 100 mg OM on alternate days, ramipril 10 mg OM, aspirin 75 mg OM (withheld 7 days prior to surgery), co-dydramol 10/500 TT QDS, salbutamol 100 micrograms T-TT PRN QDS, Qvar® Autohaler® 50 micrograms T BD; she had a trial of warfarin therapy for stroke prophylaxis in the past, which was stopped because of a persistently unstable INR; allergies: NKDA

SH: ex-smoker (gave up 6 years ago), occasional alcohol

On Examination

Temperature 36.6°C, HR 82/min and irregular, BP 133/75 mmHg, RR 13/min, O_2 sat 98% on air

Weight: 92 kg; height: 1.64 m

Investigations

WBC 5.6×10^9/L (4–11), Neut 4.1×10^9/L (2.0–7.5), Plt 322×10^9/L (150–400), Hb 13.6 g/dL (11.5–16.5), APTT 25 s (23–31), INR 1.0

Na⁺ 140 mmol/L (135–146), K⁺ 3.7 mmol/L (3.5–5.0), U 5.8 mmol/L (2.5–6.7), Cr 142 μmol/L (79–118), eGFR 35 mL/min/1.73 m², albumin 45 g/L (35–50), ALP 43 U/L (39–117), ALT 14 U/L (5–40), total bilirubin 6 μmol/L (<17)

Mrs ME had a 40 mg dose of enoxaparin 12 hours before surgery. The SHO asks you to initiate the post-operative pharmacological venous thromboembolism prophylaxis as appropriate.

Write a prescription for ONE thromboprophylactic medicine that is most suitable for Mrs ME.

(Use the hospital 'regular medicines' prescription chart provided in Appendix 1)[84]

QUESTION 47

Mark, a 14-year-old boy who suffers from cystic fibrosis, is admitted to the paediatric respiratory ward with fever, shortness of breath and increased sputum production.

PMH: cystic fibrosis

DH: Nutrizym® 10 capsules T with meals and snacks, Forceval® Junior capsules TT OM, Fresubin Energy® one bottle BD, dornase alfa 2.5 mg OM, sodium chloride 3% nebs 4 mL TDS; allergies/intolerances: ciprofloxacin – joint pain

On Examination

Temperature 39.3°C, HR 119/min and regular, BP 98/65 mmHg, RR 32/min, O$_2$ sat 93% on air, FEV$_1$ 42% predicted

Weight: 40 kg; height: 1.52 m

Crepitations bibasally on chest auscultation; heart sounds normal

Investigations

WBC 15.7 × 10^9/L (4–11), Neut 8.6 × 10^9/L (2.0–7.5), Plt 178 × 10^9/L (150–400), Hb 11.6 g/dL (11.5–16.5)

Na$^+$ 129 mmol/L (135–146), K$^+$ 2.7 mmol/L (3.5–5.0), U 8.3 mmol/L (2.5–6.7), Cr 86 μmol/L (79–118), CRP 183 mg/L (<10)

Chest X-ray: diffuse interstitial disease

MRSA screen: negative

Sputum and blood cultures: *Pseudomonas aeruginosa* (sensitive to tobramycin)

Mark is treated with a combination of IV piperacillin/tazobactam and tobramycin for 2 weeks. He recovers fully, and the consultant suggests that he should be prescribed an eradication course for previously unrecognised chronic *P. aeruginosa* infection.

Write a prescription for ONE antimicrobial that is most suitable for Mark.

(Use the hospital 'regular medicines' prescription chart provided in Appendix 1)[85–89]

QUESTION 48

Molly is a 26-year-old university student who was diagnosed with HIV 6 months ago. Today she comes to your community psychiatry clinic for some advice. Ever since the diagnosis her life seems to have got out of hand. Molly failed all five of her exams and had to 'wave goodbye' to her part-time job. To make things worse, her partner has recently left her and she had to move out of their apartment. Molly has lost her appetite and finds it difficult to fall asleep. She thinks her life is just a 'mess' and 'not worth living anymore'.

PMH: HIV, epilepsy (last seizure 6 years ago)
DH: Kaletra® tablets TT BD, Combivir® tablets T BD, sodium valproate E/C tablets 600 mg BD; allergies: NKDA

On Examination

Temperature 36.5°C, HR 74/min and regular, BP 126/83 mmHg, RR 14/min; weight: 66 kg; height: 1.74 m

Molly has been seeing a psychologist and attending group activities for the last 3 months; however, that did not appear to have any positive effect. You decide to give pharmacological treatment a go.

Write a prescription for ONE medicine that is most suitable for Molly to help improve her symptoms.

(Use the general practice prescription form provided in Appendix 1)[90–92]

REFERENCES

1. Medusa Injectable Medicines Guide Online: National Health Service. Available at: www.injguide.nhs.uk

2. Trissel LA. *Handbook on Injectable Drugs* [Online]. London: Pharmaceutical Press; 2013. Available at: www.medicinescomplete.com

3. National Institute for Health and Clinical Excellence. *Type 2 Diabetes: NICE guideline 87 – quick reference guide*. London: NICE; 2010. Available at: www.nice.org.uk/nicemedia/live/12165/44322/44322.pdf

4. National Institute for Health and Clinical Excellence. *Chronic Obstructive Pulmonary Disease: NICE guideline 101 – quick reference guide*. London: NICE; 2010. Available at: www.nice.org.uk/nicemedia/live/13029/49399/49399.pdf

5. Ballinger A, Patchett S. Heart failure. In: Kumar P, Clark M, editors. *Pocket Essentials of Clinical Medicine*. 4th ed. London: Saunders Elsevier; 2007. pp. 423–34.

6. National Institute for Health and Clinical Excellence. *Chronic Heart Failure: NICE guideline 108 – quick reference guide*. London: NICE; 2010. Available at: www.nice.org.uk/nicemedia/live/13099/50526/50526.pdf

7. McAnaw J, Hudson SA. Chronic heart failure. In: Walker R, Whittlesea C, editors. *Clinical Pharmacy and Therapeutics*. 4th ed. London: Churchill Livingstone Elsevier; 2007. pp. 298–318.

8. National Institute for Health and Clinical Excellence. *Osteoarthritis: NICE guideline 59 – quick reference guide*. London: NICE; 2008. Available at: www.nice.org.uk/nicemedia/live/11926/39554/39554.pdf

9. Ballinger A, Patchett S. Osteoarthritis. In: Kumar P, Clark M, editor. *Pocket Essentials of Clinical Medicine*. 4th ed. London: Saunders Elsevier; 2007. pp. 258–62.

10. National Institute for Health and Clinical Excellence. *Alendronate, etidronate, risedronate, raloxifene, strontium ranelate and teriparatide for the secondary prevention of osteoporotic fragility fractures in postmenopausal women: NICE guideline 161 – quick reference guide*. London: NICE; 2008. Available at: www.nice.org.uk/nicemedia/live/11748/42508/42508.pdf

11. National Institute for Health and Clinical Excellence. *Denosumab for the prevention of osteoporotic fractures in postmenopausal women: NICE guideline 204 – quick reference guide*. London: NICE; 2010. Available at: http://guidance.nice.org.uk/TA204/QuickRefGuide/pdf/English

12. Nicoll D, McPhee SJ, Pignone M, *et al*. *Pocket Guide to Diagnostic Tests*. 3rd ed. London: McGraw-Hill; 2000.

13. Watson M, Lucas C, Hoy A, *et al*. Palliative Care Guidelines Plus [Online]; 2011. Available at: http://book.pallcare.info/index.php?wpage=3

14. Clinical Knowledge Summaries. *How do I manage nausea and vomiting in people with Parkinson's disease?* [Online]; 2009 [cited 30 November 2013]. Available at: http://cks.nice.org.uk/parkinsons-disease#!scenariorecommendation:13

15. *Antimicrobial Policies and Guidelines*. Redhill: Surrey and Sussex Healthcare NHS Trust; 2012.

16. Ballinger A, Patchett S. Skin and soft tissue infections. In: Kumar P, Clark M, editors. *Pocket Essentials of Clinical Medicine*. 4th ed. London: Saunders Elsevier; 2007. pp. 21–2.

17. Cooper-Brown L, Copeland S, Dailey S, *et al*. Feeding and swallowing dysfunction in genetic syndromes. *Dev Disabil Res Rev*. 2008; **14**(2): 147–57.

18. White R, Bradnam V. *Handbook of Drug Administration via Enteral Feeding Tubes* [Online]; 2013. Available at: www.medicinescomplete.com

19. Ballinger A, Patchett S. Addison's disease – primary hypoadrenalism. In: Kumar P, Clark M, editors. *Pocket Essentials of Clinical Medicine*. 4th ed. London: Saunders Elsevier; 2007. pp. 621–3.

20. Saeed S, Body R. Towards evidence based emergency medicine: best BETs from the Manchester Royal Infirmary. Auscultating to diagnose pneumonia. *Emerg Med J*. 2007; **24**(4): 294–6.

21. National Institute for Health and Clinical Excellence. *Atrial Fibrillation: NICE guideline 36 – quick reference guide*. London: NICE; 2006. Available at: www.nice. org.uk/nicemedia/live/10982/30054/30054.pdf

22. *Croup* [Online]. Clinical Knowledge Summaries; 2012 [cited 30 November 2013]. Available at: http://cks.nice.org.uk/croup

23. National Institute for Health and Care Excellence. *Feverish illness in children: NICE guideline 160*. London: NICE; 2013. Available at: www.nice.org.uk/nicemedia/ live/14171/63908/63908.pdf

24. *Diagnosing Croup* [Online]. London: NHS Choices; 2012 [cited 15 November 2012]. Available at: www.nhs.uk/Conditions/Croup/Pages/Diagnosis.aspx

25. Wykrzykowska JJ, Arbab-Zadeh A, Godoy G, *et al*. Assessment of in-stent restenosis using 64-MDCT: analysis of the CORE-64 Multicenter International Trial. *AJR Am J Roentgenol*. 2010; **194**(1): 85–92.

26. *Guidelines for Percutaneous Coronary Intervention* [Online]. European Society of Cardiology; 2005 [cited 18 November 2012]. Available at: www.bcis.org.uk/ resources/documents/esc_pci2005.pdf

27. *Summary of Product Characteristics Nexplanon 68 mg Implant for Subdermal Use* [Online]. Electronic Medicines Compendium; 2012 [cited 18 November 2012]. Available at: www.medicines.org.uk/EMC/medicine/23824/SPC/Nexplanon+68 +mg+implant+for+subdermal+use/#INTERACTIONS

28. Sweet DG, Carnielli V, Greisen G, *et al*.; European Association of Perinatal Medicine. European consensus guidelines on the management of neonatal respiratory distress syndrome in preterm infants – 2010 update. *Neonatology*. 2010; **97**(4): 402–17.

29. *Neonatal Respiratory Distress Syndrome* [Online]. PubMed Health; 2011 [cited 21 November 2012]. Available at: www.ncbi.nlm.nih.gov/pubmedhealth/ PMH0002530/

30. *Assessments for Newborn Babies* [Online]. Palo Alto, CA: Lucile Packard Children's Hospital at Stanford; 2012 [cited 21 November 2012]. Available at: www.lpch.org/ DiseaseHealthInfo/HealthLibrary/hrnewborn/assess.html

31. *Neonatal Handbook: blood pressure* [Online]. Melbourne: The Royal Children's Hospital (Australia); 2012 [cited 21 November 2012]. Available at: www.netsvic. org.au/nets/handbook/index.cfm?doc_id=450

32. Tinnion R, Vasey N. Neonatal care: the sick neonate. *Clin Pharm*. 2012; **4**: 165–9.

33. McMurray JJ, Adamopoulos S, Anker SD, *et al.*; ESC Committee for Practice Guidelines. ESC Guidelines for the diagnosis and treatment of acute and chronic heart failure 2012: the Task Force for the Diagnosis and Treatment of Acute and Chronic Heart Failure 2012 of the European Society of Cardiology. *Eur Heart J*. 2012; **33**(14): 847–1787.

34. Ballinger A, Patchett S. Investigations in cardiac disease. In: Kumar P, Clark M, editors. *Pocket Essentials of Clinical Medicine*. 4th ed. London: Saunders Elsevier; 2007. pp. 397–408.

35. National Institute for Health and Clinical Excellence. *Bipolar Disorder: NICE guideline 38 – quick reference guide*. London: NICE; 2006. Available at: www.nice. org.uk/nicemedia/live/10990/30191/30191.pdf

36. Pratt JP. Affective disorders. In: Walker R, Whittlesea C, editors. *Clinical Pharmacy and Therapeutics*. 4th ed. London: Churchill Livingstone Elsevier; 2007. pp. 424–37.

37. *Chlamydia – Uncomplicated Genital* [Online]. Clinical Knowledge Summaries; 2009 [cited 30 November 2013]. Available at: http://cks.nice.org.uk/ chlamydia-uncomplicated-genital

38. *Gonorrhoea* [Online]. Clinical Knowledge Summaries; 2011 [cited 30 November 2013]. Available at: http://cks.nice.org.uk/gonorrhoea

39. *Myasthenia Gravis – Treatment* [Online]. London: NHS Choices; 2011 [cited 24 November 2012]. Available at: www.nhs.uk/Conditions/Myasthenia-gravis/Pages/ Treatment.aspx

40. *Chlamydia – Symptoms* [Online]. London: NHS Choices; 2011 [cited 24 November 2012]. Available at: www.nhs.uk/Conditions/Chlamydia/Pages/Symptoms.aspx

41. Bacterial vaginosis – Symptoms [Online]. NHS Choices; 2012 [cited 24 November 2012]. Available at: www.nhs.uk/Conditions/Bacterialvaginosis/Pages/Symptoms. aspx

42. *Syphilis – Symptoms* [Online]. London: NHS Choices; 2012 [cited 24 November 2012]. Available at: www.nhs.uk/Conditions/Syphilis/Pages/Symptomspg.aspx

43. *Acute Pelvic Inflammatory Disease: tests and treatment* [Online]. Royal College of Obstetricians and Gynaecologists; 2010 [cited 24 November 2012]. Available at: www.rcog.org.uk/files/rcog-corp/Acute%20Pelvic%20Inflammatory%20 Disease%20%28PID%29_0.pdf

44. National Institute for Health and Clinical Excellence. *Hypertension: NICE guideline 127 – quick reference guide*. London: NICE; 2011. Available at: www.nice.org.uk/ nicemedia/live/13561/56015/56015.pdf

45. *How Is Cardiomyopathy Diagnosed?* [Online]. National Heart, Lung and Blood Institute; 2012 [cited 25 November 2012]. Available at: www.nhlbi.nih.gov/ health//dci/Diseases/cm/cm_diagnosis.html

46. *New Diagnostic Criteria for Diabetes (Jan 2011)* [Online]. Diabetes UK; 2011 [cited 25 November 2012]. Available at: www.diabetes.org.uk/About_us/What-we-say/ Diagnosis-prevention/New_diagnostic_criteria_for_diabetes/

47. *Vitamin K and Vitamin K Deficiency Bleeding of the Newborn* [Online]. Royal Free Hampstead NHS Trust; 2008 [cited 25 November 2012]. Available at: www.royal free.nhs.uk/pip_admin/docs/vitamin_K_1057.pdf

48. Hey E. Vitamin K: what, why, and when. *Arch Dis Child Fetal Neonatal Ed.* 2003; **88**(2): F80–3.

49. *Gout* [Online]. Clinical Knowledge Summaries; 2012 [cited 30 November 2013]. Available at: http://cks.nice.org.uk/gout

50. Jordan KM, Cameron JS, Snaith M, *et al.* British Society for Rheumatology and British Health Professionals in Rheumatology guideline for the management of gout. *Rheumatology (Oxford).* 2007; **46**(8): 1372–4.

51. Roddy E. Gout: presentation and management in primary care. *Reports on the Rheumatic Diseases (Hands On).* 2011; **6**(9): 1–8.

52. *Summary of Product Characteristics Buccastem 3mg* [Online]. Electronic Medicines Compendium; 2011 [cited 1 December 2012]. Available at: www.medicines.org. uk/EMC/medicine/22805/SPC/Buccastem+3mg/#INDICATIONS

53. *Summary of Product Characteristics Metoclopramide Tablets BP 10mg* [Online]. Electronic Medicines Compendium; 2011 [cited 1 December 2012]. Available at: www.medicines.org.uk/EMC/medicine/24123/SPC/Metoclopramide+Tablets +BP+10mg/

54. *Dehydration – Symptoms* [Online]. London: NHS Choices; 2011 [cited 1 December 2012]. Available at: www.nhs.uk/Conditions/Dehydration/Pages/Symptoms.aspx

55. *Blepharitis* [Online]. Clinical Knowledge Summaries; 2012 [cited 30 November 2013]. Available at: http://cks.nice.org.uk/blepharitis

56. *Summary of Product Characteristics Boots Infected Eyes 1% w/w Eye Ointment* [Online]. Electronic Medicines Compendium; 2011 [cited 27 March 2013]. Available at: www.medicines.org.uk/EMC/medicine/26610/SPC/Boots+Infected+Eyes+1 ++w+w+Eye+Ointment/#CONTRAINDICATIONS

57. Rees DC, Olujohungbe AD, Parker NE, *et al.* Guidelines for the management of the acute painful crisis in sickle cell disease. *Br J Haematol.* 2003; **120**(5): 744–52.

58. Brambilla F, Garcia CS, Fassino S, *et al.* Olanzapine therapy in anorexia nervosa: psychobiological effects. *Int Clin Psychopharmacol.* 2007; **22**(4): 197–204.

59. Taylor C, Carter F, Poulose J, *et al.* Clinical presentation of acute chest syndrome in sickle cell disease. *Postgrad Med J.* 2004; **80**(944): 346–9.

60. Ballinger A, Patchett S. Sickle cell disease. In: Kumar P, Clark M, editors. *Pocket Essentials of Clinical Medicine.* 4th ed. London: Saunders Elsevier; 2007. pp. 202–3.

61. Acomb C, Holden J. Anaemia. In: Walker R, Whittlesea C, editors. *Clinical Pharmacy and Therapeutics.* 4th ed. London: Churchill Livingstone Elsevier; 2007. pp. 699–714.

62. National Institute for Health and Clinical Excellence. *Lung Cancer: NICE guideline 121*. London: NICE; 2011. Available at: www.nice.org.uk/nicemedia/live/13465/54202/54202.pdf

63. Hassan I. *Lung Metastases Imaging* [Online]. Medscape; 2011 [cited 6 December 2012]. Available at: http://emedicine.medscape.com/article/358090-overview#a19

64. Ballinger A, Patchett S. Malignant oesophageal tumours. In: Kumar P, Clark M, editors. *Pocket Essentials of Clinical Medicine*. 4th ed. London: Saunders Elsevier; 2007. pp. 73–4.

65. Ballinger A, Patchett S. Carcinoma of the lung. In: Kumar P, Clark M, editors. *Pocket Essentials of Clinical Medicine*. 4th ed. London: Saunders Elsevier; 2007. pp. 538–43.

66. *Cisplatin/5-Fluorouracil + Radiotherapy (Herskovic)* [Online]. Surrey, West Sussex and Hampshire Cancer Network; 2000 [cited 30 November 2013]. Available at: www.royalsurrey.nhs.uk/Default.aspx?DN=2bde55ee-c499-4d30-a1f7-877cef08e67e

67. National Institute for Health and Clinical Excellence. *Induction of Labour: NICE guideline 70 – quick reference guide*. London: NICE; 2008. Available at: www.nice.org.uk/nicemedia/live/12012/41266/41266.pdf

68. *Summary of Product Characteristics Prostin E2 Vaginal Gel 1mg, 2mg* [Online]. Electronic Medicines Compendium; 2011 [cited 8 December 2012]. Available at: www.medicines.org.uk/EMC/medicine/1562/SPC/Prostin+E2+Vaginal+Gel+1mg%2c+2mg/

69. *Martindale: the complete drug reference* [Online]. Available at: www.medicinescomplete.com/

70. Tenore JL. Methods for cervical ripening and induction of labor. *Am Fam Physician*. 2003; **67**(10): 2123–8.

71. *Incontinence – Urinary, In Women* [Online]. Clinical Knowledge Summaries; 2009 [cited 30 November 2013]. Available at: http://cks.nice.org.uk/incontinence-urinary-in-women

72. *Urinary Tract Infection (Lower) – Women* [Online]. Clinical Knowledge Summaries; 2009 [cited 30 November 2013]. Available at: http://cks.nice.org.uk/urinary-tract-infection-lower-women

73. Pai MP, Paloucek FP. The origin of the 'ideal' body weight equations. *Ann Pharmacother*. 2000; **34**(9): 1066–9.

74. Holmes S. How to assist in the care of stoma patients. *Clin Pharm*. 2012; **4**: 327–9.

75. Ballinger A, Patchett S. Inflammatory bowel disease. In: Kumar P, Clark M, editors. *Pocket Essentials of Clinical Medicine*. 4th ed. London: Saunders Elsevier; 2007. pp. 96–104.

76. Cripps SE, Beresford S. Inflammatory bowel disease. In: Walker R WC, editor. *Clinical Pharmacy and Therapeutics*. 4th ed. London: Churchill Livingstone Elsevier; 2007. pp. 169–86.

77. Arnell TD. Surgical management of acute colitis and toxic megacolon. *Clin Colon Rectal Surg*. 2004; **17**(1): 71–4.

78. Ballinger A, Patchett S. Acute disturbances of haemodynamic function (shock). In: Kumar P, Clark M, editors. *Pocket Essentials of Clinical Medicine*. 4th ed. London: Saunders Elsevier; 2007. pp. 552–62.

79. Sedrakyan A, Gondek K, Paltiel D, *et al*. Volume expansion with albumin decreases mortality after coronary artery bypass graft surgery. *Chest*. 2003; **123**(6): 1853–7.

80. Schumacher J, Klotz KF. Fluid therapy in cardiac surgery patients. *Cardiopulmonary Pathophysiology*. 2009; **13**: 138–42.

81. Magder S, Potter BJ, Varennes BD, *et al*. Fluids after cardiac surgery: a pilot study of the use of colloids versus crystalloids. *Crit Care Med*. 2010; **38**(11): 2117–24.

82. Floss K, Borthwick M, Clark C. Intravenous fluids – principles of treatment. *Clin Pharm*. 2011; **3**(9): 27483.

83. Staples A, Dade J, Acomb C. Intravenous fluids – practical aspects of therapy. *Clin Pharm*. 2011; **3**(9): 285–91.

84. National Institute for Health and Clinical Excellence. *Venous thromboembolism – reducing the risk: NICE guideline 92 – quick reference guide* [Online]. London: NICE; 2011. Available at: www.nice.org.uk/nicemedia/live/12695/47197/47197.pdf

85. British Medical Association; Royal Pharmaceutical Society. *British National Formulary for Children* [Online]. London: Pharmaceutical Press; 2012. Available at: www.medicinescomplete.com

86. *Nutritional Management of Cystic Fibrosis* [Online]. UK Cystic Fibrosis Trust; 2002 [cited 30 November 2013]. Available at: https://www.cysticfibrosis.org.uk/media/82052/CD_Nutritional_Management_Apr_02.pdf

87. *Standards for the Clinical Care of Children and Adults with Cystic Fibrosis in the UK* [Online]. UK Cystic Fibrosis Trust; 2011 [cited 30 November 2013]. Available at: www.cysticfibrosis.org.uk/media/82070/CD_Standards_of_Care_Dec_11.pdf

88. *Antibiotic Treatment for Cystic Fibrosis* [Online]. UK Cystic Fibrosis Trust; 2009 [cited 30 November 2013]. Available at: https://www.cysticfibrosis.org.uk/media/82010/CD_Antibiotic_treatment_for_CF_May_09.pdf

89. Flume PA, O'Sullivan BP, Robinson KA, *et al*. Cystic fibrosis pulmonary guidelines: chronic medications for maintenance of lung health. *Am J Respir Crit Care Med*. 2007; **176**(10): 957–69.

90. *Summary of Product Characteristics Edronax 4mg Tablets* [Online]. Electronic Medicines Compendium; 2011 [cited 27 March 2013]. Available at: www.medicines.org.uk/EMC/medicine/8386/SPC/Edronax+4mg+Tablets/

91. National Institute for Health and Clinical Excellence. *Depression in Adults: NICE guideline 90 – quick reference guide*. London: NICE; 2009. Available at: www.nice.org.uk/nicemedia/live/12329/45890/45890.pdf

92. *Stockley's Drug Interactions* [Online]. Available at: www.medicinescomplete.com/

Chapter 2

Prescription Review

QUESTION 1

Mrs TA, a 58-year-old woman, presents to the A&E department with a recent-onset painful maculopapular rash on her trunk. The rash started a few days ago together with some flu-like symptoms that have already resolved.

PMH: T2DM, hypertension, GORD and hypothyroidism
DH: metformin 1 g OM, 500 mg midday and 500 mg at night, sitagliptin 100 mg OM, lisinopril 5 mg OM, nifedipine modified-release 10 mg BD, paracetamol 1 g QDS PRN, omeprazole 20 mg OM and levothyroxine 125 micrograms OM; her current medicines are listed in the table presented below

Mrs TA is diagnosed with shingles and is prescribed a 7-day course of aciclovir. While in hospital she develops acute kidney injury (AKI) with Cr 253 µmol/L (79–118) and eGFR 17 mL/min/1.73 m^2.

Current Prescriptions			
Drug Name	**Dose**	**Route**	**Frequency**
Metformin	1 g OM, 500 mg midday, 500 mg ON	ORAL	As per dose
Sitagliptin	100 mg	ORAL	Daily
Lisinopril	5 mg	ORAL	Daily
Adalat® Retard	10 mg	ORAL	12-hourly
Paracetamol	1 g PRN	ORAL	6-hourly
Omeprazole	20 mg	ORAL	Daily
Levothyroxine	125 micrograms	ORAL	Daily
Aciclovir	800 mg	ORAL	Five times daily

Question A

Select TWO prescriptions that are the *most likely* cause of the AKI experienced by Mrs TA.

Question B

Select TWO prescriptions (other than the ones in Question A) that are *most likely* to be temporarily withheld or have their dose reduced because of this AKI.[2]

QUESTION 2

James, a 62-year-old former long-distance runner, underwent a total hip replacement. However, 5 days later he started developing some pain, swelling and erythema around the surgical site, which was accompanied by fever (39°C) and general malaise.

PMH: atrial fibrillation, TIA, heart failure, depression and musculoskeletal neuropathic pain
DH: carvedilol 6.25 mg BD, ramipril 10 mg OM, warfarin 4 mg OD (INR 2.2 4 days after restarting warfarin following surgery), citalopram 20 mg OM, paracetamol 1 g PRN QDS and amitriptyline 10 mg ON; his current medicines are listed in the table presented below

Following the microbiologist's advice, James was started on a 6-week course of vancomycin and rifampicin for MRSA-confirmed osteomyelitis. He was also prescribed some extra painkillers. Nevertheless, a week later he suddenly deteriorated with severe confusion, hallucinations, shivering and notable tachycardia (INR 1.6). Your registrar suspected that some of James' medicines might have induced CNS toxicity.

Current Prescriptions			
Drug Name	Dose	Route	Frequency
Carvedilol	6.25 mg	ORAL	12-hourly
Ramipril	10 mg	ORAL	Daily
Warfarin	4 mg	ORAL	Daily
Citalopram	20 mg	ORAL	Daily
Paracetamol	1 g PRN	ORAL	6-hourly
Amitriptyline	10 mg	ORAL	Daily
Tramadol	100 mg	ORAL	6-hourly
Vancomycin	1 g	IV	12-hourly
Rifampicin	300 mg	ORAL	12-hourly

Question A

Select THREE prescriptions that have *most likely* contributed to the CNS toxicity experienced by James in hospital.

Question B

Select ONE prescription that has *most likely* caused a loss of the therapeutic anticoagulant effect in this case.[3,4]

QUESTION 3

Mrs Roberts, a 78-year-old confused lady, fell while walking in the park. Her lying and standing BP on admission was 125/75 mmHg and 95/55 mmHg, respectively. Clinical investigations demonstrated: glucose 3.2 mmol/L (4–9), HbA_{1c} 36 mmol/mol (48–59), Na^+ 159 mmol/L (135–146), K^+ 4.9 mmol/L (3.5–5.0) and Cr 124 μmol/L (79–118). Her urine dipstick was positive for protein and negative for nitrites.

PMH: T2DM, stroke, dementia, vertigo, anxiety
DH: her current and repeat medicines are listed in the table presented below; intolerances: metformin (severe gastrointestinal effects)
SH: ex-smoker, widow, lives independently
Weight: 85 kg; height: 1.61 m

Current Prescriptions			
Drug Name	**Dose**	**Route**	**Frequency**
Glibenclamide	10 mg	ORAL	Daily
Liraglutide	1.2 mg	S/C	Daily
Galantamine	8 mg	ORAL	12-hourly
Prochlorperazine	5 mg	ORAL	8-hourly
Lorazepam	0.5–1 mg	ORAL	8-hourly
Clopidogrel	75 mg	ORAL	Daily
Trimethoprim	200 mg	ORAL	12-hourly
Paracetamol	1 g	ORAL	6-hourly
Movicol®	T	ORAL	12-hourly

Question A

Select THREE prescriptions that are *most* inappropriate for Mrs Roberts, considering her old age and the medical history.

Question B

Select ONE prescription that has *most likely* been prescribed inappropriately taking into account her current clinical condition.[5]

QUESTION 4

A 7-year-old boy is admitted to hospital with a complicated soft-tissue infection that has been treated with oral flucloxacillin by his GP. He is started on an IV infusion of moxifloxacin 400 mg daily.

PMH: tonic–clonic seizures, ADHD, acute porphyria; weight: 22 kg
DH: carbamazepine 200 mg BD, lamotrigine 300 mg BD and methylphenidate 50 mg BD; his current medicines are listed in the table presented below

Current Prescriptions			
Drug Name	Dose	Route	Frequency
Carbamazepine	200 mg	ORAL	12-hourly
Lamotrigine	300 mg	ORAL	12-hourly
Methylphenidate	50 mg	ORAL	12-hourly
Paracetamol	250 mg	ORAL	6-hourly
Moxifloxacin	400 mg	IV	Daily

Question A

Select TWO prescriptions that are *most* inappropriate for this child considering his current clinical condition and his past medical history.

Question B

Select TWO prescriptions that have been prescribed using incorrect doses (assuming that the doses indicated in the BNF are the ones recommended for children of his age).

QUESTION 5

Mr BT, a 55-year-old, was brought to A&E by his sister following a sudden onset of ataxia, dysarthria, tremor and muscle twitching. His BP and HR on admission were 74/50 mmHg and 110 bpm, respectively. Blood investigations demonstrated: Na$^+$ 125 mmol/L (135–146), K$^+$ 5.2 mmol/L (3.5–5.0) and Cr 175 µmol/L (79–118).

PMH: osteoarthritis, mania, schizophrenia, hypertension, heart failure
DH: his current medicines are listed in the table presented below
Weight: 72 kg

Current Prescriptions			
Drug Name	**Dose**	**Route**	**Frequency**
Diclofenac	50 mg	ORAL	8-hourly
Sodium valproate MR (Episenta®)	1 g	ORAL	12-hourly
Lithium carbonate MR (Liskonium®)	450 mg	ORAL	12-hourly
Aripiprazole	10 mg	ORAL	Daily
Temazepam	20 mg	ORAL	Daily (ON)
Perindopril	4 mg	ORAL	Daily
Bumetanide	1 mg	ORAL	Daily
Bisoprolol	5 mg	ORAL	Daily

Question A

Select ONE prescription that has *most likely* induced the symptoms of toxicity experienced by Mr BT on admission.

Question B

Select THREE prescriptions that have *most likely* aggravated the toxicity of the medicine identified in Question A.

QUESTION 6

Mrs YG is brought into hospital suffering from new-onset pain in her left calf that started approximately 2 days after flying back home from Hong Kong. Her husband is very worried as Mrs YG is 28 weeks into her pregnancy.

PMH: T1DM, asthma
DH: her current and repeat medicines are listed in the table presented below
Weight (on week 6 of pregnancy): 78 kg

Your house officer colleague on call believes that Mrs YG has developed a deep vein thrombosis and initiates her on warfarin together with enoxaparin cover until her INR becomes therapeutic.

Current Prescriptions			
Drug Name	**Dose**	**Route**	**Frequency**
NovoMix® 30	18 units OM, 24 units ON	SC	12-hourly
Gliclazide	80 mg	ORAL	Daily
Ventolin® Evohaler® 100 micrograms	T-TT PRN	INH	6-hourly
Pulmicort® Turbohaler® 100 micrograms	TT	INH	12-hourly
Warfarin	10 mg for 2 days, then 5 mg (then according to INR)	ORAL	Daily
Enoxaparin	120 mg (until warfarin therapeutic)	SC	Daily
Folic acid	5 mg	ORAL	Daily

Question A

Select THREE prescriptions that are *most* inappropriate for Mrs YG considering her stage of pregnancy and the medical history.

Question B

Select ONE prescription the dose of which has NOT been prescribed correctly.

QUESTION 7

Victor is a 75-year-old gentleman who presents to your clinic at the surgery complaining of some yellow-orange discolouration of his arms. In addition, Victor finds it really hard to fall asleep at night these days, and even when he succeeds, he often suffers from nightmares. Blood investigations demonstrate a normal liver and renal function.

PMH: ulcerative colitis, hypertension, AF, adrenocortical insufficiency, neuropathic pain
DH: his current medicines are listed in the table presented below
SH: alcohol, one to two glasses of red wine a week

Current Prescriptions			
Drug Name	Dose	Route	Frequency
Propranolol	80 mg	ORAL	12-hourly
Ramipril	10 mg	ORAL	Daily
Warfarin	3 mg	ORAL	Daily
Amiodarone	200 mg	ORAL	Daily
Sulfasalazine	500 mg	ORAL	6-hourly
Hydrocortisone	20 mg (8 a.m.), 10 mg (6 p.m.)	ORAL	10-hourly
Lansoprazole	30 mg	ORAL	Daily
Atorvastatin	20 mg	ORAL	Daily
Amitriptyline	25 mg	ORAL	Daily

Question A

Select ONE prescription that is *most likely* to have caused the skin discolouration reported by Victor.

Question B

Select THREE prescriptions that are *most likely* contributing to Victor's disturbed sleeping patterns.

QUESTION 8

Mrs Robinson, an 82-year-old lady, was found confused at home by her son.

PMH: polymyalgia rheumatica, osteoporosis, epilepsy, breast cancer, asthma
DH: her repeat medicines are listed in the table presented below
SH: fully independent, non-smoker, nil alcohol

On Examination

Temperature 38.3°C, HR 103/min and regular, BP 98/62 mmHg; GCS 10/15
Red, diffuse, exfoliative, purpuric rash is noted on her trunk together with profound cervical
    lymphadenopathy

Investigations

WBC 14.2×10^9/L (4–11), Neut 8.4×10^9/L (2.0–7.5), eosinophils 2.4×10^9/L (0.04–0.4)
Na^+ 127 mmol/L (135–146), K^+ 5.3 mmol/L (3.5–5.0), Cr 178 µmol/L (79–118), eGFR 25 mL/
    min/1.73 m², CRP 47 mg/L (<10), albumin 28 g/L (35–50), ALP 198 U/L (39–117), ALT
    102 U/L (5–40), total bilirubin 24 µmol/L (<17)
Chest X-ray: bilateral pulmonary infiltration; ECG: sinus tachycardia

Current Prescriptions			
Drug Name	**Dose**	**Route**	**Frequency**
Prednisolone	3 mg	ORAL	Daily
Calcichew D3 Forte® tablets	TT	ORAL	Daily
Co-dydramol 10/500	T-TT PRN	ORAL	6-hourly
Omeprazole	20 mg	ORAL	Daily
Phenytoin	150 mg	ORAL	12-hourly
Strontium ranelate	2 g	ORAL	At night
Letrozole	2.5 mg	ORAL	Daily
Symbicort 200/6®	T-TT	INH	12-hourly
Ventolin® 100 micrograms Evohaler®	T-TT PRN	INH	6-hourly

Question A

Select TWO prescriptions that have *most likely* caused the serious rash experienced by Mrs Robinson.

Question B

Select TWO prescriptions that are *most likely* to carry an increased risk of toxicity in the presence of hypoalbuminaemia.[6,7]

QUESTION 9

Mr Chiew, a 67-year-old retired pharmacist, is urgently taken to hospital after developing sudden right-sided hemisensory loss.

PMH: NSTEMI (5 years ago), depression
DH: his current and repeat prescriptions are listed in the table presented below
SH: lives with his wife in a private house

Mr Chiew is confirmed to have suffered a TIA. Following a 14-day course of aspirin 300 mg OM, he is switched to aspirin 75 mg OM and clopidogrel 75 mg OM.

Current Prescriptions			
Drug Name	**Dose**	**Route**	**Frequency**
Aspirin	75 mg	ORAL	Daily
Clopidogrel	75 mg	ORAL	Daily
Omeprazole	20 mg	ORAL	Daily
Ramipril	5 mg	ORAL	Daily
Simvastatin	10 mg	ORAL	At night
Bisoprolol	2.5 mg	ORAL	Daily
Fluoxetine	20 mg	ORAL	Daily
Glyceryl trinitrate 400 micrograms spray	T-TT PRN	S/L	For angina pain

Question A

Select TWO prescriptions that are not prescribed correctly according to the latest NICE and BNF guidance.

Question B

Select TWO prescriptions that are *most likely* to interact with clopidogrel reducing its antiplatelet effect.[8–12]

QUESTION 10

Mrs PM, a 62-year-old Greek lady, is taken to hospital by her son. He explains that while walking around London his mum started complaining of some generalised muscle aches. He didn't think it was anything serious, so they just decided to have a coffee break. During this time Mrs PM became very lethargic, confused and started to become less responsive.

PMH: T2DM, hypertension, recurrent UTIs, leg cramps, rheumatoid arthritis
DH: her current and repeat prescriptions are listed in the table presented below
SH: occasional red wine

On Examination

Temperature 35.8°C, HR 110/min and regular, BP 94/54 mmHg; GCS 9/15; jaundice noted
Abdominal, cardiovascular and chest examination unremarkable

Investigations

Glucose 17.8 mmol/L (4–9), Na$^+$ 127 mmol/L (135–146), K$^+$ 6.7 mmol/L (3.5–5.0), Cr 476 µmol/L (79–118), CRP 7 mg/L (<10), Hb 6.8 g/dL (11.5–16.5), MCV 105 fL (80–96), ALP 105 U/L (39–117), ALT 94 U/L (5–40), total bilirubin 37 µmol/L (<17), creatinine kinase 3589 µmol/L (24–170)
Chest X-ray: clear; ECG: sinus tachycardia

Mrs PM is suspected to have developed acute kidney injury secondary to rhabdomyolysis. She is also reviewed by the haematologist who, on further investigation, confirms haemolytic anaemia due to glucose 6-phosphate dehydrogenase (G6PD) deficiency.

Current Prescriptions			
Drug Name	**Dose**	**Route**	**Frequency**
Aspirin	75 mg	ORAL	Daily
Eucreas® 50/850 tablets	T	ORAL	12-hourly
Gliclazide	80 mg	ORAL	Daily
Amlodipine	10 mg	ORAL	Daily
Perindopril	4 mg	ORAL	Daily
Simvastatin	40 mg	ORAL	At night

Current Prescriptions			
Drug Name	Dose	Route	Frequency
Nitrofurantoin	100 mg	ORAL	At night
Quinine sulphate	300 mg	ORAL	At night
Methotrexate	15 mg	SC	Fridays
Folic acid	5 mg	ORAL	Sundays

Question A

Select THREE prescriptions that should be used with the greatest caution in G6PD-deficient patients.

Question B

Select ONE prescription that has most likely precipitated the statin-related rhabdomyolysis experienced by Mrs PM.[7,13–17]

QUESTION 11

Mr Rasmussen, an 88-year-old gentleman, is brought in by ambulance from his nursing home with a high fever, shortness of breath and confusion.

PMH: AF, CCF, MI (two stents), hypertension, diverticular disease, anaemia
DH: his current and repeat prescriptions are listed in the table presented below
SH: non-smoker
Temperature 39.7°C, HR 142/min, irregular, JVP raised, BP 102/69 mmHg; GCS 10/15; bilateral crepitations on chest auscultation; bilateral ankle oedema noted

Mr Rasmussen is treated empirically for severe community-acquired pneumonia with co-amoxiclav and clarithromycin. He is also prescribed 240 mg of IV furosemide over 30 minutes as treatment for heart failure. Mr Rasmussen is given an extra dose of digoxin and his warfarin is switched to the treatment dose of enoxaparin. The next morning his antibiotic regimen is replaced by IV vancomycin and PO rifampicin as per microbiology advice for suspected MRSA chest sepsis.

Three days later, the staff nurse looking after Mr Rasmussen asks you to prescribe some laxatives as he is having difficulty opening his bowels. You decide to speak to Mr Rasmussen about his bowel problem and notice a marked decrease in his hearing ability.

Current Prescriptions			
Drug Name	**Dose**	**Route**	**Frequency**
Digoxin	125 micrograms	ORAL	Daily
Enoxaparin	100 mg	SC	Daily
Furosemide	80 mg	IV	8 a.m., 2 p.m.
Atorvastatin	80 mg	ORAL	At night
Eplerenone	25 mg	ORAL	Daily
Enalapril	10 mg	ORAL	12-hourly
Buscopan® tablets	20 mg	ORAL	6-hourly
Ferrous fumarate	210 mg	ORAL	8-hourly
Rifampicin	300 mg	ORAL	12-hourly
Vancomycin	750 mg	IV	12-hourly

Question A

Select TWO prescriptions that have *most likely* caused Mr Rasmussen's hearing impairment.

Question B

Select TWO prescriptions that have *most likely* contributed to constipation in Mr Rasmussen's case.[18,19]

QUESTION 12

You are a house officer on the urology ward. Mr Rees, a 59-year-old coach driver, is on the morning list for a transurethral resection of his prostate (TURP). It is now 20 hours before his procedure and you have been asked to carry out a final medication review prior to surgery. Mr Rees is to be kept nil by mouth from midnight.

PMH: hypertension, PE (3 months ago), COPD, BPH, mania

DH: his current and repeat prescriptions are listed in the table presented below; allergies: ramipril – dry cough

SH: gave up smoking 4 years ago, occasional alcohol

On Examination

Temperature 36.5°C, HR 67/min and regular, BP 132/86 mmHg, O_2 sat 97% on air, RR 13/min
Weight: 114 kg, height: 5'7"

Investigations

Hb 13.6 g/dL (13.5–17.7), WBC 6.7×10^9/L (4–11), Neut 4.1×10^9/L (2.0–7.5), Plt 312×10^9/L (150–400)

Na^+ 137 mmol/L (135–146), K^+ 4.8 mmol/L (3.5–5.0), Cr 93 µmol/L (79–118), APTT 26 seconds (23–31), INR 1.4, ALP 43 U/L (39–117), ALT 28 U/L (5–40), total bilirubin 9 µmol/L (<17)

Chest X-ray: clear; ECG: sinus rythmn

Current Prescriptions			
Drug Name	**Dose**	**Route**	**Frequency**
Olmesartan	20 mg	ORAL	Daily
Enoxaparin (omit the night before surgery)	170 mg	SC	Daily
Amlodipine	10 mg	ORAL	Daily
Indapamide	2.5 mg	ORAL	Daily
Seretide® 500 Accuhaler®	T	ORAL	12-hourly
Salbutamol 100 micrograms Evohaler®	T-TT PRN	ORAL	6-hourly
Tamsulosin MR	400 micrograms	ORAL	Daily
Priadel®	400 mg	ORAL	Daily
Tolterodine MR	4 mg	ORAL	Daily

Question A

Select TWO prescriptions that should be stopped in preparation for his TURP.

Question B

Select TWO prescriptions that may be permanently discontinued after the procedure.[20–22]

QUESTION 13

Mrs Gomez, a 47-year-old, undergoes a laparotomy to enable resection of a recently diagnosed liver cancer affecting the right lobe. Unfortunately, post-operative recovery is not smooth, and Mrs Gomez develops intra-abdominal sepsis. This is complicated by paralytic ileus. An NG tube is inserted and IV fluids commenced.

PMH: schizophrenia, Raynaud's disease, trigeminal neuralgia; allergies: amoxicillin – angioedema

DH: her current and repeat prescriptions are listed in the table presented below

SH: smokes 25 cigarettes a day, no alcohol

On Examination

Temperature 38.6°C, HR 110/min and regular, BP 90/65 mmHg, O_2 sat 95% on air, RR 24/min; a distended abdomen with absent bowel sounds is noted on examination; weight: 63 kg

Investigations

WBC 15.7×10^9/L (4–11), Neut 11.3×10^9/L (2.0–7.5), Plt 350×10^9/L (150–400), APTT 31 seconds (23–31), INR 1.1, ALP 322 U/L (39–117), ALT 89 U/L (5–40), total bilirubin 22 μmol/L (<17), CRP 243 mg/L (<10)

Mrs Gomez is prescribed a course of teicoplanin, ciprofloxacin and metronidazole.

Current Prescriptions			
Drug Name	**Dose**	**Route**	**Frequency**
Carbamazepine liquid	100 mg	NG	At night
Clozapine suspension	100 mg OM, 125 mg ON	NG	Daily
Amitriptyline tabs	10 mg	NG	At night
Hyoscine patches	1 mg	TOP	72-hourly
Paracetamol	1 g	IV/NG	6-hourly
Senna liquid	15 mg	NG	At night
Teicoplanin (pre-loaded)	400 mg	IV	24-hourly
Metronidazole	500 mg	IV	8-hourly
Ciprofloxacin liquid	750 mg	NG	12-hourly

Question A

Select THREE prescriptions that should be avoided in the presence of paralytic ileus.

Question B

Select ONE prescription that has been prescribed incorrectly considering Mrs Gomez's clinical status.[19,23,24]

QUESTION 14

Mrs Lebedeva, a 48-year-old lady, is due for elective nephrectomy of stage II renal cell carcinoma under general anaesthesia. You see her in the pre-assessment clinic 4 weeks before the procedure.

PMH: relapsing/remitting multiple sclerosis, adrenocortical insufficiency
DH: her current and repeat prescriptions are listed in the table presented below
SH: non-smoker, nil alcohol

On Examination

Temperature 36.5°C, HR 65/min and regular, BP 123/78 mmHg, O₂ sat 98% on air, RR 13/min

You decide to review and plan her peri-operative pharmaceutical care.

Current Prescriptions			
Drug Name	**Dose**	**Route**	**Frequency**
FemSeven Conti®	50 micrograms/24 hours/ 7 micrograms/24 hours	TOP	Weekly
Diazepam	2 mg	ORAL	8-hourly
Lansoprazole	15 mg	ORAL	Daily
Paracetamol	1 g PRN	ORAL	6-hourly
Baclofen	10 mg OM, 5 mg lunchtime, 5 mg ON	ORAL	8-hourly
Hydrocortisone	10 mg OM, 10 mg lunchtime, 5 mg ON	ORAL	8-hourly
Laxido® sachets	T	ORAL	12-hourly
Domperidone	10 mg	ORAL	8-hourly
Alendronic acid	70 mg	ORAL	Weekly
Adcal-D3® tablets	T	ORAL	12-hourly

Question A

Select ONE prescription that should be withheld before Mrs Lebedeva is admitted for her surgery.

Question B

Select THREE prescriptions that should not be stopped abruptly prior to Mrs Lebedeva's surgery.[20,25–27]

QUESTION 15

Mr YR, a 55-year-old, suffers an acute intracerebral haemorrhage (ICH) and is urgently referred for decompressive hemicraniectomy.

PMH: stable angina, hypertension, hypercholesterolaemia
DH: simvastatin 20 mg ON, ramipril 5 mg OM, escitalopram 20 mg OM, isosorbide mononitrate MR 30 mg OM, atenolol 50 mg OM, aspirin 75 mg OM (stopped on admission); his current prescriptions are listed in the table presented below
SH: smokes 19 cigarettes a day, social drinker

He recovers successfully after the procedure and is being prepared for discharge 3 weeks later. One night you are bleeped by the sister in charge and asked to come see Mr YR, who has become very confused and developed some 'serious palpitations'.

On Examination

Temperature 36.5°C, HR 189/min and irregular, BP 136/87 mmHg, O_2 sat 96% on air, RR 15/min; GCS 9/15

Investigations

Na$^+$ 136 mmol/L (135–146), K$^+$ 3.4 mmol/L (3.5–5.0), Cr 105 µmol/L (79–118), U 6.5 mmol/L (2.5–6.7), Mg^{2+} 0.4 mmol/L (0.7–1.1), corrected Ca^{2+} 2.4 mmol/L (2.20–2.67), Plt 201 × 10^9/L (150–400), APTT 27 seconds (23–31), INR 1.0
ECG: VT with QTc of 460 ms

Mr YR is appropriately resuscitated and undergoes cardioversion followed by a STAT dose of IV magnesium.

Current Prescriptions			
Drug Name	Dose	Route	Frequency
Simvastatin	20 mg	ORAL	At night
Ramipril	5 mg	ORAL	Daily
Escitalopram	20 mg	ORAL	Daily
Paracetamol	1 g PRN	QDS	6-hourly
Domperidone	10 mg	ORAL	8-hourly
Ondansetron	4 mg PRN	IV	8-hourly

Current Prescriptions			
Drug Name	Dose	Route	Frequency
Senna	15 mg	ORAL	At night
Oramorph® liquid 10 mg/5 mL	2.5–5 mg PRN	ORAL	6-hourly
Isosorbide mononitrate MR	30 mg	ORAL	Daily
Atenolol	50 mg	ORAL	Daily

Question A

Select THREE prescriptions that could have precipitated the type of arrhythmia encountered by Mr YR.

Question B

Select ONE prescription that could have increased the risk of bleeding associated with aspirin (stopped on admission) and led to ICH.[11,28-31]

QUESTION 16

Mr CE, an 88-year-old, is admitted to hospital with progressive shortness of breath and significant limitation of daily activities. He is treated aggressively for an exacerbation of chronic heart failure and demonstrates a rapid recovery.

PMH: STEMI (10 years ago), COPD, CHF, gout, CKD
DH: his current and repeat prescriptions are listed in the table presented below
SH: smokes 19 cigarettes a day, social drinker

During one of the ward rounds Mr CE asks you to have a look at his ankles which according to him are the usual site of his gout attacks.

On Examination

Temperature 36.6°C, HR 78/min and regular, BP 129/65 mmHg, RR 15/min, O_2 sat 93% on air
Weight: 82 kg; height: 1.76 m
Red, swollen, tender right ankle

Investigations

WBC 4.6×10^9/L (4–11), Neut 2.7×10^9/L (2.0–7.5), Na$^+$ 137 mmol/L (135–146), K$^+$ 4.2 mmol/L (3.5–5.0), Cr 162 μmol/L (79–118), eGFR 28 mL/min/1.73 m^2, CRP 6 mg/L (<10), urate 0.7 mmol/L (0.18–0.42)
Arterial blood gas on room air confirms: P_aO_2 9.6 kPa (10–13.3), P_aCO_2 5.9 kPa (4.8–6.1)

Mr CE is treated with colchicine for an acute attack of gout. His atorvastatin is withheld for the duration of treatment.

Current Prescriptions			
Drug Name	**Dose**	**Route**	**Frequency**
Colchicine	500 micrograms	ORAL	12-hourly
Aspirin	75 mg	ORAL	Daily
Allopurinol	100 mg	ORAL	Daily
Ramipril	2.5 mg	ORAL	12-hourly
Alfacalcidol	250 micrograms	ORAL	Daily
Seretide® 500 Accuhaler®	T	INH	12-hourly
Salbutamol	2.5–5 mg PRN	NEB	6-hourly

Current Prescriptions			
Drug Name	**Dose**	**Route**	**Frequency**
Furosemide	80 mg OM, 40 mg lunchtime	ORAL	As per dose
Oxygen 40%	2 L/min PRN	INH	Daily
Isosorbide mononitrate	10 mg at 8 a.m. and 8 p.m.	ORAL	12-hourly

Question A

Select ONE prescription that could have contributed to the development of an acute gout attack experienced by Mr CE.

Question B

Select THREE prescriptions that have not been prescribed correctly on the drug card.[32,33]

QUESTION 17

Mrs LA, a 90-year-old, is taken to hospital by her nursing home manager, who could not cope with her anymore. She has become very unwell and has been having delusions about taking her children to school. The manager thinks she probably has a UTI or new-onset dementia.

PMH: hypertension, AF, Parkinson's disease, depression, osteoporosis
DH: her current and repeat prescriptions are listed in the table presented below
SH: gave up smoking and alcohol 50 years ago

A urine dip taken in A&E is positive for nitrites and Mrs LA is prescribed a course of trimethoprim for a suspected UTI. However, 3 days later she remains delirious with little clinical improvement. Her inflammatory markers are not raised and the microbiological culture results are negative. Her routine observations are normal.

You decide to review her medicines. The nurse also asks you to prescribe something for a dry mouth that Mrs LA has been suffering from ever since admission.

Current Prescriptions			
Drug Name	Dose	Route	Frequency
Felodipine	5 mg	ORAL	Daily
Aspirin	75 mg	ORAL	Daily
Metoprolol	50 mg	ORAL	12-hourly
Sinemet Plus® 25/100 tablets	T	ORAL	At 8 a.m., 12 p.m. and 10 p.m.
Paracetamol	1 g PRN	ORAL	6-hourly
Nortriptyline	75 mg	ORAL	At night
Risedronate	35 mg	ORAL	Weekly
Calcichew D3 Forte®	T	ORAL	12-hourly
Risperidone	0.5 mg	ORAL	Daily

Question A

Select TWO prescriptions that have *most likely* contributed to Mrs LA's hallucinations.

Question B

Select TWO prescriptions that have *most likely* caused the dry mouth symptoms experienced by Mrs LA.[34]

QUESTION 18

Lucas, a 13-year-old, is taken to a hospital walk-in centre by his mum after developing a terrible earache in his right ear. For the last couple of days he has been feeling generally unwell and has also been coughing a lot, so she bought him some codeine linctus and some Night Nurse® from the local chemist.

PMH: spina bifida, eczema

DH: Movicol Paediatric Plain® TT OD, tolterodine 2 mg BD, Tears Naturale® (0.4 mL single use) T both eyes PRN TDS, Oilatum® cream T PRN TDS, Betnovate-RD® cream T PRN BD; OTC: Night Nurse® (paracetamol 1 g, promethazine 20 mg and dextromethorphan 15 mg per 20 mL) 20 mL PRN ON, codeine linctus 15 mg/5 mL PRN 5 mL TDS; current medicines are listed in the table presented below; allergies: benzalkonium chloride

SH: parents divorced, lives with his mother

On Examination

Temperature 38.7°C, HR 101/min and regular, BP 105/75 mmHg, RR 19/min, O_2 sat 98% on air

Weight: 33 kg; height: 1.36 m

Bulging, red and cloudy tympanic membrane of the right ear; some otorrhoea in the external auditory canal

Lucas is prescribed antibiotics for complicated acute otitis media.

Current Prescriptions			
Drug Name	**Dose**	**Route**	**Frequency**
Tolterodine	2 mg	ORAL	12-hourly
Movicol Paediatric Plain®	TT	ORAL	Daily
Betnovate® cream	T to affected areas PRN	TOP	12-hourly
Oilatum® cream	T to affected areas PRN	TOP	8-hourly
OTC Night Nurse®	20 mL PRN	ORAL	At night
OTC codeine linctus	5 mL PRN	ORAL	8-hourly
Co-amoxiclav	1.2 g	IV	8-hourly for 48 hours
Gentamicin 0.3% ear drops	TT to T-TT drops	RIGHT EAR	6-hourly for 7/7
Tears Naturale® eye drops	T PRN	BOTH EYES	8-hourly

Question A

Select THREE prescriptions that have not been prescribed correctly, taking into account Lucas' past medical and pharmaceutical histories as well as his current clinical condition.

Question B

Select ONE medicine that Lucas should not receive considering his age.[35-38]

QUESTION 19

After developing a fever and failing to get out of bed, Miss UC, a 43-year-old, is taken to hospital by the manager of her sheltered accommodation.

PMH: schizophrenia, major depression, heroin addiction, sciatica, vertigo
DH: her current and repeat prescriptions are listed in the table presented below; allergies: penicillin (anaphylaxis)
SH: smokes 27 cigarettes a day, alcohol one bottle of vodka/day

On Examination

Temperature 38.9°C, HR 124/min and regular, BP 101/74 mmHg, RR 23/min, O_2 sat 96% on air
Weight: 43 kg; height: 5'0"

Investigations

WBC 1.7×10^9/L (4–11), Neut 0.3×10^9/L (2.0–7.5), Plt 321×10^9/L (150–400), Na^+ 152 mmol/L (135–146), K^+ 2.7 mmol/L (3.5–5.0), Cr 95 μmol/L, U 7.3 mmol/L (2.5–6.7), CRP 187 mg/L (<10)

Miss UC is prescribed necessary fluid support and antibiotics for the treatment of neutropenic sepsis.

Current Prescriptions			
Drug Name	**Dose**	**Route**	**Frequency**
Methadone liquid 1 mg/mL	45 mL	ORAL	Daily
Clozapine	100 mg OM, 125 mg ON	ORAL	12-hourly
Hyoscine patches	1 mg/72 hours	TOP	72-hourly
Co-codamol 30/500 tablets	T-TT	ORAL	6-hourly
Mirtazapine	45 mg	ORAL	Daily
Teicoplanin	400 mg	IV	Daily
Gentamicin	215 mg	IV	Daily
Ciprofloxacin	750 mg	ORAL	12-hourly
Chlordiazepoxide	According to protocol	ORAL	6-hourly
Pabrinex®	One pair	IV	12-hourly

Question A

Select TWO prescriptions that have *most likely* contributed to the development of the signs and symptoms experienced by Miss UC.

Question B

Select TWO prescriptions that are *most likely* to cause a prolonged QT interval during ECG monitoring for Miss UC.[7,39]

QUESTION 20

Mrs BC, a 67-year-old retired primary school teacher, is brought to A&E following a fit at home.

PMH: epilepsy, depression, amyloidosis, T2DM, peripheral neuropathy
DH: her current and repeat prescriptions are listed in the table presented below; allergies:
   pregabalin and gabapentin (rash), fluconazole (stomach upset)
SH: non-smoker, nil alcohol; lives with her husband in a bungalow

On Examination

Temperature 36.5°C, HR 78/min and regular, BP 125/64 mmHg, RR 12/min, O_2 sat 98% on
   air; weight: 88 kg; height: 162 cm; systems examination unremarkable
Glucose 6.8 mmol/L (4–9)

While in hospital she suffers another episode of tonic–clonic seizures, which is relieved by rectal diazepam. Mrs BC is seen by the neurologist, who increases her dose of phenytoin accordingly.

Current Prescriptions			
Drug Name	**Dose**	**Route**	**Frequency**
Phenytoin capsules	300 mg OM, 200 mg ON	ORAL	12-hourly
Cyclophosphamide	500 mg	ORAL	Weekly
Thalidomide	100 mg	ORAL	Daily
Dexamethasone	20 mg	ORAL	Weekly
Itraconazole liquid 10 mg/mL	200 mg	ORAL	12-hourly
Esomeprazole	20 mg	ORAL	Daily
Citalopram	40 mg	ORAL	Daily
Amitriptyline	20 mg	ORAL	At night
Metformin	1 g OM, 1 g evening	ORAL	12-hourly
Tramadol	50 mg	ORAL	6-hourly

Question A

Select THREE prescriptions that have most likely lowered the seizure threshold for Mrs BC, precipitating tonic–clonic seizures.

Question B

Select ONE prescription that exceeds the maximum dose recommended for this patient.[40,41]

QUESTION 21

Mrs GU, a 38-year-old lady, and her husband are trying for a baby and come to the prenatal clinic for a review.

PMH: asthma, hypertension, T2DM, insomnia
DH: her current and repeat prescriptions are listed in the table presented below
SH: smokes 10 cigarettes a day; occasional glass of wine

On Examination

Temperature 36.8°C, HR 67/min and regular, BP 131/75 mmHg, RR 14/min, O_2 sat 97% on air; weight: 85 kg; height: 169 cm
Glucose 4.5 mmol/L (4–9), HbA_{1c} 40 mmol/mol (48–59)

You decide to review her regular medicines for use during pregnancy. During the review Mrs GU also mentions having had some strange taste disturbances in the last couple of months and wonders if that could be linked to any of her medications.

Current Prescriptions			
Drug Name	**Dose**	**Route**	**Frequency**
Symbicort® Turbohaler® 200/6	TT	ORAL	12-hourly
Salbutamol 100 micrograms Evohaler®	T-TT PRN	ORAL	6-hourly
Losartan	50 mg	ORAL	Daily
Aspirin	75 mg	ORAL	Daily
Metformin	500 mg	ORAL	12-hourly
Folic acid	400 micrograms	ORAL	Daily
Halibut liver oil capsules	T	ORAL	Daily
Zopiclone (prescribed last week)	3.75 mg PRN	ORAL	At night

Question A

Select TWO prescriptions that should be completely avoided in pregnancy as far as possible.

Question B

Select TWO prescriptions that are *most likely* the cause of taste disturbances experienced by Mrs GU.[42]

QUESTION 22

Mrs OP, a 27-year-old who gave birth 2 weeks ago, is admitted to hospital with suspected pyelonephritis. There have been no concerns regarding her new born baby who is currently being breastfed.

PMH: epilepsy, PE (3 months ago), polymyalgia rheumatica
DH: her current and repeat prescriptions are listed in the table presented below; allergies: penicillin (rash, pruritus)
SH: smokes 15 cigarettes a day; social drinker

On Examination

Temperature 38.7°C, HR 99/min and regular, BP 101/65 mmHg, RR 15/min, O_2 sat 98% on air; weight: 68 kg; height: 165 cm

Investigations

Urine dipstick positive for protein and nitrites
Chest X-ray: clear

Mrs OP is prescribed a STAT dose of gentamicin and oral ciprofloxacin.

Current Prescriptions			
Drug Name	**Dose**	**Route**	**Frequency**
Ciprofloxacin	750 mg	ORAL	12-hourly for 7/7
Tegretol® Prolonged Release	400 mg	ORAL	12-hourly
Epilim Chrono®	1 g OM, 500 mg ON	ORAL	12-hourly
Warfarin	4 mg	ORAL	Daily
St John's wort capsules (OTC)	T OM, T afternoon	ORAL	6 hours apart
Prednisolone	2 mg	ORAL	Daily
Adcal-D3® tablets	T	ORAL	12-hourly
Ibuprofen	400 mg PRN	ORAL	8-hourly
Norinyl-1® tablets (taken as a 'tricyclic' regimen)	T	ORAL	Daily

Question A

Select TWO prescriptions that are *most inappropriate* for Mrs OP considering her past medical history and breastfeeding status.

Question B

Select TWO prescriptions that are *most likely* to reduce the effectiveness of the COC taken by Mrs OP.[19,43-47]

QUESTION 23

Mr XV, a 38-year-old soft contact lens wearer, comes to see you complaining of some eye inflammation and impaired vision. He has tried chloramphenicol eye drops bought from the chemist for a week, but that did not seem to have done much.

PMH: epilepsy, severe acne, chronic perennial allergy, eczema
DH: his current and repeat prescriptions are listed in the table presented below
SH: non-smoker, nil alcohol

On Examination

Temperature 36.5°C, HR 88/min and regular, BP 123/76 mmHg, RR 13/min, O_2 sat 99% on air
Weight: 73 kg; height: 175 cm
Bilateral conjunctival inflammation, reduced visual fields and acuity, small amount of watery discharge present

Current Prescriptions			
Drug Name	Dose	Route	Frequency
Chlorphenamine	4 mg PRN	ORAL	6-hourly
Celluvisc® 0.5% eye drops	T PRN	BOTH EYES	8-hourly
Epilim Chrono®	1 g	ORAL	12-hourly
Vigabatrin	1.5 g OM, 1 g ON	ORAL	12-hourly
Isotretinoin	40 mg	ORAL	Daily
Beconase® nasal spray	100 micrograms	EACH NOSTRIL	12-hourly
Diprobase® cream	T	AFFECTED AREAS	12-hourly
Aveeno® bath additive	T	ALL BODY	Daily
Dermovate® cream	T PRN	AFFECTED AREAS	Daily

Question A

Select TWO prescriptions that have *most likely* caused the visual symptoms experienced by Mr XV.

Question B

Select TWO prescriptions that are *most likely* to affect the contact lens wear.[48,49]

QUESTION 24

Mr JH, a 66-year-old retired journalist, complains of persistent dizziness, fatigue, breathlessness and puffy ankles.

PMH: COPD, AF, osteoarthritis
DH: his current and repeat prescriptions are listed in the table presented below
SH: ex-smoker (25 pack-years), occasional can of beer

On Examination

Temperature 36.6°C, HR 79/min and irregular, BP 164/93 mmHg, RR 18/min, O_2 sat 96% on air, JVP raised
Weight: 67 kg; height: 169 cm
Bilateral peripheral oedema present, some bilateral basal lung crackles heard on auscultation

Mr JH is prescribed furosemide and ramipril to help with his pulmonary congestion, puffy ankles and high blood pressure. During the consultation he also mentions that he has recently been finding it hard to drive at night because of the appearance of dazzling lights. He wonders if that could be drug-related since he takes so many tablets.

Current Prescriptions			
Drug Name	**Dose**	**Route**	**Frequency**
Salbutamol 100 micrograms Evohaler®	T-TT PRN	INH	6-hourly
Seretide® 500 Accuhaler®	T	INH	12-hourly
Prednisolone	10 mg	ORAL	Daily
Carbocysteine	750 mg	ORAL	8-hourly
Warfarin	3.5 mg	ORAL	Daily
Amiodarone	100 mg	ORAL	Daily
Naproxen	500 mg	ORAL	12-hourly
Day Nurse® capsules OTC (paracetamol 500 mg, pseudoephedrine 30 mg, pholcodine 5 mg) – (NB has been taking for a few weeks since he thought he had a cold)	TT PRN	ORAL	4-hourly
Furosemide	40 mg	ORAL	Daily
Ramipril	1.25 mg	ORAL	Daily

Question A

Select THREE prescriptions that have *most likely* contributed to the oedema and hypertension experienced by Mr JH.

Question B

Select ONE prescription that is *most likely* responsible for the visual symptoms reported by Mr JH.[50-53]

REFERENCES

1. *Prescribing Safety Assessment: resources* [Online]. Medical Schools Council, British Pharmacological Society [27 March 2013]. Available at: www.prescribe.ac.uk/psa/?page_id=14

2. *Shingles* [Online]. Clinical Knowledge Summaries; 2013 [cited 30 November 2013]. Available at: http://cks.nice.org.uk/shingles

3. *Osteomyelitis* [Online]. London: NHS Choices; 2012 [cited 27 March 2013]. Available at: www.nhs.uk/conditions/Osteomyelitis/Pages/Introduction.aspx

4. *SSRIs (Selective Serotonin Reuptake Inhibitors) – Side Effects* [Online]. London: NHS Choices; 2012 [cited 27 March 2013]. Available at: www.nhs.uk/Conditions/SSRIs-%28selective-serotonin-reuptake-inhibitors%29/Pages/Side-effects.aspx

5. Ballinger A, Patchett S. Urinary tract infection. In: Kumar P, Clark M, editors. *Pocket Essentials of Clinical Medicine*. 4th ed. London: Saunders Elsevier; 2007. pp. 354–7.

6. *Erythema multiforme* [Online]. PubMed Health; 2012 [cited 1 January 2013]. Available at: www.ncbi.nlm.nih.gov/pubmedhealth/PMH0001854/

7. *Martindale: the complete drug reference* [Online]. Available at: www.medicinescomplete.com/

8. Ballinger A, Patchett S. Transient ischaemic attacks. In: Kumar P, Clark M, editors. *Pocket Essentials of Clinical Medicine*. 4th ed. London: Saunders Elsevier; 2007. pp. 732–3.

9. National Institute for Health and Clinical Excellence. *Clopidogrel and modified-release dipyridamole for the prevention of occlusive vascular events (review of technology appraisal guidance 90): NICE guideline 210 – quick reference guide*. London: NICE; 2010. Available at: www.nice.org.uk/nicemedia/live/13285/52189/52189.pdf

10. National Institute for Health and Clinical Excellence. *Lipid Modification: NICE guideline 67 – quick reference guide*. London: NICE; 2010. Available at: www.nice.org.uk/nicemedia/live/11982/40675/40675.pdf

11. *Stockley's Drug Interactions* [Online]. Available at: www.medicinescomplete.com/

12. *Clopidogrel and Proton Pump Inhibitors: interaction – updated advice* [Online]. Medicines and Healthcare Products Regulatory Agency; 2010 [cited 21 September 2013]. Available at: www.mhra.gov.uk/Safetyinformation/DrugSafetyUpdate/CON087711

13. Ballinger A, Patchett S. Haemolytic anaemia. In: Kumar P, Clark M, editors. *Pocket Essentials of Clinical Medicine*. 4th ed. London: Saunders Elsevier; 2007. pp. 196–9.

14. Ballinger A, Patchett S. Renal failure. In: Kumar P, Clark M, editors. *Pocket Essentials of Clinical Medicine*. 4th ed. London: Saunders Elsevier; 2007. pp. 369–82.

15. Acomb C, Holden J. Anaemia. In: Walker R, Whittlesea C, editors. *Clinical Pharmacy and Therapeutics*. 4th ed. London: Churchill Livingstone Elsevier; 2007. pp. 699–714.

16. *Rhabdomyolysis* [Online]. PubMed Health; 2011 [cited 4 January 2013]. Available at: www.ncbi.nlm.nih.gov/pubmedhealth/PMH0001505/

17. *Simvastatin: updated advice on drug interactions – updated contraindications* [Online]. Medicines and Healthcare Products Regulatory Agency; 2012 [cited 4 January 2013]. Available at: www.mhra.gov.uk/Safetyinformation/DrugSafetyUpdate/CON180637

18. Ballinger A, Patchett S. Pneumonia. In: Kumar P, Clark M, editors. *Pocket Essentials of Clinical Medicine*. 4th ed. London: Saunders Elsevier; 2007. pp. 516–23.

19. *Antimicrobial Policies and Guidelines*. Redhill: Surrey and Sussex Healthcare NHS Trust; 2012.

20. Blood S. Medication considerations before surgery. *Pharm J*. 2012; **288**: 179.

21. Rahman MH, Beattie J. Peri-operative medication in patients with cardiovascular disease. *Pharm J*. 2004; **272**: 352–4.

22. Wu ZL, Geng H. Combination of tolterodine and tamsulosin for benign prostatic hyperplasia [Chinese]. *Zhonghua Nan Ke Xue*. 2009; **15**(7): 639–41.

23. Cagir B. *Ileus* [Online]. Medscape; 2013 [cited 27 March 2013]. Available at: http://emedicine.medscape.com/article/178948-overview#a0199

24. White R, Bradnam V. *Handbook of Drug Administration via Enteral Feeding Tubes* [Online] 2013. Available at: www.medicinescomplete.com

25. Rahman MH, Beattie J. Medication in the peri-operative period. *Pharm J*. 2004; **272**: 287–9.

26. *Kidney Cancer – Renal Cell Carcinoma (RCC)* [Online]. Weill Cornell Medical College James Buchanan Brady Foundation Department of Urology; 2013 [cited 6 January 2013]. Available at: www.cornellurology.com/clinical-conditions/kidney-cancer/renal-cell-carcinoma/

27. National Institute for Health and Clinical Excellence. *Multiple Sclerosis: NICE guideline 8*. London: NICE; 2003. Available at: www.nice.org.uk/nicemedia/live/10930/46699/46699.pdf

28. *Domperidone: small risk of serious ventricular arrhythmia and sudden cardiac death* [Online]. Medicines and Healthcare Products Regulatory Agency; 2012 [cited 6 January 2013]. Available at: www.mhra.gov.uk/Safetyinformation/DrugSafetyUpdate/CON152725

29. Yap YG, Camm AJ. Drug induced QT prolongation and torsades de pointes. *Heart*. 2003; **89**(11): 1363–72.

30. *Intravenous Ondansetron: important new dose restriction* [Online]. Medicines and Healthcare Products Regulatory Agency; 2012 [cited 6 January 2013]. Available at: www.mhra.gov.uk/Safetyinformation/Safetywarningsalertsandrecalls/Safetywarningsandmessagesformedicines/CON178189

31. *Torsade de Pointes* [Online]. Patient.co.uk (via NHS Evidence); 2010 [cited 6 January 2013]. Available at: www.patient.co.uk/doctor/Torsades-de-Pointes.htm

32. *Gout* [Online]. Clinical Knowledge Summaries; 2012 [cited 30 November 2013]. Available at: http://cks.nice.org.uk/gout

33. O'Driscoll BR, Howard LS, Davison AG; British Thoracic Society. BTS guideline for emergency oxygen use in adult patients. *Thorax* [Online]. 2008; **63**(6): vi1–68. Available at: www.brit-thoracic.org.uk/portals/0/guidelines/emergency%20 oxygen%20guideline/appendix%201%20summary%20of%20recommendations. pdf

34. Lee A. Mental health disorders. In: *Adverse Drug Reactions*. 2nd ed. London: Pharmaceutical Press; 2006. pp. 352–5.

35. Proprietary Association of Great Britain. *OTC Directory 2010/2011*. London: Communications International Group; 2010.

36. *Otitis Media – Acute* [Online]. Clinical Knowledge Summaries; 2009 [cited 30 November 2013]. Available at: http://cks.nice.org.uk/otitis-media-acute

37. British Medical Association; Royal Pharmaceutical Society. *British National Formulary for Children* [Online]. London: Pharmaceutical Press; 2012. Available at: www.medicinescomplete.com

38. *Summary of Product Characteristics Night Nurse* [Online]. Electronic Medicines Compendium; 2012 [cited 22 September 2013]. Available at: www.medicines.org. uk/emc/medicine/19915/SPC/Night+Nurse/#INDICATIONS

39. *Summary of Product Characteristics Mirtazapine 15mg Tablets* [Online]. Electronic Medicines Compendium; 2010 [cited 26 January 2013]. Available at: www.medicines. org.uk/EMC/medicine/23038/SPC/Mirtazapine+15mg+Tablets/#MACHINE OPS

40. *CTD/CTDa* [Online]. Surrey, West Sussex and Hampshire Cancer Network; 2012 [cited 10 February 2013]. Available at: www.royalsurrey.nhs.uk/Default. aspx?DN=f3d12e47-c273-48b3-8023-35572a2e8e00

41. *Citalopram and Escitalopram: QT interval prolongation – new maximum daily dose restrictions (including in elderly patients), contraindications, and warnings* [Online]. Medicines and Healthcare Products Regulatory Agency; 2011 [cited 10 February 2013]. Available at: www.mhra.gov.uk/Safetyinformation/DrugSafetyUpdate/ CON137769

42. *Summary of Product Characteristics Zopiclone 3.75mg Tablets* [Online]. Electronic Medicines Compendium; 2009 [cited 10 February 2013]. Available at: www.medicines. org.uk/EMC/medicine/24285/SPC/Zopiclone+3.75mg+Tablets./

43. Burgess A. *Is It Safe for Breast Feeding Women to Take Herbal Medicines?* [Online]. NHS Evidence; 2012 [cited 30 November 2013]. Available at: www.evidence.nhs. uk/search?q=%22Is+it+safe+for+breastfeeding+women+to+take+herbal+medici nes%22

44. *Summary of Product Characteristics Epilim Chrono 200mg* [Online]. Electronic Medicines Compendium; 2012 [cited 10 February 2013]. Available at: www.medicines. org.uk/EMC/medicine/26124/SPC/Epilim+Chrono+200mg/

45. *Summary of Product Characteristics Tegretol Prolonged Release 200mg and 400mg Tablets (Formerly Tegretol Retard)* [Online]. Electronic Medicines Compendium; 2012 [cited 10 February 2013]. Available at: www.medicines.org.uk/EMC/

medicine/24201/SPC/Tegretol+Prolonged+Release+200mg+and+400mg+Tablet
s+%28formerly+Tegretol+retard%29/

46. *Summary of Product Characteristics Ciprofloxacin 500mg Film-Coated Tablets* [Online]. Electronic Medicines Compendium; 2012 [cited 10 February 2013]. Available at: www.medicines.org.uk/EMC/medicine/25756/SPC/Ciprofloxacin+500mg++Film-Coated+Tablets/#PREGNANCY

47. *Summary of Product Characteristics Norinyl-1 Tablets* [Online]. Electronic Medicines Compendium; 2007 [cited 10 February 2013]. Available at: www.medicines.org.uk/EMC/medicine/1920/SPC/Norinyl-1+Tablets/#INTERACTIONS

48. *Conjunctivitis – Infective* [Online]. Clinical Knowledge Summaries; 2012 [cited 30 November 2013]. Available at: http://cks.nice.org.uk/conjunctivitis-infective

49. *Summary of Product Characteristics Isotretinoin 20mg Capsules* [Online]. Electronic Medicines Compendium; 2012 [cited 10 February 2013]. Available at: www.medicines.org.uk/EMC/medicine/15655/SPC/Isotretinoin+20mg+capsules/

50. *Summary of Product Characteristics Amiodarone 100mg Tablets* [Online]. Electronic Medicines Compendium; 2012 [cited 10 February 2013]. Available at: www.medicines.org.uk/EMC/medicine/25743/SPC/Amiodarone+100mg+Tablets/

51. *Summary of Product Characteristics Prednisolone 1mg Tablets* [Online]. Electronic Medicines Compendium; 2012 [cited 10 February 2013]. Available at: www.medicines.org.uk/EMC/medicine/24113/SPC/Prednisolone+1mg+Tablets/

52. *Summary of Product Characteristics Day Nurse Capsules* [Online]. Electronic Medicines Compendium; 2012 [cited 10 February 2013]. Available at: www.medicines.org.uk/EMC/medicine/20671/SPC/Day+Nurse+Capsules/

53. Ballinger A, Patchett S. Heart failure. In: Kumar P, Clark M, editors. *Pocket Essentials of Clinical Medicine*. 4th ed. London: Saunders Elsevier; 2007. pp. 423–34.

Chapter 3

Planning Management

---

* Note that you will be asked to select a single most appropriate option from a list of five during the PSA.

QUESTION 1

Mr BT, a 61-year-old man, is admitted with a 3-day history of severe epigastric pain, nausea and haematemesis. He was recently treated for a chest infection.

PMH: hypertension, dyspepsia
DH: felodipine MR 5 mg OM, indapamide MR 1.5 mg OM, omeprazole 20 mg OM, erythromycin 250 mg QDS (2 weeks ago) for a chest infection; NKDA
SH: one to two cans of beer a day, non-smoker

On Examination

Temperature 36.5°C, HR 120/min and regular, BP 90/85 mmHg, JVP not elevated, RR 18/min, O_2 sat 97% on air
No audible murmurs noted, chest clear with epigastric tenderness on abdominal palpation
Maelena detected on PR
Conjunctival pallor noted

Investigations

WBC 8.4×10^9/L (4–11), Neut 5.1×10^9/L (2.0–7.5), Plt 256×10^9/L (150–400), Hb 9.1 g/dL (11.5–16.5), INR 1.1, PT 13 s (12–16), Na^+ 149 mmol/L (135–146), K^+ 5.1 mmol/L (3.5–5.0), Cr 69 µmol/L (79–118), U 5.8 mmol/L (2.5–6.7), CRP 4 mg/L (<10)

Mr BT is kept nil by mouth, started on IV fluids and a 72-hour continuous IV infusion of omeprazole.

He undergoes an OGD, which shows an active bleeding duodenal ulcer. This is immediately treated with adrenaline.

A rapid urease test on biopsy confirms *Helicobacter pylori*.

After 72 hours, Mr BT is stepped down to omeprazole 20 mg BD for 7 days, with plan for outpatient review.

Select the TWO *most appropriate* management options at this stage.[20]

Management Options	
A	Amoxicillin 500 mg TDS
B	Amoxicillin 1 g BD
C	Metronidazole 400 mg TDS
D	Clarithromycin 250 mg BD
E	Clarithromycin 500 mg BD

QUESTION 2

Gemma is a 58-year-old teacher who is brought in by ambulance after her husband found her unresponsive in the bathroom. He informs you that his wife was going to have a bath just before he left home to meet some friends in town (3–4 hours ago) and that she had been complaining of hearing difficulties.

PMH: NSTEMI (4 years ago), depression (anti-depressant overdose one year ago)
DH: aspirin 75 mg OM, bisoprolol 10 mg OM, atorvastatin 40 mg ON, citalopram (stopped after she had an overdose)
SH: smokes 20 cigarettes a day

On Examination

Temperature 35.6°C, HR 94/min and regular, BP 124/75 mmHg, JVP not elevated, RR 37/min, O_2 sat 94% on air; abdominal, cardiovascular and respiratory examination unremarkable

Investigations

Na^+ 138 mmol/L (135–146), K^+ 2.8 mmol/L (3.5–5.0), PO_4^{3-} 0.69 mmol/L (0.8–1.5), Mg^{2+} 0.8 mmol/L (0.7–1.1), corrected Ca^{2+} 2.03 mmol/L (2.20–2.67), HCO_3^- 13 mmol/L (22–30), glucose 6.4 mmol/L (4–9), Cr 110 μmol/L (79–118), U 7.9 mmol/L (2.5–6.7)

Arterial blood gas on room air: pH 7.05 (7.35–7.45), P_aO_2 9.4 kPa (10–13.3), P_aCO_2 3.2 kPa (4.8–6.1), base excess –4 mmol/L (–2 to +2)

Select the TWO *most appropriate* management options at this stage.[3]

	Management Options
A	Activated charcoal 50 g STAT
B	100 mL of 10% calcium gluconate in 1 L of NaCl 0.9% IV infusion over 12 hours
C	500 mL of KCl 0.15% (20 mmol) with NaCl 0.9% IV infusion over 2–3 hours
D	500 mL of sodium bicarbonate 1.26% in NaCl IV infusion over 3–4 hours
E	45 mL of phosphate Polyfusor® (9 mmol PO_4^{3-}) IV infusion over 12 hours

QUESTION 3

Tom, a 45-year-old engineer, is admitted with a severe flare of Crohn's disease. An abdominal X-ray demonstrates toxic megacolon. He is scheduled for an urgent colectomy with ileoanal anastomosis.

PMH: Crohn's disease
DH: mercaptopurine 50 mg OD, infliximab 350 mg IV every 2 months; NKDA
SH: one glass of wine a week

On Examination

Temperature 37.6°C, HR 123/min and regular, BP 100/80 mmHg, JVP not elevated, RR 14/min, O_2 sat 98% on air

Investigations

WBC 15.4 × 10^9/L (4–11), Neut 9.5 × 10^9/L (2.0–7.5), Plt 450 × 10^9/L (150–400), Hb 10.6 g/dL (11.5–16.5), INR 1.3, PT 14 s (12–16), Na^+ 131 mmol/L (135–146), K^+ 3.4 mmol/L (3.5–5.0), glucose 7.4 mmol/L (4–9), Cr 83 µmol/L (79–118), U 5.6 mmol/L (2.5–6.7), CRP 45 mg/L (<10)
Weight: 70 kg; height: 173 cm

Select the TWO *most appropriate* single prophylactic antibiotic doses for Tom to be administered before surgery.[4,5]

Management Options	
A	Co-amoxiclav 1.2 g IV STAT
B	Teicoplanin 400 mg IV STAT
C	Metronidazole 500 mg IV STAT
D	Cefuroxime 750 mg IV STAT
E	Gentamicin 100 mg IV STAT

QUESTION 4

Jennifer is a 26-year-old pregnant lady who goes into labour under lumbar epidural blockade with bupivacaine. Twenty minutes after induction of the block she becomes drowsy and less responsive.

PMH: asthma

DH: salbutamol 100-microgram Evohaler® T-TT PRN QDS, beclomethasone 100-microgram Evohaler® (Clenil Modulite®) TT BD

SH: non-smoker, occasional alcohol

On Examination

Temperature 35.4°C, HR 45/min and regular, BP 86/60 mmHg, JVP not elevated, RR 9/min, O_2 sat 87% on air

Investigations (Pre-labour)

WBC 4.5×10^9/L (4–11), Neut 3.4×10^9/L (2.0–7.5), Plt 254×10^9/L (150–400), Hb 12.3 g/dL (11.5–16.5), INR 1.2, PT 12 s (12–16), Na+ 136 mmol/L (135–146), K+ 3.8 mmol/L (3.5–5.0), Cr 89 μmol/L (79–118), U 3.2 mmol/L (2.5–6.7), CRP 5 mg/L (<10)

Weight: 55 kg; height: 162 cm

Select the TWO *most appropriate* management options at this stage.[6]

Management Options	
A	Ephedrine 3–6 mg by slow IV injection repeated every 3–4 minutes according to response
B	Noradrenaline 40 micrograms (base)/mL by IV infusion at a rate of 0.16–0.33 mL/min, adjusted according to response
C	Phenylephrine 100–500 micrograms by slow IV injection repeated as necessary after at least 15 minutes
D	Oxygen 28% via simple face mask at the rate of 2–10 L/min
E	Oxygen 40% via simple face mask at the rate of 5–10 L/min

QUESTION 5

Mr GH, a 55-year-old gentleman, is brought into hospital following a sudden onset of headache preceded by nausea and vomiting. While being examined in A&E he becomes less responsive.

PMH: T2DM, angina, TIA, AF

DH: metformin 1 g OM, 500 mg at midday, 500 mg in the evening, atorvastatin 40 mg OD, sitagliptin 100 mg OM, atenolol 50 mg BD, warfarin 4 mg daily (5 mg on Sundays), amiodarone 200 mg OM (started 3 weeks ago)

SH: gave up smoking 4 years ago following a TIA

On Examination

Temperature 36.7°C, HR 87/min irregular, BP 180/110 mmHg, JVP raised, RR 22/min, O_2 sat 95% on air

Weight: 98 kg; height: 182 cm

Investigations

WBC 4.5×10^9/L (4–11), Neut 3.4×10^9/L (2.0–7.5), Plt 254×10^9/L (150–400), Hb 11.2 g/dL (11.5–16.5), INR 3.5, PT 18 s (12–16); Na$^+$ 131 mmol/L (135–146), K$^+$ 4.5 mmol/L (3.5–5.0), Cr 110 μmol/L (79–118), U 5.9 mmol/L (2.5–6.7), CRP 5 mg/L (<10)

ECG: AF

He undergoes an urgent CT head, which shows intraventricular bleeding. An MRI demonstrates an aneurysm of the middle cerebral artery. As a result, Mr GH is planned for craniotomy and surgical clipping to prevent re-bleeding.

Select the TWO *most appropriate* management options at this stage.[7]

Management Options	
A	GTN IV infusion in sodium chloride 0.9% at 200 micrograms/min and adjust according to BP response
B	Nimodipine 1 mg/hr by IV infusion increased after 2 hours to 2 mg/hr if no severe fall in BP
C	Stop warfarin; give 5 mg of phytomenadione IV and 2500 units of dried prothrombin complex
D	Stop warfarin; give 50 mg of phenindione PO and 2500 units of dried prothrombin complex
E	Stop warfarin; give 3 mg of phytomenadione IV; repeat dose of phytomenadione if INR still too high after 24 hours

QUESTION 6

Miss FU is a 19-year-old who has come to the A&E department following a week-long history of progressive lower abdominal pain. She has recently also noticed some mucopurulent discharge PV and sexual intercourse has become increasingly more unpleasant.

PMH: nil
DH: OTC ibuprofen 200 mg PRN for menstrual pain; allergies: severe allergy to beta-lactam antibiotics (anaphylaxis)
SH: non-smoker, social drinker

On Examination

Temperature 38.2°C, HR 101/min and regular, BP 125/76 mmHg, JVP normal, RR 14/min, O_2 sat 98% on air
Lower abdominal tenderness on palpation noted, bowel sounds audible; cervical tenderness noted on vaginal examination
Weight: 63 kg; height: 168 cm

Investigations

WBC 12.3 × 10^9/L (4–11), Neut 8.1 × 10^9/L (2.0–7.5), Plt 210 × 10^9/L (150–400), Hb 12.4 g/dL (11.5–16.5); Na$^+$ 137 mmol/L (135–146), K$^+$ 4.6 mmol/L (3.5–5.0), Cr 82 μmol/L (79–118), U 3.5 mmol/L (2.5–6.7), CRP 13 mg/L (<10)
Endocervical swabs: negative for *Chlamydia trachomatis* and *Neisseria gonorrhoeae*
Pregnancy test: negative

Select the TWO *most appropriate* management options at this stage.[8]

Management Options	
A	Metronidazole 400 mg BD PO for 14 days
B	Ceftriaxone 500 mg STAT IM
C	Doxycycline 100 mg BD PO for 14 days
D	Azithromycin 1 g PO STAT
E	Ofloxacin 400 mg BD PO for 14 days

QUESTION 7

Jamie, a 7-year-old, was brought in to hospital after he suddenly became very breathless and wheezy following a football match. This was not relieved by his salbutamol inhaler. Jamie's mother thinks that her son has been using his asthma pump more often than normal, particularly before playing football.

PMH: asthma
DH: Ventolin® 100-microgram Evohaler® T-TT PRN QDS
SH: nil relevant

On Examination

Temperature 36.6°C, HR 130/min and regular, BP 123/82 mmHg, JVP not elevated, RR 35/min, O_2 sat 90% on air, peak flow 40% of predicted
You observe Jamie has difficulty talking during your consultation; GCS 13/15
Weight: 23 kg; height: 122 cm

Investigations

WBC 5.4×10^9/L (4–11), Neut 4.3×10^9/L (2.0–7.5), Plt 180×10^9/L (150–400), Hb 14.5 g/dL (11.5–16.5), Na$^+$ 141 mmol/L (135–146), K$^+$ 4.2 mmol/L (3.5–5.0), Cr 74 µmol/L (79–118), U 2.7 mmol/L (2.5–6.7), CRP 2 mg/L (<10)

Select the TWO *most appropriate* management options at this stage.

Management Options	
A	Ipratropium bromide 250 micrograms via oxygen-driven nebuliser repeated every 20–30 minutes for the first 2 hours, then every 4–6 hours as necessary
B	Prednisolone 40 mg PO for 3 days
C	Prednisolone 50 mg PO for 3 days
D	Salbutamol 5 mg via oxygen-driven nebuliser repeated at 20- to 30-minute intervals if necessary
E	Terbutaline 10 mg via oxygen-driven nebuliser repeated at 10- to 15-minute intervals if necessary

QUESTION 8

Louise, a 16-year-old, is taken to hospital by her dad who is very worried about his daughter. She has been complaining of severe tummy pain and has spent 'the entire morning' in the bathroom. He has also noticed that she has terrible breath and thinks that unfortunately Louise might have had too much to drink at her friend's birthday party last night.

PMH: T1DM
DH: Levemir® via Flexpen® 14 units SC in the evening, NovoRapid® via Flexpen® SC before meals adjusted according to insulin requirements
SH: nil relevant

On Examination

Temperature 35.3°C, HR 120/min and regular, BP 100/65 mmHg, JVP not elevated, RR 31/min, O_2 sat 94% on air
Sunken eyes, deep rapid breathing
GCS 11/15
Weight: 52 kg; height: 156 cm

Investigations

WBC 12.1×10^9/L (4–11), Neut 6.8×10^9/L (2.0–7.5), Plt 365×10^9/L (150–400), Hb 12.5 g/dL (11.5–16.5), Na^+ 152 mmol/L (135–146), K^+ 5.2 mmol/L (3.5–5.0), HCO_3^- 15 mmol/L (22–30), glucose 23 mmol/L (4–9), Cr 142 µmol/L (79–118), U 10.9 mmol/L (2.5–6.7), CRP 4 mg/L (<10), pH 7.14 (7.35–7.45), P_aO_2 10.2 kPa (10–13.3), P_aCO_2 3.4 kPa (4.8–6.1), base excess −4 mmol/L (−2 to +2)
CXR: clear; urine dipstick: ketones+++, leukocytes nil, nitrites nil

Select the TWO *most appropriate* management options at this stage (assuming that adult dosages apply in this case).[3,9,10]

Management Options	
A	Give 10–20 mL of calcium gluconate 10% by slow IV injection, titrated and adjusted to ECG improvement, to temporarily protect against myocardial excitability
B	Stop regular long-acting insulin and initiate IV infusion of soluble insulin in NaCl 0.9% at the rate of 5 units/hour

Management Options	
C	Maintain the patient on long-acting insulin and initiate IV infusion of soluble insulin in NaCl 0.9% at the rate of 5 units/hour
D	Maintain the patient on long-acting insulin, initiate IV infusion of soluble insulin in NaCl 0.9% at the rate of 5 units/hour together with an IV infusion of glucose 10% at a rate of 125 mL/hour
E	Give 1000 mL of NaCl 0.9% with 40 mmol of K+ as IV infusion over 60 minutes, adjusted to plasma U&Es

QUESTION 9

Mrs O'Neill, an 81-year-old lady, is admitted to hospital with a suspected chest infection and diarrhoea. Blood investigations demonstrate neutropenia. Stool cultures for *Clostridium difficile* are negative. Mrs O'Neill is put on piperacillin/tazobactam 4.5 g IV QDS and gentamicin 150 mg IV OD for suspected neutropenic sepsis. She is also prescribed an adequate fluid regimen and 3 days of lenograstim 263 micrograms SC.

PMH: rheumatoid arthritis, dementia, recurrent UTIs
DH: methotrexate 20 mg weekly, co-codamol 30/500 T-TT PRN QDS, donepezil 5 mg ON, trimethoprim 100 mg ON
SH: a widow living in Surrey; weight: 49 kg; height: 156 cm

Three days later, Mrs O'Neill is still unwell and very confused.

On Examination

GCS 9/15, temperature 36.4°C, HR 99/min and regular, BP 95/63 mmHg, JVP not elevated, RR 21/min, O_2 sat 95% on air

Investigations

On Admission	Today
Cr 253 µmol/L (79–118)	263 µmol/L
U 18.4 mmol/L (2.5–6.7)	19.3 mmol/L
CRP 67 mg/L (<10)	35 mg/L
WBC 1.5×10^9/L (4–11)	1.1×10^9/L
Neut 0.5×10^9/L (2.0–7.5)	0.1×10^9/L
Plt 163×10^9/L (150–400)	89×10^9/L
Hb 11.4 g/dL (11.5–16.5)	9.6 g/dL

Select the TWO *most appropriate* management options at this stage.[11]

	Management Options
A	Stop methotrexate and trimethoprim
B	Stop methotrexate and donepezil
C	Give calcium folinate 20 mg by IV infusion, repeated as needed

Management Options	
D	Switch piperacillin/tazobactam and gentamicin to an alternative regimen for neutropenic sepsis, such as teicoplanin 400 mg IV BD for three doses, then 400 mg OD + meropenem 1 g BD
E	Continue lenograstim 263 micrograms SC for another 7 days

QUESTION 10

Mr McKee, an 82-year-old who is well known to the palliative care team, is brought into hospital following a fall. He is treated with trimethoprim 200 mg BD for a probable urinary tract infection at the same time withholding his bendroflumethiazide due to suspected dehydration.

PMH: metastatic prostate cancer, hypertension

DH: lisinopril 20 mg OM, bendroflumethiazide 2.5 mg OM, Zoladex® LA 10.8 mg SC every 12 weeks (last time 7 weeks ago), zoledronic acid 4 mg IV every 4 weeks (last time 3 weeks ago), co-codamol 30/500 TT QDS, MST Continus® 10 mg BD, Oramorph® liquid 10 mg/5 mL 1.25–2.5 mL PRN 4–6 hourly, cyclizine 50 mg TDS, metoclopramide 10–20 mg TDS

SH: lives alone with a twice-daily social care package

Weight: 56 kg; height: 167 cm

Two days later the staff nurse looking after Mr McKee tells you that he has been unable to keep his morphine down despite taking antiemetics and that he has also been feeling extremely dizzy soon after taking it. His blood pressure would also temporarily drop soon after having a dose. You check Mr McKee's drug history, which indicates that MST Continus® and Oramorph® have only been started a week before hospital admission.

On Examination

GCS 12/15, temperature 36.6°C, HR 65/min and regular, BP 124/85 mmHg, JVP not elevated, RR 15/min, O_2 sat 97% on air

Select the TWO *most appropriate* management options at this stage.

Management Options	
A	Switch MST Continus® to continuous diamorphine SC infusion 20 mg over 24 hours
B	Switch MST Continus® to OxyContin® 5 mg BD
C	Switch MST Continus® to fentanyl 12 µg/hour patch every 72 hours
D	Switch Oramorph® to OxyNorm® liquid 5 mg/5 mL 1.0–1.5 mg every 4–6 hours
E	Switch Oramorph® to diamorphine 2 mg SC PRN every 4–6 hours

QUESTION 11

Mrs King, a 66-year-old, is taken to A&E following a sudden significant loss of vision and severe pain in her left eye, which she describes as excruciating. She denies any recent trauma or injury to her eye, infection or travel abroad.

PMH: sciatica (following a car accident 10 years ago), perennial rhinitis (allergy to cat fur?)
DH: amitriptyline 10 mg ON, co-codamol 30/500 TT QDS, ibuprofen 400 mg TDS, OTC chlorphenamine 4 mg every 4–6 hours PRN (up to six tablets/day)
SH: lives with her husband and three children in Bethnal Green, London

On Examination

GCS 15/15, temperature 36.5°C, HR 73/min and regular, BP 132/76 mmHg, JVP not elevated, RR 16/min, O_2 sat 98% on air
Ciliary flush seen in the affected eye; the pupil is oval and unreactive to light

Select the TWO *most appropriate* management options at this stage.[12–16]

Management Options	
A	Stop amitriptyline; consider alternatives, such as pregabalin 75 mg BD, following surgery
B	Stop amitriptyline and chlorphenamine; consider alternatives, such as pregabalin 75 mg BD and loratadine 10 mg OD, following surgery
C	Stop chlorphenamine; consider alternatives, such as cetirizine 10 mg OD, following surgery
D	Prescribe betaxolol 0.5% eye drops to left eye BD, thereafter reviewed as appropriate
E	Prescribe mannitol 20% (up to 500 mL) by slow IV infusion, thereafter reviewed as appropriate

QUESTION 12

Mr Landgren, a 69-year-old, presents to hospital with a recent onset of facial numbness preceded by vomiting and vertigo. He is found to have suffered an infarct in the region supplied by the posterior inferior cerebellar artery. During the recovery period Mr Landgren develops severe diarrhoea, and tests positive for *Clostridium difficile*. He is treated with vancomycin 125 mg PO QDS.

PMH: epilepsy, depression, trigeminal neuralgia
DH: Epanutin® Infatabs® 150 mg BD, Tegretol® tablets 200 mg TDS, citalopram 20 mg OM, aspirin 300 mg OM for 14 days (started post infarction)
SH: retired social worker; non-smoker, occasional whisky drinker
Weight: 86 kg; height: 179 cm

Despite input from the team Mr Landgren deteriorates further and becomes dysphagic. Four days later, the decision is made to insert an NG tube and commence feeding. One of the ward sisters asks you to kindly adjust Mr Landgren's pharmaceutical therapies as appropriate.

On Examination

GCS 11/15, temperature 37.6°C, HR 84/min and regular, BP 139/87 mmHg, JVP not elevated, RR 17/min, O_2 sat 95% on air

Investigations

Cr 121 µmol/L (79–118), U 9.6 mmol/L (2.5–6.7), CRP 89 mg/L (<10), WBC 15.7 × 10⁹/L (4–11), Neut 8.7 × 10⁹/L (2.0–7.5)

Select the TWO *most appropriate* management options at this stage.[17–19]

	Management Options
A	Switch citalopram tablets to eight citalopram oral drops of 40 mg/mL strength OM via the NG tube
B	Switch Epanutin® Infatabs® to Epanutin® capsules (175 mg of powder from the capsules mixed with 10 mL of water and 9.3 mL of this dispersion administered via the NG tube BD)
C	Switch oral vancomycin to IV vancomycin infusion 500 mg every 12 hours
D	Switch oral vancomycin to IV metronidazole 500 mg TDS
E	Switch Tegretol® tablets to Tegretol® suppositories 250 mg TDS for up to 7 days, to be reviewed later

QUESTION 13

Mr PO, a 71-year-old retired carpenter, comes to your clinic complaining of a frequent night-time need to void that is often accompanied by urgency. However, whenever he does void, his flow is rather poor and leaves him with a sense of 'incompleteness'. This has been gradually getting worse over the last couple of months.

PMH: postural hypotension, Parkinson's disease, cataract surgery of the left eye (scheduled for right eye cataract surgery in a month's time), restless legs syndrome

DH: fludrocortisone 50 micrograms OM, oxybutynin 5 mg MR T OM, Stalevo® 200/50/200 mg T at 8 a.m., 12 noon, 3 p.m., 6 p.m. and 10 p.m., ropinirole 2 mg ON

SH: gave up smoking 25 years ago; lives on his own, independent; weight: 76 kg; height: 174 cm

On Examination

Temperature 36.4°C, HR 68/min and regular, BP 115/74 mmHg, RR 14/min
Abdominal and external genitalia examination: normal
Digital rectal examination demonstrates an enlarged prostate (estimated at 30–35 g)

Investigations

Urine dip: negative

Select the TWO *most appropriate* management options at this stage.[20,21]

	Management Options
A	Initiate a trial of tamsulosin 400 micrograms MR OM for 4–6 weeks
B	Reduce the dose of Stalevo® to 200/50/200 mg four times a day, thereafter monitored and adjusted as appropriate
C	Initiate a trial of finasteride 5 mg OM for 3–6 months
D	Discontinue fludrocortisone 50 micrograms OM
E	Discontinue oxybutynin 5 mg MR T OM

REFERENCES

1. *Prescribing Safety Assessment: resources* [Online]. Medical Schools Council; British Pharmacological Society [27 March 2013]. Available at: www.prescribe.ac.uk/psa/?page_id=14

2. Ballinger A, Patchett S. *Helicobacter pylori* and the upper gastrointestinal tract. In: Kumar P, Clark M, editors. *Pocket Essentials of Clinical Medicine.* 4th ed. London: Saunders Elsevier; 2007. pp. 76–80.

3. Ballinger A, Patchett S. Disorders of the acid-base balance. In: Kumar P, Clark M, editors. *Pocket Essentials of Clinical Medicine.* 4th ed. London: Saunders Elsevier; 2007. pp. 327–32.

4. Ballinger A, Patchett S. Inflammatory bowel disease. In: Kumar P, Clark M, editors. *Pocket Essentials of Clinical Medicine.* 4th ed. London: Saunders Elsevier; 2007. pp. 96–104.

5. Cripps SE, Beresford S. Inflammatory bowel disease. In: Walker R, Whittlesea C, editors. *Clinical Pharmacy and Therapeutics.* 4th ed. London: Churchill Livingstone Elsevier; 2007. pp. 169–86.

6. *Martindale: the complete drug reference* [Online]. Available at: www.medicines complete.com/

7. Ballinger A, Patchett S. Primary intracranial haemorrhage. In: Kumar P, Clark M, editors. *Pocket Essentials of Clinical Medicine.* 4th ed. London: Saunders Elsevier; 2007. pp. 733–6.

8. *Pelvic Inflammatory Disease* [Online]. London: Clinical Knowledge Summaries; 2013 [cited 2 December 2013]. Available at: http://cks.nice.org.uk/pelvic-inflammatory-disease

9. Ballinger A, Patchett S. Diabetic ketoacidosis. In: Kumar P, Clark M, editors. *Pocket Essentials of Clinical Medicine.* 4th ed. London: Saunders Elsevier; 2007. pp. 658–62.

10. *The Management of Diabetic Ketoacidosis in Adults* [Online]. Joint British Diabetes Societies Inpatient Care Group; 2010 [cited 22 September 2013]. Available at: www.bsped.org.uk/clinical/docs/DKAManagementOfDKAinAdultsMarch20101.pdf

11. *Summary of Product Characteristics Methotrexate 2.5 mg Tablets* [Online]. Electronic Medicines Compendium; 2012 [cited 28 March 2013]. Available at: www.medicines.org.uk/EMC/medicine/12033/SPC/Methotrexate+2.5+mg+Tablets/#PHARMA COKINETIC_PROPS

12. Titcomb LC, Andrew SD. Glaucoma. In: Walker R, Whittlesea C, editors. *Clinical Pharmacy and Therapeutics.* 4th ed. London: Churchill Livingstone Elsevier; 2007. pp. 789–806.

13. National Institute for Health and Clinical Excellence. *Neuropathic Pain – pharmacological management: NICE guideline 96 – quick reference guide.* London: NICE; 2010. Available at: www.nice.org.uk/nicemedia/pdf/CG96QuickRefGuide.pdf

14. *Summary of Product Characteristics Lyrica Capsules* [Online]. Electronic Medicines Compendium; 2009 [cited 29 March 2013]. Available at: www.medicines.org.uk/EMC/medicine/14651/SPC/Lyrica+Capsules/

15. *Summary of Product Characteristics Amitriptyline 10mg Film-coated Tablets* [Online]. Electronic Medicines Compendium; 2005 [cited 29 March 2013]. Available at: www.medicines.org.uk/EMC/medicine/25741/SPC/Amitriptyline+10mg+Film-coated+Tablets/

16. *Summary of Product Characteristics Piriton Allergy Tablets* [Online]. Electronic Medicines Compendium; 1997 [cited 29 March 2013]. Available at: www.medicines.org.uk/EMC/medicine/16103/SPC/Piriton+Allergy+Tablets/

17. *Summary of Product Characteristics Vancomycin 1g Powder for Solution for Infusion* [Online]. Electronic Medicines Compendium; 2008 [cited 29 March 2013]. Available at: www.medicines.org.uk/EMC/medicine/20835/SPC/Vancomycin+1g+Powder+for+Solution+for+Infusion+%28Wockhardt+UK+Ltd%29/#PHARMACOKINETIC_PROPS

18. White R, Bradnam V. *Handbook of Drug Administration via Enteral Feeding Tubes* [Online] 2013. Available at: www.medicinescomplete.com

19. *Antimicrobial Policies and Guidelines*. Redhill: Surrey and Sussex Healthcare NHS Trust; 2012.

20. Gower RL. Benign prostatic hyperplasia. In: Walker R, Whittlesea C, editor. *Clinical Pharmacy and Therapeutics*. 4th ed. London: Churchill Livingstone Elsevier; 2007. pp. 691–8.

21. National Institute for Health and Clinical Excellence. *The Management of Lower Urinary Tract Symptoms in Men: NICE guideline 97 – quick reference guide*. London: NICE; 2010. Available at: www.nice.org.uk/nicemedia/live/12984/48575/48575.pdf

Chapter 4

Communicating Information

---

* Note that you will be asked to select a single most appropriate option from a list of five during the PSA.

QUESTION 1

Stephen, a 56-year old type 2 diabetic, was found to have impaired long-term blood sugar control during his admission for a suspected right diabetic foot infection. Unfortunately, he also has a significant history of hypoglycaemic episodes. Following review, the specialist diabetes nurse initiated pioglitazone 15 mg OD. Stephen was not found to have any medication adherence problems. You decide to briefly counsel him on his new medicine before he goes home.

PMH: T2DM

DH: metformin 1 g OM, 500 mg lunchtime, 500 mg evening, flucloxacillin 500 mg QDS and phenoxymethylpenicillin 500 mg QDS for 7 days

SH: alcohol, one to two cans of beer a day

On the day of consultation: blood sugar 14.5 mmol/L (4–9), HbA$_{1c}$ 65 mmol/mol (48–59)

Select the TWO *most appropriate* information options that should be communicated to the patient.[2]

Information Options	
A	He should avoid alcohol during treatment with pioglitazone
B	He should discontinue treatment and seek immediate medical help if his skin or whites of the eyes turn yellow
C	When taken with metformin, pioglitazone increases the risk of heart failure and he should promptly report any symptoms of breathlessness or fatigue
D	Pioglitazone carries a small increased risk of prostate cancer and he should report any difficulty in urination
E	He should report any haematuria, dysuria, or urinary urgency during treatment

QUESTION 2

Mrs GH is a 62-year-old who has just been initiated on methotrexate 7.5 mg and folic acid 5 mg once weekly for rheumatoid arthritis. The rheumatologist asks you to go over the main points of methotrexate therapy with Mrs GH before she starts taking the medicine.

PMH: rheumatoid arthritis, gout
DH: allopurinol 300 mg OM, diclofenac 50 mg TDS, OTC paracetamol 500 mg – 1 g QDS PRN
SH: nil relevant

Select the TWO *most appropriate* information options that should be communicated to the patient.

Information Options	
A	She should stop taking diclofenac, as NSAIDs increase the risk of methotrexate toxicity
B	She should stop taking paracetamol, as it increases the risk of methotrexate toxicity
C	She should take methotrexate and folic acid on the same day each week
D	She should seek immediate medical help if symptoms, such as dyspnoea or cough, develop while on methotrexate
E	She should report any onset of nausea or abdominal discomfort while on methotrexate immediately

QUESTION 3

Mrs UR, a 65-year-old, is admitted for emergency total left hip replacement.

PMH: CKD, anaemia, hypertension
DH: ferrous fumarate 322 mg BD, alfacalcidol 1 microgram OD, NeoRecormon® 2000 units three times a week (last given 2 days before the operation), losartan 50 mg OD, UFH 5000 units BD
SH: smokes 15 cigarettes a day

On the morning of the third day after the operation, the ward sister rings to tell you that Mrs UR has rapidly deteriorated and there are some significant abnormalities in her latest blood test results.

You check Mrs UR's blood test results:

WBC 7×10^9/L (4–11), Plt 243×10^9/L (150–400), Hb 12.4 g/dL (11.5–16.5), INR 1.2, PT 15 s (12–16), Na^+ 139 mmol/L (135–146), K^+ 6.6 mmol/L (3.5–5.0), HCO_3^- 21 mmol/L (22–30), corrected Ca^{2+} 2.43 mmol/L (2.20–2.67), Cr 185 μmol/L (79–118), U 8.6 mmol/L (2.5–6.7) pH 7.34 (7.35–7.45), base excess –2 mmol/L (–2 to +2)

Select the TWO *most appropriate* information options that should be communicated to the ward sister.

Information Options	
A	Withhold heparin and give a STAT dose of NeoRecormon®
B	Withhold heparin and losartan until repeat blood test results are available
C	Withhold UFH and give a dose of enoxaparin 20 mg at 6 p.m.
D	Give 10–20 mL of calcium gluconate 10% IV together with 500 mL of sodium bicarbonate 1.26% in NaCl IV infusion
E	Give 10–20 mL of calcium gluconate 10% IV together with 5–10 units of soluble insulin in 50 mL of 50% glucose

QUESTION 4

Peter, your SHO colleague from the care of the elderly ward, comes to you for some advice on a new medicine called Didronel PMO®, which his consultant is so passionate about. Peter is going to see Mrs TG, an 83-year-old, at the fracture clinic today. She was started on once-weekly alendronate following her hip fracture 2 weeks ago; however, she has not been tolerating this medicine well at all. Peter's consultant is very keen on trying Didronel PMO® and vitamin D supplements instead of alendronic acid + Cacit D3® before moving to other options.

PMH: iron-deficiency anaemia, orthostatic hypotension, falls, osteoporosis, fractured neck of femur

DH: ferrous sulphate 200 mg OM, fludrocortisone 50 micrograms OM, Cacit D3® T BD, alendronic acid 70 mg once weekly

SH: nil relevant

Select the TWO *most appropriate* information options that should be communicated to your SHO colleague about how this lady should take the new medicine.[3]

Information Options	
A	She should take one pink tablet daily for 14 days, followed by one white tablet for 76 days
B	She should swallow each tablet whole with plenty of water while sitting or standing at least 30 minutes before breakfast or another oral medicine
C	She should have a regular dental check-up, maintain good oral hygiene and should immediately report any oral symptoms while on Didronel PMO®
D	She should avoid food at least 2 hours before and an hour after taking the white tablet
E	She should leave a 2- to 3-hour gap between taking her white 'bone' tablet and her regular iron tablet

QUESTION 5

Lesley is a 6-year-old who suffers from cystic fibrosis. He was admitted to hospital with worsening tummy upset and steatorrhoea a few days ago. The specialist team concluded that Lesley's pancreatic insufficiency had progressed and he required Creon® 10 000 therapy (to be started as one capsule with each meal). Lesley's mother catches you in the middle of the ward round and asks you to kindly explain how to give the new medicine that Lesley has just been prescribed.

PMH: cystic fibrosis
DH: dornase alfa 2500 units via jet nebuliser OD 1 hour before physiotherapy, flucloxacillin 500 mg OM, Ketovite® tablets T TDS, Ketovite® liquid 5 mL OD
SH: nil relevant
Weight: 11 kg; height: 1.04 cm

Select the TWO *most appropriate* information options that should be communicated to Lesley's mum.[4–11]

	Information Options
A	Creon® should be given before, with or immediately after food
B	She should avoid mixing Creon® with hot fluids or foods and giving it with concurrent antacids
C	She should aim for Lesley to drink at least 1–2 L of fluids/day because it is essential to ensure adequate hydration with higher-strength pancreatin preparations
D	Once mixed with liquids or food, Creon® should be given immediately and the resulting mixture should not be kept for more than 1 hour
E	She should immediately report any symptoms of constipation or lower abdominal pain, since all pancreatin preparations have been associated with the development of large bowel strictures

QUESTION 6

Debbie is a 25-year-old who survived a road traffic accident 4 months ago. Unfortunately, her dad suffered severe injuries during the crash and died in hospital. Ever since the accident and her dad's funeral, Debbie has felt like her life has 'lost meaning'. She has found it impossible to fall asleep and started developing chronic headaches throughout the day. On the advice of the psychiatrist, you prescribe paroxetine 20 mg OM and decide to counsel her on the new medicine before she leaves the clinic.

PMH: insomnia, migraine? (self-medicating)
DH: temazepam 20 mg ON, sumatriptan 50 mg PRN for migraine (OTC), paracetamol 500 mg T-TT QDS PRN for migraine
SH: nil relevant

Select the TWO *most appropriate* information options that should be communicated to Debbie before she leaves the clinic today.

Information Options	
A	She should stop taking temazepam because it interacts with paroxetine; paroxetine alone is likely to improve her sleeplessness in the long run
B	She should stop taking sumatriptan and make an appointment with the GP to review her self-diagnosed migraine
C	She should report back to you or the GP if she experiences any suicidal, self-harm or hostile thoughts, particularly at the beginning of the treatment
D	She should stop the treatment and seek immediate medical advice if she experiences any dizziness, tingling in her limbs or tinnitus
E	Angle-closure glaucoma is rather common with paroxetine and she should seek immediate medical advice if she develops any visual disturbances or pain in her eyes

QUESTION 7

Miss AP, a 19-year-old, is admitted to hospital with severe dehydration secondary to persistent vomiting. It started after she began taking erythromycin, which was prescribed by her GP to treat a possible chest infection.

PMH: nil relevant
DH: erythromycin 500 mg QDS (started 2 days ago), Microgynon 30 ED®; allergies: penicillin
SH: smoker, 10–15 cigarettes/day

Miss AP is a little bit worried because she was not able to take her 'pill' for the last 2 days due to vomiting. She would like to get some advice from you as to what to do next. Miss AP has just started her cycle. She has not had any unprotected sexual intercourse in the last 2 days.

Select the TWO *most appropriate* information options that should be communicated to Miss AP.

	Information Options
A	Erythromycin decreases the efficacy of Microgynon 30 ED®, and therefore she must either abstain from sex or use an additional method of contraception such as a condom for the next 7 days
B	Erythromycin increases the efficacy of Microgynon 30 ED® and, since she has not had any unprotected sexual intercourse in the last 2 days, she can carry on taking her 'pill' as normal without any extra precautions or methods of contraception
C	She should resume taking her 'pill' as soon as possible and use a 'tricycling' regimen for the next 3 cycles, followed by a shortened tablet-free interval of 4 days
D	She should resume taking her 'pill' as soon as possible and then must either abstain from sex or use an additional method of contraception such as condoms for the next 7 days
E	She should stop taking her 'pill' immediately and seek medical help if she experiences severe chest pain, sudden breathlessness or unexplained swelling/severe pain in the calf of one leg

QUESTION 8

You are one of the doctors on the cardiology ward. The GP rings you regarding Paul, a 58-year-old bus driver, who was discharged from hospital with newly diagnosed AF about a month ago. Today Paul presented to him complaining of stiffness and coldness in both of his legs. He has no other complaints and is otherwise fine.

PMH: T2DM, AF

DH: metformin 1 g OM, 500 mg midday and 500 mg ON, insulin detemir 16 units ON, amiodarone 200 mg OM, warfarin 3 mg OD, atorvastatin 20 mg ON, and carvedilol 6.25 mg BD (the latter four started a month ago)

SH: alcohol, 16 units/week

On Examination

Temperature 36.6°C, HR 79/min and regular, BP 135/82 mmHg

Investigations

Glucose 13.8 mmol/L (4–9), HbA_{1c} 63 mmol/mol (48–59)

His GP is concerned and would like your opinion on what could be causing Paul's problems. You call the cardiology SpR and explain the situation. In turn, she tells you what message to pass on to the GP.

Select the TWO *most appropriate* information options that should be communicated to the GP.

Information Options	
A	The stiffness and coldness of the extremities are likely to be the result of amiodarone-induced peripheral neuropathy; amiodarone should be temporarily withheld and the patient should be monitored as appropriate
B	The stiffness and coldness of the extremities are likely to be the result of atorvastatin-induced myopathy; atorvastatin should be temporarily withheld and the patient should be monitored as appropriate
C	The stiffness and coldness of the extremities are likely to be caused by carvedilol; a beta blocker with intrinsic sympathomimetic activity, such as acebutolol, may be an alternative option if this cannot be tolerated
D	Impaired T2DM control is likely to be caused by carvedilol; a cardioselective beta blocker, such as bisoprolol, may cause less fluctuation in T2DM control

Communicating Information

Information Options	
E	Impaired T2DM control is likely to be caused by carvedilol; a more water-soluble beta blocker, such as celiprolol, may cause less fluctuation in T2DM control

QUESTION 9

Betty is a 52-year-old lady who was admitted to hospital with excruciating pain in her left calf. She was diagnosed with a DVT and loaded on warfarin with bridging enoxaparin therapy.

PMH: sciatica, menopausal symptoms

DH: paracetamol 1 g QDS, pregabalin 150 mg BD, Oramorph® liquid 10 mg/5 mL 2.5–5 mL PRN QDS, warfarin 4 mg OD (adjusted according to the INR at the clinic) for 6 months, Premique® 625 micrograms OD

SH: alcohol – two to three glasses of red wine/week

Weight: 65 kg; height: 158 cm
INR (on the day in question): 2.3

You stop her Premique®, which was thought to have contributed to the development of a DVT. Betty is now fit for discharge and you decide to briefly counsel her on warfarin therapy.

Select the TWO *most appropriate* information options that should be communicated to the patient.

Information Options	
A	She should take one brown and one blue tablet of warfarin until reviewed at the clinic
B	She should stop taking vitamin K-containing green vegetables because vitamin K antagonises the anticoagulant effect of warfarin
C	She should avoid drinking alcohol because it may affect the anticoagulant control with warfarin
D	She should avoid drinking grapefruit juice because it may enhance the anticoagulant effect of warfarin
E	She should avoid self-medicating with over-the-counter medicines, particularly aspirin, ibuprofen, diclofenac and related products

QUESTION 10

It is Saturday morning, and the Fletcher family are bringing their 2-month-old baby Thomas to receive a round of vaccinations.

PMH: full-term, healthy baby with no clinical abnormalities
Weight: 5.2 kg; height: 56 cm

You decide to provide the parents with some information about the vaccinations scheduled.

Select the TWO *most appropriate* information options that should be communicated to the parents.[4]

Information Options	
A	Baby Thomas is due for Synflorix®, a pneumococcal vaccine
B	Baby Thomas is due for Pediacel®, a 'high dose' diphtheria toxoid-containing vaccine
C	Should baby Thomas suffer from post-immunisation fever (pyrexia), he may have a paracetamol dose of 60 mg, which can be repeated 6 hours later if needed
D	Should baby Thomas suffer from post-immunisation fever (pyrexia), he may have an ibuprofen dose of 60 mg which can be repeated 6 hours later if needed
E	Live attenuated vaccines, such as polio, which baby Thomas is due for, produce a durable immunity, but are not always as long-lasting as that resulting from natural infection

QUESTION 11

Janette, a 16-year-old, has just been initiated on oral isotretinoin for severe acne unresponsive to oral antibacterials and associated with psychological problems.

PMH: acne vulgaris
DH: doxycycline 100 mg OM
SH: parents are divorced; lives with her mother in Elephant & Castle, London
Weight: 56 kg; height: 167 cm

Janette asks you for some further information about the treatment and potential adverse effects.

Select the TWO *most appropriate* information options that should be communicated to the patient.[12]

Information Options	
A	Janette should take ONE 10 mg and ONE 20 mg capsule once a day until a further review
B	Janette should avoid blood donation during the treatment and for at least 6 months after stopping isotretinoin
C	Isotretinoin can cause congenital malformations and therefore Janette should use at least 2 methods of contraception, such as oral progestogen-only contraceptives, during the treatment
D	Janette should be tested for pregnancy every 3 months during the treatment, preferably in the first 3 days of the menstrual cycle
E	Similar to doxycycline, isotretinoin can cause sensitivity to light (photosensitivity); Janette should wear long sleeves and trousers, and should use a sunscreen and emollient from the start of the treatment

QUESTION 12

Layla, a lady who is 19 weeks pregnant, is admitted to hospital with an acute exacerbation of asthma. She markedly improves during her stay and is being discharged with Qvar®, a new pressurised metered-dose inhaler recommended by the respiratory consultant.

PMH: asthma

DH: salbutamol Evohaler® 100 micrograms T-TT PRN QDS and Clenil Modulite® 100 micrograms TT BD both via the AeroChamber® Plus

SH: non-smoker, vegetarian

Weight: 48 kg; height: 154 cm

The consultant asks you to prescribe an appropriate dose of Qvar® (instead of Clenil Modulite®) and to go over the main counselling points for this inhaler with Layla. She is to be followed up in his clinic in 4 weeks' time.

Select the TWO *most appropriate* information options that should be communicated to the patient.[13]

Information Options	
A	Layla should take one puff of Qvar® 100-microgram inhaler twice a day
B	Qvar® must be used regularly for maximum benefit; the alleviation of symptoms usually occurs about 12 hours after initiation
C	Qvar® is relatively safe for use during pregnancy and breastfeeding
D	The risk of Qvar®-induced oral candidiasis can be reduced by using AeroChamber® Plus and by mouth rinsing with water after each inhalation
E	AeroChamber® Plus should be cleaned after each inhalation by washing it in mild detergent and allowing it to dry in air without rinsing

QUESTION 13

Mr Ahmed, a 76-year-old gentleman, comes in for a 6-monthly diabetes review.

PMH: T2DM, hypertension, dry eyes, bilateral primary open-angle glaucoma (diagnosed a week ago)

DH: gliclazide 80 mg OM and 80 mg in the evening, ramipril 10 mg OM, Tears Naturale® 0.3%/0.1% eye drops T to affected eyes PRN

SH: lives with his wife and son's family

Mr Ahmed has recently been prescribed latanoprost eye drops 0.005% by the hospital ophthalmologist. He has found it hard to understand the patient information leaflet; therefore, he would like you to provide him with some information about the use of these eye drops and any problems that may arise during the treatment.

Select the TWO *most appropriate* information options that should be communicated to the patient.[14,15]

Information Options	
A	Latanoprost may cause darkening, thickening and lengthening of the eyelashes
B	Latanoprost may make the colour of the eyes turn blue
C	Pressing the finger against the inner corner of the eye (by the nose) for at least a minute after applying the drop reduces its drainage into the mouth and down the throat
D	Mr Ahmed should apply at least two drops of latanoprost to each eye at a time, preferably in the evening
E	Mr Ahmed should leave at least a 15-minute gap between the application of Tears Naturale® and latanoprost eye drops

REFERENCES

1. *Prescribing Safety Assessment: resources* [Online]. Medical Schools Council; British Pharmacological Society [27 March 2013]. Available at: www.prescribe.ac.uk/psa/?page_id=14

2. National Institute for Health and Clinical Excellence. *Type 2 Diabetes: NICE guideline 87 – quick reference guide*. London: NICE; 2010. Available at: www.nice.org.uk/nicemedia/live/12165/44322/44322.pdf

3. *Stockley's Drug Interactions* [Online]; 2013. Available at: www.medicines complete.com/mc/stockley/current/x07-3726.htm?q=diltiazem%20phenytoin &t=search&ss=text&p=1#_hit

4. British Medical Association; Royal Pharmaceutical Society. *British National Formulary for Children* [Online]. London: Pharmaceutical Press; 2012. Available at: www.medicinescomplete.com

5. *Summary of Product Characteristics Pulmozyme 2500 U/2.5ml, Nebuliser Solution* [Online]. Electronic Medicines Compendium; 2010 [cited 14 July 2012]. Available at: www.medicines.org.uk/EMC/medicine/1723/SPC/Pulmozyme+2500+U++2.5 ml%2c+nebuliser+solution/

6. *Summary of Product Characteristics Creon 10000 Capsules* [Online]. Electronic Medicines Compendium; 2013 [cited 29 March 2013]. Available at: www.medicines. org.uk/EMC/medicine/2068/SPC/Creon+10000+Capsules/#POSOLOGY

7. *Standards for the Clinical Care of Children and Adults with Cystic Fibrosis in the UK* [Online]. UK Cystic Fibrosis Trust; 2011 [cited 30 November 2013]. Available at: https://www.cysticfibrosis.org.uk/media/82070/CD_Standards_of_Care_Dec_11. pdf

8. *Nutritional Management of Cystic Fibrosis* [Online]. UK Cystic Fibrosis Trust; 2002 [cited 30 November 2013]. Available at: https://www.cysticfibrosis.org.uk/ media/82052/CD_Nutritional_Management_Apr_02.pdf

9. *Antibiotic Treatment for Cystic Fibrosis* [Online]. UK Cystic Fibrosis Trust; 2009 [cited 30 November 2013]. Available at: https://www.cysticfibrosis.org.uk/ media/82010/CD_Antibiotic_treatment_for_CF_May_09.pdf

10. Flume PA, O'Sullivan BP, Robinson KA, *et al*. Cystic fibrosis pulmonary guidelines: chronic medications for maintenance of lung health. *Am J Respir Crit Care Med*. 2007; **176**(10): 957–69.

11. Ballinger A, Patchett S. Cystic fibrosis. In: Kumar P, Clark M, editors. *Pocket Essentials of Clinical Medicine*. 4th ed. London: Saunders Elsevier; 2007. pp. 505–8.

12. *Summary of Product Characteristics Isotretinoin 20mg Capsules* [Online]. Electronic Medicines Compendium; 2012 [cited 10 February 2013]. Available at: www.medicines. org.uk/EMC/medicine/15655/SPC/Isotretinoin+20mg+capsules/.

13. *Summary of Product Characteristics Qvar MDI 100 micrograms* [Online]. Electronic Medicines Compendium; 2012 [cited 28 October 2012]. Available at: www.medicines. org.uk/EMC/medicine/23274/SPC/Qvar+MDI+100+micrograms.

14. *Patient Information Leaflet Latanoprost 50mcg/ml Eye Drops* [Online]. Electronic Medicines Compendium; 2012 [cited 28 October 2012]. Available at: www.medicines.org.uk/EMC/medicine/25680/PIL/Latanoprost+50mcg+ml+eye+drops/

15. *Patient Information Leaflet Tears Naturale* [Online]. Electronic Medicines Compendium; 2010 [cited 28 October 2012]. Available at: www.medicines.org.uk/EMC/medicine/17865/PIL/Tears+Naturale/

Chapter 5

Calculation Skills

QUESTION 1

A 43-year-old woman is due for her first cycle of FEC chemotherapy following breast cancer surgery.

FEC:
- 5-fluorouracil 600 mg/m^2
- Epirubicin 75 mg/m^2
- Cyclophosphamide 600 mg/m^2

Weight: 10 stone
Height: 5'8"

What dose of epirubicin should be prescribed (assuming no biochemical or physical abnormalities were found pre-chemotherapy)?[2]

(Round your answer to the nearest 10 mg)
Body Surface Area = (weight in kg × height in cm / 3600)$^{1/2}$

QUESTION 2

Mr TA, a 56-year-old gentleman, suffered a severe myocardial infarction and is due for CABG surgery. He is hypotensive secondary to cardiogenic shock, and an IV dopamine infusion (3 micrograms/kg/min) is chosen in an attempt to restore his blood pressure. Dopamine is available as 1.6 mg/mL in glucose 5% (250 mL bags).
Weight: 83 kg; height: 1.85 m

What rate (expressed as mL/hour) should dopamine be given to Mr TA?[3,4]

(Round your answer to the nearest 0.1 mL)

QUESTION 3

Deborah is an 88-year-old woman with a history of atrial fibrillation for which she takes digoxin tablets 125 micrograms daily. However, she finds it increasingly more difficult to swallow tablets, and the nurse asks you to prescribe her digoxin liquid (50 micrograms/mL) instead.

F (bioavailability) of digoxin tablets = 63%
F of digoxin elixir = 75%

What dose of digoxin elixir (in mL) should you prescribe for this lady?[5]

(Round your answer to the nearest mL)

QUESTION 4

Thomas, a 24-year-old, has just been diagnosed with mild eczema, which has spread to both of his hands and arms. You decide to prescribe him a 2-week trial of E45 lotion for twice-daily application.

What is the total amount (in mL) of E45 lotion you should prescribe for Thomas?

(Round your answer to the nearest container pack size available)
E45 lotion is available in 200 and 500 mL pump packs.

QUESTION 5

Newly born baby Jerome (38 weeks) is suspected to have developed neonatal sepsis. The microbiology team have advised to initiate the extended interval IV tobramycin infusion. You are asked to prescribe the dose as appropriate. Tobramycin (available as 40 mg/mL vials) is to be diluted with sodium chloride 0.9% to 50 mL and is to be given over 60 minutes. The ideal body weight is 3.5 kg.

What volume of tobramycin solution from the vial(s) is required for the first infusion to be given to baby Jerome?

(Round your answer to the nearest 0.1 mL)

Adapted BNF-C guidance for neonatal sepsis (extended interval dose regimen of tobramycin):
- neonate less than 32 weeks postmenstrual age, 4 mg/kg every 36 hours
- neonate 32 weeks and over postmenstrual age, 5 mg/kg every 24 hours.[6,7]

QUESTION 6

Miss UG suffered a psychotic relapse while on chlorpromazine 100 mg TDS, and the consultant psychiatrist decides to switch her to an equivalent dose of clozapine.

What is the total daily dose of clozapine that the consultant psychiatrist should prescribe for Miss UG?

QUESTION 7

Sandy, a 20-year-old who is 30 weeks pregnant, is diagnosed with pre-eclampsia. She is to be given an immediate IV injection of 16 mmol of magnesium followed by an IV infusion of 4 mmol of magnesium/hour over a 24-hour period.

To prepare this infusion magnesium sulphate 50% is to be diluted to 10% with glucose 5% and infused at 10 mL/hour.

What volume of glucose 5% is needed to produce the infusion described?[6]

Magnesium sulphate is available as 10 mL 50% vials containing approximately 2 mmol/mL of magnesium ions.

QUESTION 8

Joseph, a 19-year-old, is admitted to hospital with suspected phenytoin overdose. He normally takes 200 mg of phenytoin capsules (Epanutin®) BD. The plasma level is taken and returns as 52 mg/L; weight: 73 kg.

Assuming linear first order kinetics, how soon is phenytoin concentration likely to fall down to the middle of the optimal range for it to be restarted?[8,9]

(Round your answer to the nearest hour)

Desired optimal range: 10–20 mg/L
Phenytoin elimination constant (k) = 0.03 h^{-1}
Phenytoin volume of distribution (Vd) = 0.7 L/kg
Clearance (mL/min) = k × Vd
k (h^{-1}) = 0.693 / T$_{1/2}$

QUESTION 9

Mrs LM has been prescribed patient-controlled analgesia (PCA) following her appendectomy procedure:

Bolus dose: 1 mg of morphine sulphate
Lock-out period: 10 minutes
She was also put on a background infusion of morphine sulphate set at 2 mg/hr

24 hours later you check the PCA monitor to find out that Mrs LM has pressed the button 10 times since she was started on the PCA. There were no unsuccessful attempts recorded. Since she is now able to take medicines orally, you decide to put her on prolonged release MST Continus® for a day or two until her pain improves.

What dose of MST Continus® should you prescribe for Mrs LM, considering her pain requirements?[10]

(Round your answer to the nearest 10 mg)

QUESTION 10

Anne, an 87-year old lady, was admitted to the care of the elderly ward after she was suspected to have developed urosepsis. Your registrar asks you to initiate IV therapy of co-amoxiclav and give Anne a STAT dose of gentamicin IV as Gram-negative cover.

Her baseline serum creatinine (Cr) is 145 μmol/L (79–118)
Weight: 7 stone and 5 pounds; height: 5'4"

What dose of STAT gentamicin should you prescribe? *(For the purpose of this calculation, use the patient's actual body weight, and round your final answer to the nearest mg)*

    Gentamicin Dose in Renal Impairment (adapted from Renal Handbook[11] *for this calculation)*

GFR (mL/min):
30–70: 5 mg/kg daily and monitor levels
10–30: 3 mg/kg daily and monitor levels
5–10: 2 mg/kg every 48–72 hours according to levels
GFR (mL/min) = (140 – age) × weight (kg) × constant / Cr (μmol/L)
Constant = 1.23 for men; 1.04 for women

QUESTION 11

Mrs Jennings, a previously healthy 52-year-old, was diagnosed with uterine cancer and underwent total abdominal hysterectomy with bilateral salpingo-oophorectomy. She is now recovering and has been prescribed Evorel® '50' patches as hormone replacement therapy (HRT).

Mrs Jennings has just read the patient information leaflet for Evorel® '50' patches and has become a little concerned about the side effects this medicine may cause, particularly breast cancer. She would like to find out more about the risks of developing this type of malignancy while on Evorel® '50' patches.

What is the percentage difference in the 10-year risk of developing breast cancer with Evorel® '50' patches compared with not using HRT?

QUESTION 12

Geraldine, a 7-year-old, is brought to the paediatric ITU with refractory status epilepticus. Buccal midazolam has not been found to be effective, and she is to be initiated on an IV phenytoin infusion.

What total dose of IV phenytoin (expressed as milligrams) is Geraldine to receive in the first 24 hours of treatment?

The dose of IV phenytoin infusion (adapted for this calculation from BNF-C):
- *Neonate initially 20 mg/kg as a loading dose over 1 hour, then 2.5 mg/kg twice daily*
- *Child 1 month–12 years initially 20 mg/kg as a loading dose over 1 hour, then 5 mg/kg twice daily*
- *Child 12–18 years initially 20 mg/kg as a loading dose over 1 hour, then 100 mg three times daily.*[7]

QUESTION 13

Arjan is a 48-year-old Punjabi gentleman who attends his yearly health check-up today.

PMH: nil
DH: OTC paracetamol and Nurofen® PRN
FH: mother had a stroke at the age of 64
SH: non-smoker, occasional can of lager
Weight: 75 kg; height: 1.63 m
BP 140/84 mmHg; HR 67/min

Investigations (Random, Non-fasting Tests)

Today	12 Months Ago
Glucose 4.7 mmol/L (4.5–5.6)	5.0 mmol/L
Total cholesterol (TC) 4.7 mmol/L (<4.0)	4.8 mmol/L
LDL-cholesterol (LDL-C) 1.8 mmol/L (<2.0)	1.9 mmol/L

What is Arjan's 10-year risk of cardiovascular disease (CVD) according to Joint British Societies' charts (rounded to the nearest percentage)? Is lipid-regulating therapy indicated in his case? (1 mark for answering each part of the question.)[12]

REFERENCES

1. *Prescribing Safety Assessment: resources* [Online]. Medical Schools Council; British Pharmacological Society [27 March 2013]. Available at: www.prescribe.ac.uk/psa/?page_id=14

2. *FEC for Adjuvant Use in Breast Cancer* [Online]. Surrey, West Sussex and Hampshire Cancer Network; 2010 [cited 29 March 2013]. Available at: www.royalsurrey.nhs.uk/Default.aspx?DN=7e40a193-2b03-4ff2-9eef-f883634bec6b

3. Ballinger A, Patchett S. Ischaemic heart disease. In: Kumar P, Clark M, editors. *Pocket Essentials of Clinical Medicine*. 4th ed. London: Saunders Elsevier; 2007. pp. 434–9.

4. Ballinger A, Patchett S. Acute disturbances of haemodynamic function (shock). In: Kumar P, Clark M, editors. *Pocket Essentials of Clinical Medicine*. 4th ed. London: Saunders Elsevier; 2007. pp. 552–62.

5. *Summary of Product Characteristics Lanoxin PG Elixir* [Online]. Electronic Medicines Compendium; 2012 [cited 29 March 2013]. Available at: www.medicines.org.uk/EMC/medicine/2176/SPC/Lanoxin+PG+Elixir/

6. Medusa Injectable Medicines Guide Online: National Health Service. Available at: www.injguide.nhs.uk

7. British Medical Association; Royal Pharmaceutical Society. *British National Formulary for Children* [Online]: London: Pharmaceutical Press; 2012. Available at: www.medicinescomplete.com

8. Fitzpatrick R. Practical pharmacokinetics. In: Walker R, Whittlesea C, editors. *Clinical Pharmacy and Therapeutics*. 4th ed. London: Churchill Livingstone Elsevier; 2007. pp. 24–39.

9. *Summary of Product Characteristics Epanutin capsules 25, 50 and 100mg* [Online]. Electronic Medicines Compendium; 2012 [cited 2 December 2013]. Available at: www.medicines.org.uk/emc/medicine/25070/SPC/Epanutin+capsules+25%2c+50+and+100mg/

10. Rahman MH, Beattie J. Managing post-operative pain. *Pharm J*. 2005; **275**: 145–8.

11. Ashley C, Currie A; UK Renal Pharmacy Group. *The Renal Drug Handbook*. 3rd ed. Oxford: Radcliffe Publishing; 2009.

12. National Institute for Health and Clinical Excellence. *Lipid Modification: NICE guideline 67 – quick reference guide*. London: NICE; 2010. Available at: www.nice.org.uk/nicemedia/live/11982/40675/40675.pdf

Chapter 6

Adverse Drug Reactions

READ BEFORE YOU START

- There are eight 'Adverse Drug Reactions' (ADRs) question items in the PSA worth 2 marks each (16 marks in total).
- In this chapter, you will be asked to select two out of the five options given that are most relevant and/or appropriate for the clinical presentation described in the scenario (specific drugs/adverse effects/interactions/management actions).*
- There are four main types of ADR questions in this chapter:
  - *Type A* – asks you to identify the two most likely ADRs for specific commonly prescribed drugs, e.g. beta blockers causing bronchospasm, statins resulting in myopathy, sulfonylureas causing hypoglycaemia
  - *Type B* – asks you to identify two medicines that have most likely caused an ADR presented in that question, e.g. rifampicin/isoniazid causing hepatotoxicity, antidepressants/diuretics resulting in hyponatraemia, antimuscarinics/antipsychotics causing urinary retention
  - *Type C* – asks you to identify the potential drug–drug interaction between two medicines that has most likely caused the clinical presentation in that question, e.g. amiodarone and warfarin (increased anticoagulant effect), antiepileptics and SSRIs (lowered seizure threshold), digoxin and loop diuretics (increased risk of digoxin toxicity)
  - *Type D* – asks you to choose the two most appropriate management options for a particular ADR, e.g. opioid toxicity, methotrexate overdose, digoxin and bradycardia.[1]
- Some of the questions in this chapter may require you to read/utilise additional reference sources, such as relevant NICE guidance or the BNF.

---

* Note that you will be asked to select a single most appropriate option from a list of five during the PSA.

QUESTION 1

Ronny, a 7-year-old boy, has just been started on sodium valproate for newly diagnosed generalised absence seizures.

Select the TWO adverse effects that are *most likely* to be caused by this treatment.

Adverse Effect Options	
A	Weight gain
B	Liver toxicity
C	Blood or hepatic disorders
D	Transient hair loss
E	Pancreatitis

QUESTION 2

Mr Wilkinson is a 53-year-old type 2 diabetic gentleman who presents to hospital with a rapid onset of sharp left-sided chest pain. He subsequently undergoes coronary angiography.

PMH: T2DM, liver transplant (2 years ago)
DH: metformin 500 mg OM, 1 g lunchtime, 500 mg evening, saxagliptin 5 mg OM, Neoral® 450 mg OM, prednisolone 2.5 mg OM
SH: retired taxi driver, lives with his wife in Birmingham

Twenty-four hours later Mr Wilkinson suddenly deteriorates. U+Es are requested and demonstrate a marked increase in serum creatinine:

Cr 257 µmol/L (79–118), eGFR 24 mL/min/1.73 m^2 from a pre-admission baseline of Cr 94 µmol/L, eGFR 77 mL/min/1.73 m^2; weight: 92 kg.

Select the TWO prescriptions that have *most likely* contributed to the acute renal impairment experienced by Mr Wilkinson.[2–7]

Prescription Options	
A	Aspirin 300 mg and clopidogrel 300 mg STAT
B	Metformin 500 mg OM, 1 g lunchtime, 500 mg evening
C	Iodinated contrast media for angiography
D	Neoral® 450 mg OM
E	Prednisolone 2.5 mg OM

QUESTION 3

Mrs BU, an 84-year-old, is admitted to hospital with severe generalised muscle pain. She was previously in hospital a week ago following an acute attack of gout.

PMH: gout, heart failure

DH: ramipril 2.5 mg OM, bisoprolol 5 mg OM, furosemide 40 mg OM, digoxin 125 micrograms OM, allopurinol 300 mg OM, colchicine 500 micrograms BD for 6/7

SH: nil relevant

Blood investigations: Na^+ 132 mmol/L (135–146), K^+ 5.1 mmol/L (3.5–5.0), Cr 187 μmol/L (79–118), creatine kinase 1345 U/L (24–170 U/L)

Select the TWO prescriptions that are *most likely* to interact with each other to cause the clinical manifestation reported in Mrs BU's case.[8]

Prescription Options	
A	Ramipril
B	Furosemide
C	Allopurinol
D	Digoxin
E	Colchicine

QUESTION 4

You are asked to see a 10-year-old boy on a paediatric ward who started feeling nauseous soon after a blood transfusion. He also complains of intense 'tummy' pains and has been to the toilet three times in the past hour.

PMH: thalassaemia major
DH: regular blood transfusions, NKDA
Blood investigations: ferritin 360 micrograms/L (20–260), iron 41 µmol/L (13–32), TIBC 65 µmol/L (42–80), transferrin saturation 63%[9]

Select the TWO *most appropriate* options for the management of this adverse drug event.[10,11]

Management Options	
A	Deferiprone
B	Venesection
C	Desferrioxamine
D	Metoclopramide
E	Cyclizine

QUESTION 5

Mrs Mann, a 75-year-old lady, has just been initiated on co-beneldopa 12.5/50 capsules one TDS to help manage her newly confirmed early Parkinson's disease.

Select the TWO adverse effects that are *most likely* to be caused by this treatment.

	Adverse Effect Options
A	Oculogyric crisis
B	Neuroleptic malignant syndrome
C	Postural hypotension
D	Reddish discolouration of the urine
E	Henoch–Schönlein purpura

QUESTION 6

Mrs Nathan, a 64-year-old, presents to the GP surgery with increasingly 'puffy' ankles. She has no pain or sensitivity in either of her legs and seems to be otherwise well.

PMH: rheumatoid arthritis, hypertension
DH: methotrexate 12.5 mg weekly, sulfasalazine 500 mg BD, diclofenac 50 mg TDS PRN, felodipine MR 10 mg OM, irbesartan 150 mg OM
SH: once-daily care package at home

Select the TWO prescriptions that have *most likely* contributed to Mrs Mann's complaint.[12,13]

Prescription Options	
A	Methotrexate 12.5 mg weekly
B	Felodipine MR 10 mg OM
C	Diclofenac 50 mg TDS PRN
D	Sulfasalazine 500 mg BD
E	Irbesartan 150 mg OM

QUESTION 7

Miss GT, a 20-year-old, is admitted to hospital after she started fitting at home and subsequently lost consciousness.

PMH: epilepsy

DH: phenytoin capsules 300 mg OM (started 10 years ago), lamotrigine 100 mg BD, Yasmin® two tablets OM taken as a 'tricyclic' regimen (unlicensed), amoxicillin 250 mg TDS for 7/7 (prescribed by the GP a week ago for a periodontal abscess), paracetamol OTC 1 g PRN QDS for headaches

SH: nil alcohol, non-smoker

Select the TWO prescriptions that have *most likely* interacted with each other to induce an epileptic seizure experienced by Miss GT.

Prescription Options	
A	Paracetamol OTC 1 g PRN QDS
B	Phenytoin capsules 300 mg OM
C	Yasmin® one tablet OM in 21-day cycles
D	Amoxicillin 250 mg TDS
E	Lamotrigine 100 mg BD

QUESTION 8

You are an FY1 in a psychiatric hospital. Mr HJ, a well-known 28-year-old patient, is brought in by ambulance. His carers found him unresponsive in the bathroom. According to them, Mr HJ's bottle of Valium® was left empty on the floor next to him. Other medicines were brought in to hospital and appeared untouched.

PMH: schizophrenia, depression and generalised anxiety disorder (multiple suicide attempts)

DH: quetiapine 150 mg OM, 300 mg ON, escitalopram 20 mg OM, diazepam 4 mg TDS, zopiclone 7.5 mg ON

On examination, Mr HJ is talking but appears extremely confused.

Select the TWO *most appropriate* options for the initial management of this adverse drug event.[12]

Management Options	
A	Activated charcoal 50 g STAT
B	Lorazepam 2 mg IV STAT
C	Naloxone 2 mg IV STAT
D	Flumazenil 300 micrograms IV STAT
E	Naloxone 2 mg IM STAT

QUESTION 9

Mrs UP has been recently diagnosed with colon cancer and subsequently undergoes a left hemicolectomy. Following surgery, she is initiated on PRN morphine via the patient-controlled analgesia (PCA) system.

Select the TWO adverse effects that are *most likely* to be caused by this treatment.

	Adverse Effect Options
A	Bradypnoea
B	Hyperalgesia
C	Adrenal insufficiency
D	Urinary incontinence
E	Tachycardia

QUESTION 10

Mr Patel, a 44-year-old, underwent a successful total left knee replacement. However, in the post-operative period he started developing both localised and systemic signs of infection, and was diagnosed with septic arthritis.

PMH: osteoarthritis
DH: meloxicam 15 mg OM, esomeprazole 20 mg OM
SH: nil relevant

Mr Patel was started on a 4- to 6-week course of flucloxacillin 2 g IV QDS and sodium fusidate 1 g PO TDS. He was also prescribed some supportive care to help relieve his pain and occasional nausea: paracetamol 1 g PO QDS, codeine 60 mg PO QDS, cyclizine 50 mg SC TDS. Two weeks later his nausea suddenly got worse and he was unable to keep his food or medicines down. Mr Patel also developed a degree of jaundice with some diffuse itchiness. Blood investigations demonstrated:

Na$^+$ 150 mmol/L (135–146), K$^+$ 3.1 mmol/L (3.5–5.0), U 5.8 mmol/L (2.5–6.7), Cr 85 μmol/L (79–118), albumin 46 g/L (35–50), ALP 232 U/L (39–117), ALT 194 U/L (5–40), total bilirubin 49 μmol/L (<17).

Select the TWO prescriptions that have *most likely* contributed to the deterioration of Mr Patel's clinical condition.[12,14-17]

Prescription Options	
A	Flucloxacillin 2 g IV QDS
B	Sodium fusidate 1 g PO TDS
C	Paracetamol 1 g PO QDS
D	Codeine 60 mg PO QDS
E	Cyclizine 50 mg SC TDS

QUESTION 11

You are on call on a Sunday night and one of the nurses on the geriatric ward bleeps asking you to review Mrs Thompson, an 84-year-old who has collapsed after being transferred from the Acute Medical Unit. The nurse tells you that before 'passing out' the patient was feeling very nauseous and vomited once. Mrs Thompson also kept telling the nurse that everything, including the nursing staff, appeared yellow, but the nurse thought it was probably due to her confusion. She recorded Mrs Thompson's observations as BP 123/79 mmHg, HR 45 beats per minute, RR 10 breaths per minute, S_aO_2 on room air 97%.

PC: new-onset AF
PMH: heart failure, hypertension
Drug chart: digoxin 125 micrograms OM, furosemide 40 mg BD, simvastatin 40 mg ON, bisoprolol 5 mg OM, quinapril 10 mg BD (has been taking all five for the last 5 years), warfarin 4 mg in the evening, amiodarone 200 mg TDS

Select the TWO prescriptions that have *most likely* interacted with each other to result in the clinical signs and symptoms exhibited by Mrs Thompson.[18]

Prescription Options	
A	Warfarin 4 mg in the evening
B	Digoxin 125 micrograms OM
C	Bisoprolol 5 mg OM
D	Amiodarone 200 mg TDS
E	Quinapril 10 mg BD

QUESTION 12

Mrs GJ, a 62-year-old retired schoolteacher, is brought to A&E following a 2-day history of coffee ground vomiting and severe abdominal pain. An endoscopy (OGD) shows a major gastric ulcer actively bleeding.

PMH: dyspepsia, rheumatoid arthritis

DH: indometacin 100 mg BD, methotrexate 15 mg weekly, folic acid 5 mg weekly (on a different day than methotrexate), pantoprazole 20 mg OM

SH: nil relevant

Select the TWO *most appropriate* options for the initial management of this adverse drug event.

Management Options	
A	Pantoprazole 80 mg PO OD
B	Omeprazole 40 mg OD as an IV injection or short IV infusion
C	Omeprazole 80 mg IV over 40–60 minutes, then 8 mg/hour for 72 hours as a continuous IV infusion
D	Discontinue indometacin
E	Phytomenadione 1 mg IV STAT

QUESTION 13

Lynn, a 61-year-old, is brought into hospital with severe suprapubic pain and dysuria. She is prescribed IV co-amoxiclav (Augmentin®) for suspected urosepsis.

PMH: hypertension, COPD, liver transplantation
DH: amlodipine 10 mg OM, salbutamol nebules 2.5 mg PRN up to QDS, Seretide® 500 Accuhaler® T BD, Seebri® Breezhaler® 44 micrograms OM, Slo-Phyllin® 500 mg BD, prednisolone 5 mg OM, Neoral® 300 mg OM
SH: lives with her husband in Croydon
Weight: 55 kg; height: 1.62 m

Four days later the SHO bleeps you while reviewing this lady's blood test results. She sounds a little concerned and asks for your opinion.

Blood Test Results

Today	On Admission
Na⁺ 148 mmol/L (135–146)	Na⁺ 149 mmol/L (135–146)

Today
Na⁺ 148 mmol/L (135–146)
K⁺ 5.9 mmol/L (3.5–5.0)
U 16.5 mmol/L (2.5–6.7)
Cr 223 µmol/L (79–118)
eGFR of 21 mL/min/1.73 m²

On Admission
Na⁺ 149 mmol/L (135–146)
K⁺ 4.7 mmol/L (3.5–5.0)
U 15.6 mmol/L (2.5–6.7)
Cr 214 µmol/L (79–118)
eGFR of 22 mL/min/1.73 m²

Select the TWO prescriptions that have *most likely* contributed to Lynn's abnormal blood test results.[2,9,19,20]

Prescription Options	
A	Co-amoxiclav (Augmentin®) 1.2 g IV TDS
B	Prednisolone 5 mg OM
C	Salbutamol nebules 2.5 mg PRN up to QDS
D	Slo-Phyllin® 500 mg BD
E	Neoral® 300 mg OM

REFERENCES

1. *Prescribing Safety Assessment: resources* [Online]. Medical Schools Council; British Pharmacological Society [27 March 2013]. Available at: www.prescribe.ac.uk/psa/?page_id=14

2. Marriott J, Smith S. Acute renal failure. In: Walker R, Whittlesea C, editors. *Clinical Pharmacy and Therapeutics*. 4th ed. London: Churchill Livingstone Elsevier; 2007. pp. 250–64.

3. Thomsen HS, Morcos SK. Contrast media and the kidney: European Society of Urogenital Radiology (ESUR) guidelines. *Br J Radiol*. 2003; **76**(908): 513–18.

4. Stegall MD, Everson GT, Schroter G, *et al.* Prednisone withdrawal late after adult liver transplantation reduces diabetes, hypertension, and hypercholesterolemia without causing graft loss. *Hepatology*. 1997; **25**(1): 173–7.

5. Mathew R, Haque K, Woothipoom W. Acute renal failure induced by contrast medium: steps towards prevention. *BMJ*. 2006; **333**(7567): 539–40.

6. *Summary of Product Characteristics Aspirin Tablets BP 300mg* [Online]. Electronic Medicines Compendium; 2010 [cited 29 March 2013]. Available at: www.medicines.org.uk/EMC/medicine/23776/SPC/Aspirin+Tablets+BP+300mg/#UNDESIRABLE_EFFECTS

7. *Summary of Product Characteristics Prednisolone Tablets BP 5 mg* [Online]. Electronic Medicines Compendium; 2013 [cited 29 March 2013]. Available at: www.medicines.org.uk/EMC/medicine/26657/SPC/Prednisolone+Tablets+BP+5+mg/#UNDESIRABLE_EFFECTS

8. *Stockley's Drug Interactions* [Online]. Available at: www.medicinescomplete.com/

9. Wynne H, Edwards C. Laboratory data. In: Walker R, Whittlesea C, editors. *Clinical Pharmacy and Therapeutics*. 4th ed. London: Churchill Livingstone Elsevier; 2007. pp. 64–81.

10. Ballinger A, Patchett S. Haemoglobin abnormalities. In: Kumar P, Clark M, editors. *Pocket Essentials of Clinical Medicine*. 4th ed. London: Saunders Elsevier; 2007. pp. 199–202.

11. Mir MA. Transfusion-induced iron overload workup [Online]. *Medscape*; 2012 [cited 30 March 2013]. Available at: http://emedicine.medscape.com/article/1389732-workup

12. *Martindale: the complete drug reference* [Online]. Available at: www.medicinescomplete.com/

13. *Summary of Product Characteristics Methotrexate 2.5 mg Tablets* [Online]. Electronic Medicines Compendium; 2012 [cited 28 March 2013]. Available at: www.medicines.org.uk/EMC/medicine/12033/SPC/Methotrexate+2.5+mg+Tablets/#PHARMACOKINETIC_PROPS

14. *Summary of Product Characteristics Fucidin Tablets* [Online]. Electronic Medicines Compendium; 2012 [cited 29 March 2013]. Available at: www.medicines.org.uk/EMC/medicine/2448/SPC/Fucidin+Tablets/#UNDESIRABLE_EFFECTS

15. *Summary of Product Characteristics Cyclizine 50mg Tablets* [Online]. Electronic Medicines Compendium; 2012 [cited 30 March 2013]. Available at: www.medicines. org.uk/EMC/medicine/27036/SPC/Cyclizine+50mg+Tablets/

16. *Summary of Product Characteristics Codeine Phosphate Tablets 30mg* [Online]. Electronic Medicines Compendium; 2010 [cited 16 September 2012]. Available at: www.medicines.org.uk/EMC/medicine/23910/SPC/Codeine+Phosphate+Tab lets+30mg/#UNDESIRABLE_EFFECTS

17. Kennedy P, O'Grady J. Liver disease. In: Walker R, Whittlesea C, editors. *Clinical Pharmacy and Therapeutics*. 4th ed. London: Churchill Livingstone Elsevier; 2007. pp. 215–31.

18. *Summary of Product Characteristics Digoxin Tablets BP 125 micrograms* [Online]. Electronic Medicines Compendium; 2012 [cited 30 March 2013]. Available at: www.medicines.org.uk/EMC/medicine/23943/SPC/Digoxin+Tablets+BP+125+ micrograms/#UNDESIRABLE_EFFECTS

19. Ballinger A, Patchett S. Hyperkalaemia. In: Kumar P, Clark M, editors. *Pocket Essentials of Clinical Medicine*. 4th ed. London: Saunders Elsevier; 2007. pp. 324–5.

20. *Summary of Product Characteristics Neoral Soft Gelatin Capsules, Neoral Oral Solution* [Online]. Electronic Medicines Compendium; 2012 [cited 27 October 2012]. Available at: www.medicines.org.uk/EMC/medicine/1307/SPC/Neoral+Soft+ Gelatin+Capsules%2c+Neoral+Oral+Solution/#CLINICAL_PRECAUTIONS

Chapter 7

Drug Monitoring

---

* Note that you will be asked to select a single most appropriate option from a list of five during the PSA.

QUESTION 1

After undergoing mitral valve replacement Mr Brown, a 69-year-old, develops endocarditis of suspected enterococcal origin. He is started on amoxicillin IV 2 g every 4 hours and gentamicin 85 mg IV every 12 hours for 6 weeks.

Weight: 85 kg; height: 5'11"; Cr 234 µmol/L (79–118), eGFR 26 mL/min/1.73 m²

Select the TWO *most appropriate* monitoring options to assess the beneficial/adverse effects of this treatment.[2]

Monitoring Options	
A	Blood samples for gentamicin level should be taken 16–24 hours after the first dose and interpreted using the Hartford nomogram
B	Blood samples for gentamicin level should be taken 1 hour after the administration of each dose for the first 24 hours (considering poor renal function), thereafter adjusting the interval of dosing as appropriate
C	Blood samples for gentamicin level should be taken 1 hour after the third or fourth dose and just before the next dose; the dose and/or dosing interval should be adjusted accordingly based on these results
D	The target 'peak' serum concentration of gentamicin should be 5–10 mg/L
E	The target 'trough' serum concentration of gentamicin should be <1 mg/L

QUESTION 2

Mrs Jones is a 75-year-old lady who suffers from long-standing hypertension and COPD. She had been a smoker for over 25 years but she gave up about 10 years ago when she was diagnosed with COPD. She is brought into hospital today with worsening shortness of breath and chest tightness.

DH: amlodipine 10 mg OM, bendroflumethiazide 2.5 mg, enalapril 20 mg OM, Slo-Phyllin® 250 mg BD, Spiriva® Handihaler® 18 micrograms OM, Ventolin® Accuhaler® 200 micrograms up to QDS PRN, Seretide® 500 Accuhaler® one puff BD

On questioning, Mrs Jones admits that ever since her husband passed away about 4 months ago she has been drinking whisky and has gone back to smoking cigarettes. She does not think that she can stop any of these habits any time soon.[3,4]

Results 6 Months Ago
FEV_1 predicted 39%
FEV_1/FVC 0.65
S_aO_2 on room air 98%
P_aO_2 9.4 kPa (10–13.3)
P_aCO_2 5.8 kPa (4.8–6.1)

Results Today
FEV_1 predicted 32%
FEV_1/FVC 0.55
S_aO_2 on room air 94%
P_aO_2 7.8 kPa
P_aCO_2 6.6 kPa

Mrs Jones is treated for non-infective exacerbation of COPD. On discharge, you decide to review her COPD treatment.

Select the TWO *most appropriate* monitoring options to assess the beneficial effects of Mrs Jones' COPD treatment.

Monitoring Options	
A	Smoking and chronic alcohol inhibits the metabolism of aminophylline; aim for a pre-dose aminophylline plasma level of 10–20 mg/L after increasing the dose to 500 mg BD
B	Smoking and chronic alcohol induces the metabolism of theophylline; aim for a pre-dose theophylline plasma level of 55–110 µmol/L after increasing the dose to 500 mg BD
C	Smoking and chronic alcohol induces the metabolism of theophylline; aim for a post-dose theophylline plasma level of 10–20 mg/L after increasing the dose to 500 mg BD

Monitoring Options	
D	Aim for a target FEV_1 predicted 40% and FEV_1/FVC 0.65
E	Aim for a target P_aO_2 12 kPa and P_aCO_2 5 kPa

QUESTION 3

Benjamin, a 23-year-old, has just been diagnosed with schizophrenia and initiated on olanzapine 10 mg OM. The psychiatrist wants him to be monitored closely every 3 months for the first year.

Select the TWO *most appropriate* monitoring options to assess the beneficial and adverse effects of this treatment 6 months after the initiation.[5,6]

Monitoring Options	
A	FBC, U+Es and LFTs
B	Blood lipids
C	Weight
D	ECG
E	Physical health monitoring and symptomatic assessment using DSM-IV and/or ICD-10 tools

QUESTION 4

Miss Thompson, a 32-year-old woman, has been finding it increasingly more difficult to comply with her daily oral combined contraceptive regimen and has been recently switched to Evra® patches.

PMH: nil

DH: Evra® patches 33.9 micrograms/24 hours apply one patch once weekly for 3 weeks, followed by a 7-day patch-free interval

Weight: 88 kg; height: 167 cm; BP: 125/78 mmHg

Select the TWO *most appropriate* monitoring options to assess the beneficial and adverse effects of Miss Thompson's contraceptive patches.

	Monitoring Options
A	Weight and BMI
B	Sudden appearance of severe back pain
C	Diarrhoea and vomiting
D	Prolactin levels
E	Increase in headache frequency or onset of focal symptoms

QUESTION 5

Mrs Wang, a 78-year-old, is seen at your clinic with worsening breathlessness, cough and production of purulent sputum. You suspect a mild chest infection and prescribe some erythromycin 250 mg QDS for 5/7.

PMH: AF, TIA, hypertension

DH: CoAprovel® 150 mg/12.5 mg T OM, warfarin 4 mg on Mondays, Wednesdays and Fridays, 5 mg on other days, carvedilol 3.125 mg BD and simvastatin 40 mg ON; allergies: amoxicillin (unknown type of reaction)

Select the TWO *most appropriate* monitoring options to assess the adverse effects of erythromycin treatment in light of the patient's clinical condition and concomitant pharmaceutical therapies.

Monitoring Options	
A	Increased risk of thrombotic events (a decrease in INR)
B	Increased risk of haemorrhage (an increase in INR)
C	Increased risk of thrombotic events (an increase in INR)
D	Increased risk of myopathy; withhold the statin during the course of erythromycin
E	Increased risk of myopathy; continue statin therapy with careful monitoring for symptoms of muscle pain, tenderness or weakness

QUESTION 6

Henry, a 61-year-old, suffers a myocardial infarction and presents with ventricular tachycardia (VT). Your consultant initiates IV amiodarone 300 mg as a rapid IV infusion over an hour during which Henry's VT begins to resolve. Subsequently, Henry is loaded with 900 mg of IV amiodarone over 24 hours with a potential switch to an oral loading regimen thereafter.

PMH: T2DM
DH: metformin 500 mg OM

Select the TWO *most appropriate* monitoring options to assess the beneficial and adverse effects of amiodarone.[7–9]

	Monitoring Options
A	Amiodarone is a class II antiarrhythmic, which may increase the sinus rate
B	Amiodarone is a class III antiarrhythmic, which can broaden the QRS complex
C	Amiodarone is a class III antiarrhythmic, which can significantly prolong the QT interval
D	Amiodarone is hepatotoxic; baseline liver function tests should be requested as appropriate and should be repeated every 6 months
E	Amiodarone has been reported to cause pneumonitis; however, a baseline chest X-ray is not normally indicated unless pulmonary signs/symptoms are present

QUESTION 7

Juliet, a 10-year-old type 1 diabetic girl, is diagnosed with pulmonary tuberculosis. She is to be initiated on rifampicin 300 mg OD, ethambutol 500 mg OD, isoniazid 300 mg OD, pyrazinamide 1 g OD and pyridoxine 10 mg OD for 2 months, and then reviewed accordingly.

DH: Humalog Mix25® 15 units OM, 12 units ON
Weight: 32 kg

The registrar asks you to arrange all the necessary examination and monitoring.

Select the TWO *most appropriate* monitoring options for Juliet's new medicines.

	Monitoring Options
A	Visual acuity testing using a Snellen chart should be undertaken prior to treatment initiation to reduce the risk of isoniazid-related ophthalmic effects
B	Renal function should be checked before the treatment and appropriate dosage adjustments should be made
C	Isoniazid-induced peripheral neuropathy is more likely to occur in diabetic patients; Juliet should be monitored for symptoms of this adverse effect throughout the treatment
D	Hepatic function should be checked before the treatment and every 2 months thereafter
E	Monthly urine assessment (rifampicin imparts a brownish discolouration) may be a useful indicator of adherence to treatment

QUESTION 8

Patrick, a 6-year-old, is brought into hospital with severe wheeze and increased respiratory effort.

PMH: asthma
DH: salbutamol Evohaler® 100 micrograms T-TT up to QDS PRN

On Examination

Mildly cyanotic, using accessory muscles, warm to touch, silent chest
Temperature 37.7°C, HR 143/min and regular, BP 95/64 mmHg, RR 38/min, O_2 sat 89% on air

Investigations

PEF 30%, P_aO_2 7.8 kPa (10–13.3), P_aCO_2 6.7 kPa (4.8–6.1), pH 7.30 (7.35–7.45), K^+ 4.2 mmol/L (3.5–5.0), HCO_3^- 26 mmol/L (22–26), base excess +2 mmol/L (–2/+2)
ECG: sinus tachycardia

Patrick is treated for life-threatening acute asthma using high-flow oxygen, salbutamol and ipratropium nebules, IV aminophylline and IV hydrocortisone.

Select the TWO *most appropriate* monitoring options to assess the beneficial and harmful effects of Patrick's therapy.[10,11]

	Monitoring Options
A	Maintain K^+ below 5.0 to reduce the risk of cardiac arrhythmias; concomitant use of nebulised salbutamol, IV aminophylline and IV hydrocortisone can cause a significant rise in plasma K^+
B	Maintain K^+ above 3.5 to reduce the risk of cardiac arrhythmias; concomitant use of nebulised salbutamol, IV aminophylline and IV hydrocortisone can cause a significant decrease in plasma K^+
C	Maintain HCO_3^- above 26 to avoid the development of metabolic acidosis; concomitant use of nebulised salbutamol, IV aminophylline and IV hydrocortisone can cause a significant drop in blood pH
D	Measure plasma theophylline concentration 2 hours after the start of intravenous infusion; aim for 10–20 mg/L
E	Aim for O_2 sat 92% or higher on air and PEF of at least 50%

QUESTION 9

Mrs UM, a 48-year-old who suffers from non-valvular atrial fibrillation (AF), is admitted to hospital with persistent coffee ground vomiting. NSAID-induced active peptic ulcer bleeding is suspected, and she is prescribed IV omeprazole and fluid support until she undergoes an endoscopy.

PMH: AF, multiple TIAs, back pain

DH: rivaroxaban 20 mg OM (stopped on admission), bisoprolol 2.5 mg BD, naproxen 250 mg TDS (stopped on admission), atorvastatin 20 mg ON

Select the TWO *most appropriate* monitoring options to assess the beneficial and adverse effects of Mrs UM's pharmaceutical therapy.[12]

Monitoring Options	
A	INR
B	APTT
C	Anti-factor Xa
D	Hb
E	Repeated episodes of haematemesis

QUESTION 10

Mr Teddington, a 58-year-old gentleman, undergoes an elective laparoscopic cholecystectomy. Unfortunately, he loses about 200 mL of blood during the procedure and is prescribed 2 L of Hartmann's solution together with 1 L of glucose 5% both at 120 mL/hour as post-operative fluid replacement.

Weight: 73 kg

Select the TWO *most appropriate* monitoring options to assess the adverse effects of Mr Teddington's fluid replacement therapy.[13,14]

Monitoring Options	
A	Plasma chloride should be monitored carefully; the administration of Hartmann's solution may induce hyperchloraemic acidosis
B	Hb should be rechecked prior to discharge; excessive administration of IV fluids may lead to haemodilution
C	Renal function should be monitored carefully; excessive administration of Hartmann's solution may cause hyperoncotic acute renal failure
D	Hartmann's solution and glucose 5% leak rapidly into the interstitial space and may cause significant small bowel oedema; monitor carefully for an increase in nausea and vomiting
E	BMs should be monitored closely; glucose 5% may cause fluctuations in blood sugar

QUESTION 11

Mrs Gandhi, an 82-year-old, is admitted to hospital with worsening congestive heart failure and tachycardia (HR 115 bpm, irregular, BP 174/95 mmHg).

PMH: CHF, AF, hypertension
DH: digoxin 62.5 micrograms OM, trandolapril 500 micrograms OM, aspirin 75 mg OM and diltiazem MR (Adizem-XL®) 240 mg OM; intolerances: atenolol (gastrointestinal upset); she is switched to IV furosemide 40 mg BD, her digoxin is increased to 125 micrograms OM and she is also prescribed spironolactone 25 mg OM

Five days later Mrs Gandhi's heart rate becomes persistently low (around 45–50 bpm).

Select the TWO *most appropriate* monitoring options to assess the adverse effects of Mrs Gandhi's pharmaceutical therapy.[2,15]

Monitoring Options	
A	Digoxin plasma level; a level of <3 micrograms/L is unlikely to be associated with digoxin toxicity
B	Digoxin plasma level; a level of <1.5 micrograms/L is unlikely to be associated with digoxin toxicity
C	Digoxin plasma level; a level of <1.5 micrograms/mL is unlikely to be associated with digoxin toxicity
D	Plasma level of K⁺; spironolactone-induced hyperkalaemia may increase the risk of digoxin toxicity
E	Plasma level of K⁺; furosemide-induced hypokalaemia may increase the risk of digoxin toxicity

QUESTION 12

Mr Ayeni, a 57-year-old Nigerian gentleman, attends the GP clinic for his annual diabetes review.

PMH: T2DM (diagnosed 4 years ago)
DH: gliclazide 80 mg OM

BP 134/82 mmHg, HR 72 bpm
Glucose 11.5 mmol/L (4–9), HbA$_{1c}$ 57 mmol/mol (48–59), Cr 92 μmol/L (79–118), eGFR 95 mL/min/1.73 m^2
Urine tests (three samples): positive for microalbuminuria; albumin:creatinine ratio 2.7 mg/mmol

The dose of Mr Ayeni's gliclazide is increased to 120 mg OM and he is prescribed ramipril 1.25 mg OM.

Select the TWO *most appropriate* monitoring options to assess the beneficial and adverse effects of Mr Ayeni's pharmaceutical therapy.[16,17]

	Monitoring Options
A	Aim for blood pressure of 130/80 mmHg; titrate ramipril every 2 weeks until the target is reached (maximum 5 mg OD)
B	Monitor Cr and eGFR; ramipril is contraindicated in renal impairment
C	Monitor the patient for signs and symptoms of hypersensitivity; ramipril may cause a delayed-onset angioedema, which has a higher incidence in Afro-Caribbean patients
D	Monitor plasma K$^+$ concentration; ramipril may induce hypokalaemia
E	Monitor Cr and eGFR; titrate ramipril every 2 weeks to the maximum dose of 5 mg OD if tolerated

QUESTION 13

Miss NA, a confused 59-year-old, is brought into A&E by her partner who found her sitting on the kitchen floor.

PMH: HIV (diagnosed 7 months ago), diabetes mellitus, hypertension (both diagnosed 4 years ago), AF (diagnosed 3 weeks ago)

DH: Kivexa® tablets T OM, Kaletra® tablets TT BD, glipizide 10 mg OM, carvedilol 6.25 mg BD, bendroflumethiazide 2.5 mg OM, aspirin 75 mg OM; allergies/intolerances: amlodipine (persistently swollen ankles)

Weight: 62 kg; height: 1.72 m

On Examination

Pale, sweaty, delirious; BP 105/63 mmHg, HR 99 bpm, RR 19/min
A hump noted on the back – under further investigation
No previous episodes of hypoglycaemia

Investigations (Non-Fasting)

Today	3 Weeks Ago
Glucose 2.7 mmol/L (4–9)	5.3 mmol/L
Total cholesterol (TC) 6.3 mmol/L (<5.2)	Unavailable
LDL-C 4.6 mmol/L (<4)	Unavailable
Triglycerides (TGs) 1.5 mmol/L (0.50–1.70)	Unavailable

Miss NA is treated for hypoglycaemia. She is also initiated on simvastatin 20 mg ON.

Select the TWO *most appropriate* monitoring options to assess the adverse effects of Miss NA's pharmaceutical therapy.[18]

Monitoring Options	
A	Creatinine kinase should be monitored every 6 months; ritonavir increases the risk of simvastatin-related myopathy
B	TC, LDL-C and TGs should be measured 6-monthly; Kaletra® may cause a lipodystrophy syndrome
C	TC, LDL-C and TGs should be measured annually; Kivexa® and Kaletra® may cause a lipodystrophy syndrome
D	BMs should be rechecked at the earliest opportunity by the GP; carvedilol can contribute to the development of hypoglycaemia

Monitoring Options	
E	BMs should be rechecked at the earliest opportunity by the GP; bendroflumethiazide and glipizide can contribute to the development of hypoglycaemia

REFERENCES

1. *Prescribing Safety Assessment: resources* [Online]. Medical Schools Council; British Pharmacological Society [27 March 2013]. Available at: www.prescribe.ac.uk/psa/?page_id=14

2. Fitzpatrick R. Practical pharmacokinetics. In: Walker R, Whittlesea C, editors. *Clinical Pharmacy and Therapeutics*. 4th ed. London: Churchill Livingstone Elsevier; 2007. pp. 24–39.

3. Gibbs KP, Cripps D. Chronic obstructive pulmonary disease. In: Walker R, Whittlesea C, editors. *Clinical Pharmacy and Therapeutics*. 4th ed. London: Churchill Livingstone Elsevier; 2007. pp. 386–400.

4. National Institute for Health and Clinical Excellence. *Chronic Obstructive Pulmonary Disease: NICE guideline 101 – quick reference guide*. London: NICE; 2010. Available at: www.nice.org.uk/nicemedia/live/13029/49399/49399.pdf

5. National Institute for Health and Clinical Excellence. *Schizophrenia: NICE guideline 82 – quick reference guide*. London: NICE; 2009. Available at: www.nice.org.uk/nicemedia/live/11786/43610/43610.pdf

6. National Institute for Health and Clinical Excellence. *Schizophrenia: NICE guideline 82*. London: NICE; 2009. Available at: www.nice.org.uk/nicemedia/live/11786/43608/43608.pdf

7. Scott DK. Cardiac arrhythmias. In: Walker R, Whittlesea C, editors. *Clinical Pharmacy and Therapeutics*. 4th ed. London: Churchill Livingstone Elsevier; 2007. pp. 319–33.

8. Ballinger A, Patchett S. Ventricular arrhythmias. In: Kumar P, Clark M, editors. *Pocket Essentials of Clinical Medicine*. 4th ed. London: Saunders Elsevier; 2007. pp. 418–22.

9. *Summary of Product Characteristics Amiodarone Injection Minijet 30mg/ml (International Medication Systems)* [Online]. Electronic Medicines Compendium; 2007 [cited 6 October 2012]. Available at: www.medicines.org.uk/EMC/medicine/14156/SPC/

10. Ballinger A, Patchett S. Disorders of the acid-base balance. In: Kumar P, Clark M, editors. *Pocket Essentials of Clinical Medicine*. 4th ed. London: Saunders Elsevier; 2007. pp. 327–32.

11. Ballinger A, Patchett S. Respiratory failure. In: Kumar P, Clark M, editors. *Pocket Essentials of Clinical Medicine*. 4th ed. London: Saunders Elsevier; 2007. pp. 563–7.

12. *Summary of Product Characteristics Xarelto 20mg Film-Coated Tablets* [Online]. Electronic Medicines Compendium; 2012 [cited 30 March 2013]. Available at: www.medicines.org.uk/EMC/medicine/25586/SPC/Xarelto+20mg+film-coated+tablets/

13. Floss K, Borthwick M, Clark C. Intravenous fluids: principles of treatment. *Clin Pharm*. 2011; **3**(9): 274–83.

14. Staples A, Dade J, Acomb C. Intravenous fluids: practical aspects of therapy. *Clin Pharm*. 2011; **3**(9): 285–91.

15. *Stockley's Drug Interactions* [Online]. Available at: www.medicinescomplete.com/
16. Hackett EA, Thomas SM. Diabetes mellitus. In: Walker R, Whittlesea C, editors. *Clinical Pharmacy and Therapeutics*. 4th ed. London: Churchill Livingstone Elsevier; 2007. pp. 629–55.
17. Ballinger A, Patchett S. Complications of diabetes. In: Kumar P, Clark M, editors. *Pocket Essentials of Clinical Medicine*. 4th ed. London: Saunders Elsevier; 2007. pp. 663–8.
18. Ballinger A, Patchett S. Hypoglycaemia. In: Kumar P, Clark M, editors. *Pocket Essentials of Clinical Medicine*. 4th ed. London: Saunders Elsevier; 2007. pp. 670–2.

Chapter 8

Data Interpretation

QUESTION 1

Mrs Hopkins, a 74-year-old lady from Norwich, is admitted to hospital with persistent fatigue and decreased appetite.

PMH: AF (diagnosed 12 months ago), hypertension, depression
DH: warfarin 3 and 4 mg on alternate days, amiodarone 200 mg OM, bisoprolol 10 mg OM, candesartan 8 mg OM, mirtazapine 30 mg ON; intolerances/allergies: ramipril – persistent dry cough
SH: independent with once-a-week social care visit

On examination diffuse patches of dry skin are noted. Blood investigations demonstrate normal renal function, and thyroid function tests are as follows:

Today	12 Months Ago
Free T$_4$ 8.2 pmol/L (10–25)	17.3 pmol/L
Free T$_3$ 0.7 nmol/L (1.2–3.1)	2.7 nmol/L
TSH 4.8 mU/L (0.3–3.5)	2.5 mU/L

Select the *most appropriate* decision option with regard to Mrs Hopkin's pharmaceutical treatment based on these data.[3–5]

Decision Options	
A	Discontinue amiodarone
B	Reduce the dose of amiodarone to 100 mg OM
C	Reduce the frequency of amiodarone administration to 200 mg on alternate days
D	Discontinue amiodarone and initiate levothyroxine 25 micrograms OM
E	Continue amiodarone and initiate levothyroxine 25 micrograms OM

QUESTION 2

Mr Tselentakis, a 62-year-old, undergoes internal fixation of his fractured right tibia. A week later he presents with fever, severe pain and inflammation at the surgical site. He is confirmed to have contracted MRSA osteomyelitis and is initiated on IV vancomycin 1500 mg loading dose (LD), followed by two 750 mg maintenance doses 24 hours later. CrCl = 31 mL/min; weight: 65 kg. The 'trough' level before the third dose: 28 mg/L.

CrCl (mL/min) (Levels of Dosing)	Dose (mg)	Start Time After LD & Future Dosing Interval (hr)
40–54	500	12
30–39	750	24
20–29	500	24
<20 (no dialysis)	500	48

Pre-dose (Trough) Level	Maintenance Dose Adjustment
10–15 mg/L	Continue at current dose For MRSA pneumonia, osteomyelitis, endocarditis and bacteraemia only, move up one level
15–20 mg/L	Move down one level without omitting any doses For MRSA pneumonia, osteomyelitis, endocarditis and bacteraemia, continue at current dose
20–25 mg/L	Move down two levels without omitting any doses For MRSA pneumonia, osteomyelitis, endocarditis and bacteraemia, move down one level
25–30 mg/L	Omit next dose and decrease by 2 levels

Select the *most appropriate* decision option with regard to Mr Tselentakis' pharmaceutical treatment based on these data.[6]

Decision Options	
A	Omit one dose and reduce subsequent doses to 500 mg every 24 hours
B	Reduce subsequent doses to 500 mg every 24 hours
C	Reduce subsequent doses to 500 mg every 48 hours
D	Omit one dose and reduce subsequent doses to 500 mg every 48 hours
E	Omit one dose and continue the same dosing regimen

QUESTION 3

Mrs Costa, an 83-year-old, is brought into hospital with a 2-day history of increasing shortness of breath, fever, cough and chest pains.

PMH: hypertension (diagnosed 10 years ago), recurrent UTIs
DH: atenolol 50 mg OM, nitrofurantoin 100 mg ON
SH: non-smoker; no recent travel abroad

Investigations

U 7.6 mmol/L (2.5–6.7), CRP 25 mg/L (<10), WBC 12.4 × 10^9/L (4–11), Neut 8.1 × 10^9/L (2.0–7.5), eosinophils 2.5 × 10^9/L (0.04–0.4), Plt 215 × 10^9/L (150–400)
CXR: reticulo-alveolar infiltrates at the bases of both lungs

Mrs Costa is started on co-amoxiclav 1.2 g IV TDS and clarithromycin 500 mg IV BD for severe community-acquired pneumonia. Three days later there is still no improvement; therefore, you decide to review her pharmaceutical therapy and additional investigations.

Blood cultures/sputum: no pathogens isolated
HRCT: ground-glass opacities
Bronchoscopy: eosinophils on biopsy

Select the *most appropriate* decision option with regard to Mrs Costa's pharmaceutical treatment based on these data.[4,7]

Decision Options	
A	Discontinue current antibiotic therapy and consider piperacillin/tazobactam treatment for unresponsive septic pneumonia
B	Discontinue current antibiotic therapy and seek microbiology advice
C	Discontinue antibiotic therapy and atenolol
D	Discontinue antibiotic therapy and nitrofurantoin
E	Discontinue antibiotic therapy and consider AmBisome® treatment for suspected severe fungal infection

QUESTION 4

Mrs Ivanovic, a 37-year-old woman who is 23 weeks pregnant, is admitted with worsening abdominal pain and jaundice.

PMH: gestational hypertension (at week 13 of pregnancy), deep vein thrombosis (at week 18 of pregnancy)
DH: labetalol 200 mg BD, dalteparin 8000 units SC BD
Weight: 87 kg; height: 166 cm

Investigations

Albumin 39 g/L (35–50), ALP 232 U/L (39–117), ALT 867 U/L (5–40), total bilirubin 58 µmol/L (<17)
Hepatitis serology: negative

Select the *most appropriate* decision option with regard to Mrs Ivanovic's pharmaceutical treatment based on these data.[4,8–13]

Decision Options	
A	Discontinue dalteparin and initiate the patient on UFH
B	Discontinue labetalol and initiate the patient on methyldopa with BP monitoring
C	Discontinue labetalol and initiate the patient on nifedipine with BP monitoring
D	Discontinue dalteparin and labetalol; initiate the patient on UFH and methyldopa
E	Discontinue labetalol and monitor BP carefully; re-start labetalol cautiously once acute liver impairment resolves

QUESTION 5

Mr Scharpf, a 57-year-old, comes in for a 6-monthly health check-up.

PMH: T2DM, hypertriglyceridaemia
DH: metformin 1 g BD, tolbutamide 500 mg BD, simvastatin 80 mg ON
Weight: 114 kg; height: 1.78 m

Investigations

Glucose 6.4 mmol/L (4–9), HbA$_{1c}$ 43 mmol/mol (48–59 or less), total cholesterol (TC) 3.7 mmol/L (<4.0), HDL cholesterol (HDL-C) 1.2 mmol/L (0.8–1.8), LDL-cholesterol (LDL-C) 1.8 mmol/L (<2.0), triglycerides (TGs) 3.2 mmol/L (0.70–2.1 mmol/L)

Select the *most appropriate* decision option with regard to Mr Scharpf's pharmaceutical therapy based on these data.[14–16]

Decision Options	
A	Add ezetimibe 10 mg OD
B	Add fenofibrate 200 mg OD
C	Add gemfibrozil 0.6 g BD
D	Add colestyramine 4 g OD
E	Stop simvastatin and initiate a trial of rosuvastatin 40 mg ON

QUESTION 6

Miss Lam, a 49-year-old, undergoes triple coronary artery bypass graft surgery. Four days into the recovery period, her mental function deteriorates with a mixture of apathy and restlessness. The surgical team prescribes diazepam 2 mg TDS PRN; however, that does not turn out to be effective.

PMH: STEMI, hypertension, bipolar disorder
DH: aspirin 75 mg OM, clopidogrel 75 mg OM, bisoprolol 10 mg OM, ramipril 2.5 mg BD, atorvastatin 80 mg ON, Priadel® liquid 10 mL BD
Weight: 80 kg; height: 1.61 m

Investigations

Today	Surgical Pre-assessment
Na+ 121 mmol/L (135–146)	137 mmol/L
K+ 3.9 mmol/L (3.5–5.0)	4.2 mmol/L
eGFR 59 mL/min/1.73 m²	67 mL/min/1.73 m²

Miss Lam lost over 1 L of blood during her procedure (she received gelofusine 500 mL over 5–10 minutes immediately post procedure). You also check the daily fluid regimen she has been receiving after the procedure:

- potassium chloride 0.15% in glucose 5% 2.5 L/day
- sodium chloride 0.45% in glucose 5% 1 L/day.

Her daily urine output is about 1450 mL/day; BP 105/63 mmHg; HR 87 beats per minute.

You then request a lithium level and this comes back as 1.6 mmol/L.

Select the *most appropriate* decision option with regard to Miss Lam's pharmaceutical therapy based on these data.[2,17–19]

Decision Options	
A	Stop Priadel® and change her fluid prescription to Hartmann's solution 2 L + 1 L of potassium chloride 0.3% in glucose 5%/day
B	Stop Priadel® and change her fluid prescription to Hartmann's solution 1.5 L/day
C	Continue Priadel® and change the fluid prescription to sodium chloride 1 L of 0.18% in glucose 4% over 2 hours, thereafter adjusted as needed

Decision Options	
D	Stop Priadel® and change the fluid prescription to 1 L of sodium chloride 1.8% in glucose 4% over 2 hours, thereafter adjusted as needed
E	Stop Priadel® and change the fluid prescription to 500 mL of sodium chloride 0.9% in glucose 5% over 2 hours, thereafter adjusted as needed

QUESTION 7

Jane, a 7-year-old, is in hospital following her second exacerbation of asthma in the last 6 months. You decide to review and optimise her pharmaceutical asthma control.

PMH: asthma

DH: salbutamol 100 micrograms Evohaler® T-TT QDS PRN (has been using up to 10 times/ day lately)

Weight: 23 kg; height: 1.25 m

Chest ausculation demonstrates no evidence of wheeze

PEFR = 121 L/min

You confirm that the child possesses a sufficiently good inhaler technique.

Paediatric Normal Values					
Peak Expiratory Flow Rate					
For use with EU/EN13826 scale PEF meters only					
Height (m)	Height (ft)	Predicted EU PEFR (L/min)	Height (m)	Height (ft)	Predicted EU PEFR (L/min)
0.85	2'9"	87	1.30	4'3"	212
0.90	2'11"	95	1.35	4'5"	233
0.95	3'1"	104	1.40	4'7"	254
1.00	3'3"	115	1.45	4'9"	276
1.05	3'5"	127	1.50	4'11"	299
1.10	3'7"	141	1.55	5'1"	323
1.15	3'9"	157	1.60	5'3"	346
1.20	3'1"	174	1.65	5'5"	370
1.25	4'1"	192	1.70	5'7"	393

Normal PEF values in children correlate best with height; with increasing age, larger differences occur between the sexes. These predicted values are based on the formulae given in *Lung Function* by JE Cotes (Fourth Edition), adapted for EU scale Mini-Wright peak flow meters by Clement Clarke (date of preparation: 7 October 2004).

According to the British Thoracic Society, complete asthma control is defined as:

- no daytime symptoms

- no night-time awakening due to asthma
- no need for rescue medication
- no exacerbations
- no limitations on activity including exercise
- normal lung function (in practical terms FEV_1 and/or PEFR >80% predicted or best)
- minimal side effects from medication.

Select the *most appropriate* decision option with regard to Jane's pharmaceutical therapy based on these data.[20,21]

Decision Options	
A	Add montelukast 10 mg in the evening
B	Add mometasone 200 micrograms BD
C	Add fluticasone 50 micrograms BD
D	Add beclometasone 100 micrograms BD via the spacer
E	Add fluticasone 200 micrograms BD via the spacer

QUESTION 8

Mr Thornton, a 67-year-old gentleman, completed his first cycle of chemotherapy for stage III diffuse large B-cell lymphoma (DLBCL) a week ago and today presents to hospital with troublesome palpitations. The patient is awake and talking, and he does not appear to be confused.

PMH: gout, gallstones (removed 12 months ago)
DH: allopurinol 300 mg OM, cycle 1 of R-CHOP (rituximab, cyclophosphamide, doxorubicin, vincristine and prednisolone)
Weight: 123 kg; height: 1.84 m

Investigations

Na^+ 137 mmol/L (135–146), K^+ 6.7 mmol/L (3.5–5.0), PO_4^{3-} 2.1 mmol/L (0.8–1.5), Mg^{2+} 0.85 mmol/L (0.7–1.1), corrected Ca^{2+} 1.65 mmol/L (2.20–2.67), U 8.4 mmol/L (2.5–6.7), Cr 289 μmol/L (79–118), urate 2.3 mmol/L (0.18–0.42)

Prior to you seeing him, Mr Thornton receives immediate treatment for hyperkalaemia and vigorous hydration to maintain his urine output.

Select the *most appropriate* decision option with regard to Mr Thornton's pharmaceutical therapy based on these data.[22–25]

Decision Options	
A	Continue allopurinol, give rasburicase 25 mg as IV infusion OD (for up to 7 days) and give 100 mL of calcium gluconate 10% in 1 L of sodium chloride 0.9% IV at 50 mL/hour, adjusted to response
B	Stop allopurinol, give rasburicase 25 mg as IV infusion OD (for up to 7 days) and give 10–20 mL of calcium gluconate 10% by IV injection with ECG monitoring, adjusted to response
C	Stop allopurinol and give rasburicase 25 mg as IV infusion OD for up to 7 days
D	Stop allopurinol and give rasburicase 20 mg as IV infusion OD for up to 7 days
E	Reduce the dose of allopurinol to 100 mg OM and give rasburicase 20 mg as IV infusion OD for up to 7 days

QUESTION 9

Miss JK, a 27-year-old, is found fitting on the floor at home by her brother and is immediately brought into hospital.

PMH: epilepsy (tonic–clonic seizures; last episode 2 years ago), chronic back pain, depression

DH: carbamazepine 400 mg BD, dihydrocodeine 30–60 mg PRN QDS, diclofenac 50 mg PRN TDS, fluoxetine 20 mg OM, clarithromycin 500 mg BD for 7/7 for chest infection (started about 4 days ago); OTC (started a month or so ago on friend's advice) cranberry juice capsules T OM, St John's wort extract T OM

She gradually recovers following administration of rectal diazepam. A carbamazepine level is requested: 2.3 mg/L.

Select the *most appropriate* decision option with regard to Miss JK's pharmaceutical therapy based on these data.[26]

Decision Options	
A	Stop cranberry juice and St John's wort; increase the dose of carbamazepine to 600 mg BD, thereafter adjusted as appropriate
B	Stop St John's wort; increase the dose of carbamazepine to 600 mg BD, thereafter adjusted as appropriate
C	Stop St John's wort and fluoxetine; increase the dose of carbamazepine to 600 mg BD, thereafter adjusted as appropriate
D	Change clarithromycin to an antibiotic that does not interact with carbamazepine; increase the dose of carbamazepine to 600 mg BD, thereafter adjusted as appropriate
E	Stop fluoxetine; change clarithromycin to an antibiotic that does not interact with carbamazepine

QUESTION 10

Mr BN, a 60-year-old diabetic gentleman, is admitted to hospital with a worsening ulcer on his right foot. He also complains of persistent tiredness and generalised weakness.

PMH: T2DM, diabetic nephropathy, locally advanced prostate cancer
DH: Glucophage® SR 2g OD, exenatide 5 micrograms SC BD, bicalutamide 150 mg OM,
    ramipril 5 mg OM
Weight: 118 kg; height: 185 cm

He is treated with flucloxacillin 1 g QDS IV for 5/7 and then 1 g QDS PO for 2 more days, following which there is significant improvement in the condition of his foot. The following blood results are noted:

Hb 9.6 g/dL (13.5–17.7), serum ferritin 146 µg/L (20–260), iron 17.3 µmol/L (13–32), TIBC 75 µmol/L (42–80), MCV 76 fL (80–96), glucose 7.6 mmol/L (4–9), HbA_{1c} 51 mmol/mol (48–59 or less), Na^+ 138 mmol/L (135–146), K^+ 4.4 mmol/L (3.5–5.0), Cr 193 µmol/L (79–118), eGFR 33 mL/min/1.73 m^2, U 8.5 mmol/L (2.5–6.7)

Select the *most appropriate* decision option with regard to Mr BN's pharmaceutical therapy based on these data.[27–29]

Decision Options	
A	Stop metformin and prescribe an IV infusion of CosmoFer® at an appropriate dose to correct the iron deficiency
B	Stop exenatide and prescribe an IV infusion of MonoFer® at an appropriate dose to correct the iron deficiency
C	Review the dose of metformin and prescribe ferrous sulphate 200 mg TDS, thereafter adjusted as appropriate
D	Review the dose of metformin and prescribe NeoRecormon® 2000 units SC three times weekly, thereafter adjusted as appropriate
E	Review the dose of ramipril and prescribe Eprex® 6000 units SC three times weekly, thereafter adjusted as appropriate

QUESTION 11

Joanna, a 32-year-old business woman, comes to the walk-in centre at your hospital with severe dizziness, fatigue and muscular aches that have been getting progressively worse over the last few days.

PMH: anxiety, cluster headaches (both diagnosed 7 years ago), GORD (diagnosed about a year ago)

DH: omeprazole 20 mg OM, lorazepam 2 mg OM, 1 mg ON (dose increased 2 weeks ago), pizotifen 1.5 mg ON, co-codamol 30/500 T-TT PRN QDS

On Examination

BP 125/70 mmHg, HR 71/min, RR 13/min; power and tone grossly normal; cranial nerves intact

Investigations

Hb 13.2 g/dL (11.5–16.5), Na^+ 145 mmol/L (135–146), K^+ 3.6 mmol/L (3.5–5.0), PO_4^{3-} 1.2 mmol/L (0.8–1.5), Mg^{2+} 0.54 mmol/L (0.7–1.1), corrected Ca^{2+} 2.46 mmol/L (2.20–2.67), U 3.6 mmol/L (2.5–6.7), Cr 71 µmol/L (79–118)

Select the *most appropriate* decision option with regard to Joanna's pharmaceutical therapy based on these data.[2,30–34]

Decision Options	
A	Stop pizotifen; switch lorazepam to an equivalent dose of diazepam; give 12 mmol of magnesium sulphate as an IV infusion over 30 minutes
B	Stop pizotifen; switch omeprazole to lansoprazole; give 12 mmol of magnesium sulphate as an IM injection
C	Switch lorazepam to an equivalent dose of diazepam; give 20 mmol of magnesium sulphate as an IV injection
D	Switch omeprazole to ranitidine; give 12 mmol of magnesium sulphate as an IV infusion over 30 minutes
E	Stop lorazepam; give 12 mmol of magnesium sulphate as an IV infusion over 30 minutes

QUESTION 12

Tim, a 69-year-old retired pilot, undergoes elective partial cystectomy for bladder cancer.

PMH: T2DM, unstable angina
DH: metformin 1 g OM, 500 mg lunchtime, 500 mg in the evening, NovoRapid® 12 units OM and 8 units lunchtime, Levemir® 10 units ON, aspirin 75 mg OM, irbesartan 300 mg OM, carvedilol 25 mg BD, isosorbide mononitrate MR 30 mg OM
Weight: 95 kg; height: 178 cm

Aspirin is stopped 7 days before the procedure. Metformin is stopped 48 hours before his operation. The morning doses of NovoRapid® and irbesartan are omitted on the day of surgery. Tim is switched to sliding scale insulin comprised of Actrapid® 1 unit/mL in sodium chloride 0.9% plus adequate IV glucose and potassium supplementation (*see* the most recent overnight BM record in the table presented below). Two days later Tim begins to eat and drink. At 8.30 a.m. the consultant asks you to reintroduce his regular medicines as appropriate.

Time (24 Hours)	Blood Sugar (mmol/L)	Insulin (Units/Hour)
2300	9.4	2
0000	10.6	2
0100	15.2	4
0200	13.1	3
0300	17.4	4
0400	15.6	4
0500	12.3	3
0600	14.4	3
0700	16.5	4

Investigations

Na⁺ 138 mmol/L (135–146), K⁺ 3.9 mmol/L (3.5–5.0), U 5.8 mmol/L (2.5–6.7), Cr 86 µmol/L (79–118)

Select the *most appropriate* decision option with regard to Tim's pharmaceutical therapy based on these data.[35–39]

Decision Options	
A	Give a bolus of subcutaneous Actrapid® 20 units after breakfast and stop sliding scale insulin 30 minutes later; resume metformin with breakfast; restart his usual insulin regimen at lunchtime
B	Give a bolus of subcutaneous Actrapid® 15 units before breakfast and stop sliding scale insulin 30 minutes later; restart metformin the day after; restart his usual insulin regimen at lunchtime
C	Give a bolus of subcutaneous NovoRapid® 14 units before breakfast and stop sliding scale insulin 30 minutes later; resume metformin with breakfast; restart his usual insulin regimen at lunchtime
D	Stop the sliding scale insulin and give a bolus dose of NovoRapid® 20 units 20–30 minutes later; resume metformin with breakfast; restart his usual insulin regimen in the evening
E	Stop the sliding scale insulin and give a bolus dose of Levemir® 15 units 20–30 minutes later; resume metformin with breakfast; restart his usual insulin regimen in the evening

QUESTION 13

Mr BV, a 27-year-old, complains of two painful mouth ulcers that appeared about a week ago and have not responded to OTC Bonjela® gel. Today he is also feeling 'a bit ill' and all he wants to do is go back to bed.

PMH: schizophrenia with a deficit syndrome, anxiety, depression (three suicidal attempts), Grave's disease

DH: amisulpride 150 mg BD, duloxetine 120 mg OM, nitrazepam 10 mg ON, carbimazole 15 mg OM

SH: smokes 30 cigarettes/day

Temperature 38.4°C, BP 98/57 mmHg, HR 102/min and regular, RR 19/min, O_2 sat 97% on air

While awaiting blood test results, your registrar asks you to urgently review Mr BV's medicines.

Select the *most appropriate* 'pre-bloods' decision option with regard to MR BV's pharmaceutical therapy based on the data and information here.[40–46]

Decision Options	
A	Withhold nitrazepam and carbimazole
B	Stop carbimazole and consider a trial of propranolol once blood test results become available
C	Prescribe Difflam® oral rinse 15 mL every 1.5–3 hours PRN for up to 7 days
D	Withhold amisulpride; consider a trial of olanzapine once blood test results become available
E	Withhold duloxetine; consider a trial of fluoxetine once blood test results become available

REFERENCES

1. *Prescribing Safety Assessment: resources* [Online]. Medical Schools Council; British Pharmacological Society [27 March 2013]. Available at: www.prescribe.ac.uk/psa/?page_id=14

2. Medusa Injectable Medicines Guide Online: National Health Service. Available at: www.injguide.nhs.uk

3. Ballinger A, Patchett S. The thyroid axis. In: Kumar P, Clark M, editors. *Pocket Essentials of Clinical Medicine*. 4th ed. London: Saunders Elsevier; 2007. pp. 607–20.

4. *Martindale: the complete drug reference* [Online]. Available at: www.medicines complete.com/

5. Martino E, Bartalena L, Bogazzi F, *et al*. The effects of amiodarone on the thyroid. *Endocr Rev*. 2001; **22**(2): 240–54.

6. *Antimicrobial Policies and Guidelines*. Redhill: Surrey and Sussex Healthcare NHS Trust; 2012.

7. Twilla J, Winton J, Self TH. Nitrofurantoin pulmonary toxicity: a rare but serious complication [Online]. *Consultant*. 2010; **50**(6). Available at: www.consultant360. com/content/nitrofurantoin-pulmonary-toxicity-rare-serious-complication

8. National Institute for Health and Clinical Excellence. *Hypertension in Pregnancy: NICE guideline 107 – quick reference guide*. London: NICE; 2010. Available at: www.nice.org.uk/nicemedia/live/13098/50416/50416.pdf

9. *Summary of Product Characteristics Heparin Sodium 1,000 I.U./ml Solution for Injection or Concentrate for Solution for Infusion (Without Preservative)* [Online]. Electronic Medicines Compendium; 2009 [cited 13 October 2012]. Available at: www.medicines.org.uk/EMC/medicine/9793/SPC/Heparin+sodium+1%2c000+ I.U.+ml+Solution+for+injection+or+concentrate+for+solution+for+infusion+%2 8without+preservative%29/

10. *Summary of Product Characteristics Fragmin 10,000 IU/0.4ml Solution for Injection* [Online]. Electronic Medicines Compendium; 2013 [cited 31 March 2013]. Available at: www.medicines.org.uk/EMC/medicine/26894/SPC/Fragmin+10% 2c000+IU+0.4ml+solution+for+injection/

11. *Summary of Product Characteristics Adalat* [Online]. Electronic Medicines Compendium; 2011 [cited 13 October 2012]. Available at: www.medicines.org. uk/EMC/medicine/20901/SPC/Adalat/.

12. *Summary of Product Characteristics Methyldopa Tablets BP 125mg* [Online]. Electronic Medicines Compendium; 2007 [cited 13 October 2012]. Available at: www.medicines. org.uk/EMC/medicine/24120/SPC/Methyldopa+Tablets+BP+125mg/

13. *Drug Record: Labetalol* [Online]. US National Library of Medicine; LiverTox; 2013 [cited 31 October 2013]. Available at: http://livertox.nih.gov/Labetalol.htm

14. *Summary of Product Characteristics Ezetrol 10mg Tablets* [Online]. Electronic Medicines Compendium; 2013 [cited 31 March 2013]. Available at: www.medicines. org.uk/EMC/medicine/12091/SPC/Ezetrol+10mg+Tablets/

15. *Summary of Product Characteristics Questran Light* [Online]. Electronic Medicines Compendium; 2005 [cited 14 October 2012]. Available at: www.medicines.org.uk/ EMC/medicine/348/SPC/Questran+Light

16. *Summary of Product Characteristics Fenofibrate 200 mg Capsules* [Online]. Electronic Medicines Compendium; 2012 [cited 14 October 2012]. Available at: www.medicines. org.uk/EMC/medicine/23955/SPC/Fenofibrate+200+mg+capsules/

17. *Summary of Product Characteristics Priadel Liquid* [Online]. Electronic Medicines Compendium; 2012 [cited 14 October 2012]. Available at: www.medicines.org.uk/ emc/medicine/6981/SPC/Priadel+Liquid/

18. *Coronary Artery Bypass Graft – Recovery* [Online]. London: NHS Choices; 2012 [cited 24 November 2012]. Available at: www.nhs.uk/Conditions/Coronary-artery-bypass/Pages/Recovery.aspx

19. *Hyponatraemia (Emergency Care Guidelines)*. Version 4, Feb 2008 edition. Redhill: Surrey and Sussex Healthcare NHS Trust; 2012.

20. *Predictive Normal Values (Nomogram, EU Scale)* [Online]. Clement Clarke International; 2004 [cited 15 October 2012]. Available at: www.peakflow.com/ top_nav/normal_values/index.html

21. British Guideline on the Management of Asthma. *Thorax.* 2008; **63**(Suppl. 4): iv1–121.

22. *Guidelines for the Management of Tumour Lysis Syndrome* [Online]. Surrey, West Sussex and Hampshire Cancer Network; 2012 [cited 31 March 2013]. Available at: www. royalsurrey.nhs.uk/Default.aspx?DN=45ce893f-8494-413f-9dc6-b3c7a6e21a51

23. *Diffuse Large B-cell Lymphoma* [Online]. Lymphoma Association UK; 2011 [cited 31 March 2013]. Available at: www.lymphomas.org.uk/sites/default/files/pdfs/ Diffuse%20large%20B-cell%20lymphoma.pdf

24. Cameron L, Loughran C. Lymphomas. In: Walker R, Whittlesea C, editors. *Clinical Pharmacy and Therapeutics.* 4th ed. London: Churchill Livingstone Elsevier; 2007. pp. 731–45.

25. Ballinger A, Patchett S. Hyperkalaemia. In: Kumar P, Clark M, editors. *Pocket Essentials of Clinical Medicine.* 4th ed. London: Saunders Elsevier; 2007. pp. 324–5.

26. *Stockley's Drug Interactions* [Online]. Available at: www.medicinescomplete.com/

27. National Institute for Health and Clinical Excellence. *Anaemia Management in People with Chronic Kidney Disease: NICE guideline 114 – quick reference guide.* London: NICE; 2011. Available at: www.nice.org.uk/nicemedia/live/13329/52857/52857. pdf

28. National Institute for Health and Care Excellence. *Anaemia Management in People with Chronic Kidney Disease: NICE guideline 114.* London: NICE; 2011. Available at: www.nice.org.uk/nicemedia/live/13329/52853/52853.pdf

29. Ballinger A, Patchett S. Anaemia. In: Kumar P, Clark M, editors. *Pocket Essentials of Clinical Medicine.* 4th ed. London: Saunders Elsevier; 2007. pp. 183–96.

30. *Summary of Product Characteristics Pizotifen Tablets 0.5 mg* [Online]. Electronic Medicines Compendium; 2012 [cited 18 October 2012]. Available at: www.medicines. org.uk/EMC/medicine/24179/SPC/Pizotifen+Tablets+0.5mg

31. *Summary of Product Characteristics Losec Capsules 10mg* [Online]. Electronic Medicines Compendium; 2012 [cited 18 October 2012]. Available at: www.medicines. org.uk/EMC/medicine/7275/SPC/Losec+Capsules+10mg

32. *Summary of Product Characteristics Ranitidine 150mg Tablets* [Online]. Electronic Medicines Compendium; 2012 [cited 18 October 2012]. Available at: www.medicines. org.uk/EMC/medicine/23245/SPC/Ranitidine+150mg+tablets/

33. *Summary of Product Characteristics Lorazepam 1mg Tablets* [Online]. Electronic Medicines Compendium; 2011 [cited 18 October 2012]. Available at: www.medicines. org.uk/EMC/medicine/26011/SPC/Lorazepam+1mg+Tablets/

34. *Summary of Product Characteristics Lansoprazole 15mg Gastro-resistant Capsules* [Online]. Electronic Medicines Compendium; 2012 [cited 18 October 2012]. Available at: www.medicines.org.uk/EMC/medicine/26197/SPC/Lansoprazole+ 15mg+Gastro-resistant+Capsules/

35. Rahman MH, Beattie J. Medication in the peri-operative period. *Pharm J*. 2004; **272**: 287–9.

36. Rahman MH, Beattie J. Peri-operative care and diabetes. *Pharm J*. 2004; **272**: 323–5.

37. Rahman MH, Beattie J. Peri-operative medication in patients with cardiovascular disease. *Pharm J*. 2004; **272**: 352–4.

38. *Surgery for Bladder Cancer* [Online]. American Cancer Society; 2013 [cited 31 March 2013]. Available at: www.cancer.org/cancer/bladdercancer/detailedguide/ bladder-cancer-treating-surgery

39. *Sliding Scale – Insulin Prescription Chart*. Redhill: Surrey and Sussex Healthcare NHS Trust; 2012.

40. *Summary of Product Characteristics Amisulpride 100mg Tablets* [Online]. Electronic Medicines Compendium; 2012 [cited 27 October 2012]. Available at: www.medicines. org.uk/EMC/medicine/25318/SPC/Amisulpride+100+mg+Tablets/

41. *Summary of Product Characteristics Carbimazole 20mg tablets* [Online]. Electronic Medicines Compendium; 2011 [cited 27 October 2012]. Available at: www.medicines. org.uk/EMC/medicine/26933/SPC/Carbimazole+20+mg+tablets/.

42. *Summary of Product Characteristics Zopiclone 3.75mg Tablets* [Online]. Electronic Medicines Compendium; 2009 [cited 10 December 2013]. Available at: www. medicines.org.uk/EMC/medicine/24285/SPC/Zopiclone+3.75mg+Tablets./

43. *Summary of Product Characteristics Cymbalta 30mg Hard Gastro-resistant Capsules, Cymbalta 60mg Hard Gastro-resistant Capsules* [Online]. Electronic Medicines Compendium; 2009 [cited 27 October 2012]. Available at: www.medicines.org. uk/EMC/medicine/15694/SPC/Cymbalta+30mg+hard+gastro-resistant+capsule s%2c+Cymbalta+60mg+hard+gastro-resistant+capsules/

44. *Summary of Product Characteristics Nitrazepam Tablets 5mg* [Online]. Electronic Medicines Compendium; 2012 [cited 28 September 2013]. Available at: www. medicines.org.uk/emc/medicine/24136/SPC/Nitrazepam+Tablets+5mg/#UND ESIRABLE_EFFECTS

45. *Summary of Product Characteristics Propranolol Tablets BP 40mg* [Online]. Electronic Medicines Compendium; 2012 [cited 27 October 2012]. Available at: www.medicines. org.uk/EMC/medicine/24090/SPC/Propranolol+Tablets+BP+40mg/

46. *Hyperthyroidism – Clinical Features and Treatment* [Online]. British Thyroid Association; 2012 [cited 27 October 2012]. Available at: www.british-thyroid-association.org/info-for-patients/Docs/bta_patient_hyperthyroidism.pdf

Answers

CHAPTER 1: PRESCRIBING

Question 1

A. Drug choice

1. Gliclazide, glipizide or tolbutamide (4 marks). These are second-line antidiabetic medicines for patients who fail to control their diabetes with metformin monotherapy.[1] Short-acting sulfonylureas, such as gliclazide and tolbutamide are usually preferred over the longer-acting ones (glibenclamide and glimepiride) in elderly patients due to their lower risk of hypoglycaemia. Note that nateglinide/repaglinide are usually reserved for patients with erratic lifestyles while dipeptidyl peptidase-4 inhibitors, such as sitagliptin, are used as the second-line options in patients at a significant risk of hypoglycaemia or if sulfonylureas are contraindicated or not tolerated. Pioglitazone is less appropriate due to its cardiovascular risks (note that this patient has a history of hypertension, angina and atrial fibrillation, which may predispose him to heart failure).

2. Glibenclamide or glimepiride (3 marks). The second-line antidiabetic medicine for patients who fail to control their diabetes with metformin monotherapy. However, short-acting alternatives, such as gliclazide or tolbutamide are preferred.

B. Appropriate dose, route/pharmaceutical form, frequency of administration and duration of treatment prior to a review (1 mark for each)

1. Gliclazide: 40–80 mg PO daily with breakfast.

   Gliclazide MR: 30 mg PO daily with breakfast.

   Glipizide: 2.5–5 mg daily shortly before breakfast or lunch.

   Tolbutamide: 0.5–1.5 g (max. 2 g) PO daily in divided doses with or immediately after meals or as a single dose with or immediately after breakfast.

   Subsequently adjusted according to response; candidates are expected to issue a prescription for 14–28 days of treatment.

2. Glibenclamide: 5 mg PO daily with or immediately after breakfast.
   Glimepiride: 1 mg PO daily taken shortly before or with the first main meal.
   Subsequently adjusted according to response; candidates are expected to issue a prescription for 14–28 days of treatment.

Question 2

A. Drug choice

1. Clarithromycin IV (4 marks). Appropriate choice of antibiotic therapy for high-severity community-acquired pneumonia in combination with benzylpenicillin (see table 1, 'Summary of Antibacterial Therapy' in Chapter 5 of the BNF).
2. Clarithromycin PO (3 marks). Appropriate choice of antibiotic therapy for high-severity community-acquired pneumonia in combination with benzylpenicillin. However, initial IV clarithromycin therapy may be more appropriate.
3. Azithromycin PO (3 marks). As for PO clarithromycin.
4. Doxycycline PO (3 marks). As for PO clarithromycin.
5. Erythromycin IV (2 marks). As for PO clarithromycin; however, the (commonly used) 6-hourly administration regimen and lower activity against certain respiratory pathogens (e.g. *Haemophilus influenzae*) makes it inferior to other macrolides.
6. Erythromycin PO (1 mark). As for IV erythromycin; however, initial IV macrolide therapy may be more appropriate.

B. Appropriate dose, route/pharmaceutical form, frequency of administration and duration of treatment prior to a review (1 mark for each)

1. 500 mg IV BD for 48 hours until reviewed for a step down to oral therapy
2. 500 mg PO BD for up to 14 days (in some cases up to 21 days)
3. 500 mg PO OD for 3 days or 500 mg PO OD on first day, then 250 mg OD for 4 days
4. 200 mg PO OD for 7–10 days (in some cases up to 21 days)
5. 12.5 mg/kg (775 mg or (rounded to) 780 mg) IV QDS
6. 250–500 mg PO QDS or 0.5–1 g PO BD

Question 3

A. Fluid choice

Intravenous infusion of phosphate (monobasic potassium phosphate, Polyfusor®) providing 100 mmol PO_4^{3-} and 19 mmol K^+/L) (4 marks). The most appropriate choice of infusion fluid to treat established moderate to severe hypophosphataemia. The infusion bag also contains potassium, which may help correct mild K^+ deficiency.

B. Appropriate dose, route, volume and duration of infusion to treat moderate to severe hypophosphataemia in non-critically ill patients (1 mark for each)

Nine millimoles intravenously over 12 hours equivalent to 90 mL of fluid over 12 hours, subsequently adjusted to individual patient requirements according to plasma PO_4^{3-} and K^+. For the purpose of this exercise the regimen used for critically ill patients, i.e. 22 mmol (500 μmol/kg) intravenously over 6–12 hours, equivalent to 220 mL over 6–12 hours, subsequently adjusted to individual patient requirements according to plasma PO_4^{3-} and K^+, is considered acceptable.

Question 4

A. Fluid choice

According to the diagram of paracetamol plasma concentration against time (in the 'Emergency Treatment of Poisoning' section of the BNF), this patient should receive immediate treatment with IV acetylcysteine (plasma paracetamol concentration after 11 hours of suspected ingestion above the treatment line). Four marks are given if all three infusions are written as appropriate. Three and two marks, respectively, are given if two and one infusion(s) are written as appropriate.

B. Appropriate doses (in mL of concentrate), routes, volumes and durations of infusion (1 mark for each)

NB candidates will not be awarded 1 mark for correct doses if one of the three infusion doses is incorrect. The same principle applies to the routes, volumes and durations.

First infusion: 42 mL of 200 mg/L of acetylcysteine concentrate added to 200 mL of glucose 5% or sodium chloride 0.9% and infused IV over 1 hour.

Second infusion: 14 mL of 200 mg/mL of acetylcysteine concentrate added to 500 mL of glucose 5% or sodium chloride 0.9% and infused IV over 4 hours.

Third infusion: 28 mL of 200 mg/mL of acetylcysteine concentrate added to 1 L of glucose 5% or sodium chloride 0.9% and infused IV over 16 hours.

Question 5

A. Drug choice

1. Ispaghula husk granules or another bulk-forming laxative, such as methyl-cellulose or sterculia (4 marks). It is poorly absorbed, relatively safe to use in pregnancy and generally recommended as the first-line treatment option for constipation in pregnancy.
2. Lactulose solution (3 marks). Can be used to treat constipation in pregnancy, but bulk-forming laxatives are preferred as the first line.
3. Bisacodyl (2 marks). Can be used to treat constipation in pregnancy, but it is reserved to (more severe) cases where a stimulant effect is necessary.
4. Senna (2 marks). Can be used to treat constipation in pregnancy, but it is reserved to (more severe) cases where a stimulant effect is necessary.

B. Appropriate dose (2 marks), route/pharmaceutical form and frequency of administration (1 mark for each)

1. For Fybogel®: one sachet or two level 5 mL spoonfuls in water orally twice daily preferably after meals
2. 15 mL twice daily
3. By mouth, 5–10 mg at night; by rectum, 10 mg in the morning (2 marks)
4. Two to four tablets orally at night; 1–2 level 5 mL spoonfuls of granules at night; 10–20 mL of 7.5 mg/5 mL liquid at night

Question 6

A. Drug choice

1. Adsorbed diphtheria (low-dose), tetanus, pertussis (acellular, component) and poliomyelitis (inactivated) vaccine (4 marks). As appropriate for tetanus-prone (puncture-type, i.e. animal bite) wound where the patient is missing a booster dose of a tetanus vaccine.
2. Adsorbed diphtheria, tetanus, pertussis (acellular, component) and poliomyelitis (inactivated) vaccine (4 marks). As for (low-dose) vaccine.

B. Appropriate dose and route (2 marks each)

1. Repevax® (or generically prescribed vaccine – as per 'Drug choice') 0.5 mL IM

2. Infanrix-IPV® (or generically prescribed vaccine – as per 'Drug choice') 0.5 mL IM

Question 7

A. Drug choice

1. Salmeterol aerosol inhalation (this formulation is chosen for compliance purposes as the patient is already stabilised on salbutamol pressurised metered-dose inhaler) (4 marks for aerosol inhalation or Evohaler®, 3 marks for Accuhaler® or Diskhaler®). As per NICE guidance[2] and the BNF provided the patient who already uses short-acting beta$_2$ agonists experiences persistent breathlessness at FEV$_1$ ≥50%.

2. Formoterol aerosol inhalation (4 marks for Atimos Modulite®, i.e. aerosol inhalation, 3 marks for Easyhaler® Formoterol, Foradil® or Oxis®). As for salmeterol.

3. Tiotropium (4 marks for Spiriva Handihaler®, 1 mark for Spiriva Respimat®). As for salmeterol. Respimat® – black triangle, increase in all cause mortality[3] and restricted to patients unable to use Handihaler® (only carries 1 mark).

4. Glycopyrronium (Seebri Breezhaler®) (3 marks). As for salmeterol. A black triangle medicine.

5. Aclidinium (Eklira Genuair®) (3 marks). As for salmeterol. A black triangle medicine.

6. Indacaterol (Onbrez Breezhaler®) (3 marks). As for salmeterol. A black triangle medicine.

B. Appropriate dose (2), inhaler device and frequency of administration (1 mark for each)

1. 50 micrograms BD (one blister via Accuhaler® or Diskhaler®, two puffs via Evohaler®)

2. 12 micrograms BD (via Easyhaler® formoterol, via Atimos Modulite® or via Foradil®) or 12 micrograms OD-BD (via Oxis Turbohaler®)

3. 18 micrograms OD via Spiriva HandiHaler® or 5 micrograms (two puffs) OD via Spiriva Respimat®

4. 50 micrograms (or 44 micrograms) OD via Seebri Breezhaler®

5. 400 micrograms (or 322 micrograms) BD via Eklira Genuair®

6. 150 micrograms OD via Onbrez Breezhaler®

Question 8

A. Fluid choice

Amiodarone (3 marks) in glucose 5% (appropriate diluent 1 mark). Flecainide is an alternative option to amiodarone; however, it has to be initially given by slow IV injection rather than an infusion and therefore is not appropriate for the prescription chart provided. In contrast to the BNF, NICE guidance[4] stratifies the patients into those with or without structural heart disease. Therefore, the treatment recommended according to NICE guidance may differ to that recommended using the BNF.

B. Appropriate dose, type of infusion/route, volume and duration of administration (1 mark for each)

315 mg (5 mg/kg) or 300 mg (rounded down to make administration more convenient) over 20–120 minutes as a continuous or intermittent IV infusion. Suggested initial infusion volume 250 mL.

Question 9

A. Drug choice

1. Dalteparin (4 marks). Low-molecular-weight heparin (LMWH) – first line for venous thromboembolism (VTE) prophylaxis in adult patients (not in renal failure) undergoing orthopaedic surgery.[5]
2. Enoxaparin (4 marks). As for dalteparin.
3. Tinzaparin (4 marks). As for dalteparin.
4. UFH (3 marks). First line for VTE prophylaxis in adult patients with renal failure undergoing orthopaedic surgery. However, this patient has adequate renal function allowing LMWH to be used.[5]

B. Appropriate dose (2 marks), route and frequency (1 mark for each)

1. 2500 units 1–2 hours before surgery, then 2500 units 8–12 hours later (or 5000 units on the evening before surgery, then 5000 units on the following evening), then 5000 units every 24 hours by subcutaneous injection (5000 units every 24 hours is acceptable for the purpose of this exercise).
2. 40 mg (4000 units) 12 hours before surgery, then 40 mg (4000 units) every 24 hours by subcutaneous injection (40 mg (4000 units) every 24 hours is acceptable for the purpose of this exercise).

3. 50 units/kg (2750 or 2800 units) 2 hours before surgery, then 50 units/kg every 24 hours or 4500 units 12 hours before surgery, then 4500 units every 24 hours by subcutaneous injection (50 mg/kg or 4500 units every 24 hours is acceptable for the purpose of this exercise).
4. 5000 units 2 hours before surgery, then every 8–12 hours by subcutaneous injection (5000 units every 8–12 hours is acceptable for the purpose of this exercise).

Question 10

A. Drug choice

1. Cefotaxime (4 marks). First-line antibiotic choice for empirical treatment of suspected meningococcal disease in patients with penicillin allergy.
2. Ceftriaxone (4 marks). As for cefotaxime.
3. Chloramphenicol (3 marks). Second-line antibiotic of choice for empirical treatment of suspected meningococcal disease in patients with a history of immediate hypersensitivity reaction to penicillin or to cephalosporins. Note that the current patient is not allergic to cephalosporins (e.g. cefotaxime). It also carries a higher risk of serious side effects, such as haematological disorders and is normally reserved for life-threatening infections.

B. Appropriate dose and route (2 marks each)

1. 50 mg/kg (900 mg or 1 g) by IV or IM injection or 1–2 g by IV or IM injection if calculated based on a total daily dose of 100–200 mg/kg (in two to four divided doses)
2. 20–50 mg/kg (360–900 mg or 500–900 mg) by deep IM injection or IV injection over 2–4 minutes (answers not specifying the duration of administration accepted for the purpose of this exercise)
3. 12.5–25 mg/kg (225–450 mg or 250–450 mg) by IV injection

Question 11

A. Drug choice

Aspirin (4 marks). The antiplatelet agent of choice following an ischaemic stroke (MCA) before switching to clopidogrel monotherapy 14 days later.

B. Appropriate dose, route/pharmaceutical form, frequency of administration and duration of treatment (1 mark for each)

300 mg PO daily for 14 days.

Question 12

A. Drug choice

1. Glucagon (4 marks). First-line treatment option for hypoglycaemia that is unresponsive to oral glucose in an unconscious patient.
2. Glucose 20% (3 marks). An alternative option for a patient who does not respond to glucagon after 10 minutes or in case of prolonged hypoglycaemia. However, glucagon should be administered first in the majority of cases.
3. Glucose 10% (2 marks). As for glucose 20%, but more commonly used in children than in adults and higher volumes are usually required to be administered than with 20% solution.

B. Appropriate dose and route (2 marks for each)

1. 1 mg by SC, IM or IV injection
2. 50 mL of 20% solution for IV infusion given as an IV injection into a large vein

Question 13

A. Drug choice

Adrenaline 1 mg/mL (4 marks). First-line treatment option for anaphylaxis (anaphylactic shock). The adrenaline injection may then be followed by the injection of chlorphenamine to help counteract the histamine-mediated vasodilation and bronchoconstriction.

B. Appropriate dose and route (2 marks for each)

300 micrograms (0.3 mL) by IM injection

Question 14

A. Drug choice

1. Rivastigmine (4 marks). The first-line option acetylcholinesterase inhibitor (AChEi) for Mrs JM who is suspected to be developing Alzheimer's disease and also suffers from Parkinson's disease (rivastigmine is the only AChEi licensed for the treatment of mild to moderate dementia in Parkinson's disease).

2. Donepezil (3 marks). An AChEi licensed for the treatment of mild to moderate dementia in Alzheimer's disease; however, it is less specific than rivastgimine for Mrs JM who also suffers from Parkinson's disease.
3. Galantamine (3 marks). As for donepezil.

B. Appropriate dose (2 marks), route/pharmaceutical form and frequency of administration (1 mark for each)

1. 1.5 mg BD PO (capsules or oral solution) or 4.6 mg/24 hours transdermal patch. SMC (2007) advised that transdermal patches of rivastigmine should be restricted for use in moderately severe Alzheimer's disease, and therefore the patch would not be considered an appropriate formulation in this case (maximum of 3 rather than 4 marks)
2. 5 mg ON (or OD at bedtime) PO
3. 4 mg BD PO or 8 mg OD (MR preparation) PO

Question 15

A. Fluid choice

1. Furosemide (4 marks) in sodium chloride 0.9% (appropriate diluent 1 mark). The first-line diuretic agent (for administration via IV infusion) in reducing pulmonary oedema and pre-load (fluid overload) associated with acute heart failure or exacerbation of chronic heart failure.[6-9]
2. Bumetanide in glucose 5% or sodium chloride 0.9% (4 marks). As for furosemide.

B. Appropriate dose, type of infusion/route, volume and duration of administration (1 mark for each)

1. 50 mg (up to 1.5 g daily) by continuous IV infusion at a rate not exceeding 4 mg/min. While it is important to not cause further fluid overload, any bag size of NaCl 0.9% is acceptable for this exercise (e.g. 500 or 1000 mL) as long as the candidate prescribes the total volume of the infusion to be administered at a rate ≤4 mg/min. For example, 100 mg of furosemide can be dissolved in 100 mL of NaCl 0.9% (1 mg/mL recommended by Medusa Injectable Medicines Guide[6]) and given over at least 25 minutes at a rate of 4 mL/min (240 mL/hr). In practice, 120–240 mg are often diluted to 24–48 mL with normal saline and administered via a syringe driver at a rate of 1–2 mL/hour, typically over 24 hours.

2. 2–5 mg over 30–60 minutes by intermittent IV infusion. BNF suggests a volume of 500 mL (or concentration at or below 25 micrograms/mL, e.g. 5 mg in 200 mL).[6]

Question 16

A. Drug choice

1. Celecoxib (4 marks). A first-line NSAID (selective inhibitor of COX-2) that carries a lower risk of serious upper gastrointestinal side effects than non-selective NSAIDs (important in this case since the patient is known to have had a gastric ulcer in the past).

NB NICE guidance on osteoarthritis[10] discourages the use of etoricoxib, which is also a 'black triangle' medicine. Selective COX-2 inhibitors are also associated with an increased risk of thrombotic events compared with non-selective NSAIDs; however, Michael does not have any significant cardiovascular risk factors which would predispose him to such events.

2. Ibuprofen (3 marks). A second-line NSAID (non-selective inhibitor of COX) that is associated with the lowest risk of serious upper gastrointestinal side effects out of all non-selective COX inhibitors. Considering Michael's PMH of a gastric ulcer, recommending non-selective NSAIDs which carry an intermediate or high risk of gastrointestinal events is deemed inappropriate.

B. Appropriate dose (2 marks), route/pharmaceutical form and frequency of administration (1 mark for each)

1. 200 mg daily in one to two divided doses PO.
2. 200–400 mg TDS–QDS PO.

NB that the BNF recommends the dosage of 300–400 mg TDS–QDS; however, in practice 200–400 mg is prescribed because of the available strengths of ibuprofen dosage forms.

Question 17

A. Drug choice

1. Strontium ranelate sachets (4 marks). Generally, a third-line option for secondary prevention of osteoporotic fragility fractures in postmenopausal women. However, Mrs TY has a difficulty swallowing tablets which suggests that bisphosphonates would not be a suitable option even though they are recommended by NICE earlier in the treatment algorithm.[11] The patient is more likely to adhere to strontium ranelate therapy than to the bisphosphonate one, which therefore would not be of any benefit.
2. Teriparatide (3 marks). Usually reserved for patients who cannot take or tolerate alendronate and either risedronate, etidronate or strontium ranelate. It is also far more expensive than strontium. Given by SC injection which may be more suitable for Mrs TY who is not willing to take any more oral tablets.[11]
3. Alendronic acid (2 marks). Generally, a first-line option for secondary prevention of osteoporotic fragility fractures in postmenopausal women. However, Mrs TY has difficulty swallowing tablets, which suggests that bisphosphonates would not be a suitable option even though they are recommended by NICE early in the treatment algorithm.
4. Risedronate sodium (1 mark). Generally, a second-line option for secondary prevention of osteoporotic fragility fractures in postmenopausal women. However, Mrs TY has difficulty swallowing tablets, which suggests that bisphosphonates would not be a suitable option even though they are recommended by NICE early in the treatment algorithm.

NB denosumab is another NICE-appraised treatment option for the secondary prevention of osteoporotic fractures in postmenopausal women. Nevertheless, the question asks students to use the 'regular medicines' chart rather than a 'once-only medicines' chart which this medicine should generally be prescribed on.[12]

B. Appropriate dose (2 marks), route/pharmaceutical form and frequency of administration (1 mark for each)

1. 2 g OD PO, preferably at bedtime (ON)
2. 20 micrograms OD SC
3. 10 mg OD or 70 mg once weekly PO
4. 5 mg OD or 35 mg once weekly PO

Question 18

A. Drug choice

1. Diamorphine (4 marks). Used as first-line pain relief in suspected myocardial infarction where nitrates have not been significantly effective and immediate pain relief is required. It would also be helpful in relieving the anxiety suffered by the patient.
2. Morphine (4 marks). As for diamorphine.

B. Appropriate dose and route (2 marks for each)

1. 5 mg by slow IV injection
2. 5–10 mg by slow IV injection

Question 19

A. Fluid choice

Midazolam (2 marks) in sodium chloride 0.9% or water for injections (2 marks for appropriate diluent). The most appropriate choice of a sedative/anticonvulsant for use in addition to an antipsychotic (haloperidol) in a very restless patient with potential convulsions (twitching). Levomepromazine may be an appropriate choice of a sedative for use in a very restless patient. However, levomepromazine is unlikely to relieve the twitching experienced by Mrs LK. In fact, as an antipsychotic it may make such symptoms worse by inducing the extrapyramidal side effects (note that the patient is already on haloperidol, another antipsychotic medicine). In contrast to midazolam, levomepromazine infusion is also more likely to cause local irritation.[13,14]

B. Appropriate dose, type of infusion/route, volume and duration of administration (1 mark for each)

10–20 mg/24 hours via continuous subcutaneous infusion pump/syringe driver in 10–30 mL of sodium chloride 0.9% or water for injections (thereafter titrated according to response to the usual dose of 20–60 mg/24 hours).[13,14]

Question 20

A. Drug choice

1. Domperidone suppositories (4 marks). The first-line anti-emetic option in patients suffering from Parkinson's disease.[15] In contrast to other antidopaminergic agents, such as metoclopramide, droperidol or prochlorperazine, domperidone does not cross the blood–brain barrier and therefore does not possess the risk of causing extrapyramidal effects in patients, such as Mr Richards. Unlike antihistamine anti-emetics (e.g. cyclizine), it can also be safely used in patients with a history of glaucoma.

2. Domperidone tablets or suspension (3 marks). As for suppositories; however, suppositories may be a preferred method of administration if the patient is already feeling nauseous (the oral route of administration may be impaired).

3. Ondansetron injection (3 marks). The second-line anti-emetic option for Mr Richards. It is safe for use in patients with both Parkinson's disease and glaucoma, but it is significantly more expensive than domperidone.

4. Ondansetron tablets or oral solution (2 marks). As for ondansetron injection; however, (paradoxically) oral ondansetron preparations are much more expensive than the injection, and the parenteral route may be preferred over the oral route since the patient is already feeling nauseous.

5. Granisetron injection (3 marks). As for ondansetron injection.

6. Granisetron tablets (2 marks). As for ondansetron tablets or oral solution.

B. Appropriate dose (2 marks), route/pharmaceutical form and frequency of administration (1 mark for each)

1. 60 mg PR BD
2. 10–20 mg PO TDS-QDS (PRN)
3. 4–8 mg IM/IV up to TDS PRN (unlicensed)
4. 4–8 mg PO up to TDS PRN (unlicensed)
5. 1 mg IV OD-BD PRN (unlicensed)
6. 1 mg PO OD-BD PRN (unlicensed)

Question 21

A. Drug choice

1. Vancomycin (4 marks). The second-line treatment for confirmed *Clostridium difficile* infection (CDI) that has not responded to metronidazole and/or is severe (as indicated by WBC >15 × 10^9/L, acutely rising creatinine, pyrexia and/or signs of severe colitis). In this case the CDI was likely secondary to prolonged ciprofloxacin therapy. The fact that the patient has been on oral metronidazole for the last couple of weeks eliminates this antibiotic from the list of treatment options.

2. Metronidazole (2 marks). IV metronidazole is normally reserved for CDI that does not respond to oral vancomycin or is life-threatening. It is often used in a combination with high dose vancomycin. In Mrs da Silva's case, oral vancomycin alone should be tried first unless her condition deteriorates further.

3. Teicoplanin (2 marks). This is licensed for the treatment of CDI; however, it is rarely used other than for infections resistant to vancomycin and metronidazole.[16]

B. Appropriate dose, route/pharmaceutical form, frequency of administration and duration of treatment (1 mark for each)

1. 125 mg PO QDS for 10–14 days

NB the dose of vancomycin is usually only increased beyond 125 mg QDS where CDI fails to respond or is life-threatening.

2. 500 mg IV TDS for 10–14 days
3. 200 mg PO BD for 10 days[16]

Question 22

A. Drug choice

1. Dalteparin (4 marks). LMWHs (such as dalteparin) or fondaparinux are the first-line agents in the treatment of venous thromboembolism (such as deep vein thrombosis in Miss JH's case) in patients who are unable to take oral anticoagulants.

2. Enoxaparin (4 marks). As for dalteparin.
3. Tinzaparin (4 marks). As for dalteparin.
4. Fondaparinux (4 marks). As for dalteparin.

5. UFH (heparin sodium or calcium) (2 marks). As for dalteparin. However, in contrast to LMWH and fondaparinux, unfractionated heparin needs to be administered twice daily and requires laboratory monitoring, which may be inconvenient to both the patient and the staff. It is therefore usually reserved to patients with poor renal function.

6. Warfarin (2 marks). Miss JH has a PEG tube in place; however, warfarin administration via the PEG may result in INR fluctuations, and the use of LMWH or fondaparinux may be more justified. Warfarin can also interact with enteral feeds. In addition, warfarin dosing using a simple hospital chart provided may be complex since this medicine requires continuous dose adjustment.

5. Rivaroxaban (2 marks). Miss JH has a PEG tube in place; however, rivaroxaban administration via the PEG may result in unpredictable anti-coagulation (limited experience of rivaroxaban administration via enteral feeding tubes). Higher than LMWH or fondaparinux cost is another factor against the use of rivaroxaban.

B. Appropriate dose (2 marks), route/pharmaceutical form and frequency of administration (1 mark for each)

1. 15 000 units OD by SC injection
2. 110–115 mg (11 000–11 500 units) OD by SC injection
3. 13 000 units OD by SC injection
4. 7.5 mg OD by SC injection
5. Loading dose of 5000 units (or 6000 units) by IV injection, then 15 000 units BD by SC injection
6. 10 mg (or 5 mg) on the first day, 5 mg on the second day, 5 mg on the third day via PEG, then re-check INR and adjust the dose
7. 15 mg BD with food for 21 days, then 20 mg OD with food

Question 23

A. Drug choice

1. Fentanyl patches (4 marks). Provided patient's pain requirements remain stable, fentanyl patches can be used as a first-line alternative to oral morphine. They may reduce the gastrointestinal side effects associated with oral morphine as well as the need for PRN painkillers.

2. Buprenorphine patches (4 marks). As for fentanyl.

3. Diamorphine (2 marks). May be used as an alternative to oral morphine but it is more 'invasive' than transdermal patches. Does not provide long-lasting pain relief and is normally only used PRN. Reserved for patients whose pain requirements are rapidly changing.
4. Morphine sulphate (parenteral or rectal) (2 marks). As for diamorphine above.

B. Appropriate dose (2 marks), route/pharmaceutical form and frequency of administration (1 mark for each)

1. 75 micrograms/hour applied topically to skin on upper torso or upper arm and changed every 72 hours (the dose is based on patient's total 24-hour dose of oral morphine, i.e. 300 mg = 180 mg of MST Continus® + 120 mg of Oramorph® on average. However, according to additional guidance in the BNF (see 'Prescribing in Palliative Care'), in order to avoid possible opioid-induced hyperalgesia with the new opioid, the calculated dose should then be reduced by one-quarter to one-half, i.e. reduced to 150–225 mg of morphine. With reference to the dose equivalence table, this 24-hour dose is equivalent to a '75' patch of fentanyl changed every 72 hours).
2. 70 micrograms/hour applied to skin on upper torso and changed every 96 hours. See the earlier calculation for fentanyl patches. With reference to the dose equivalence table, 150–225 mg of 24-hour dose of oral morphine is equivalent to '70' patch of Transtec® (buprenorphine) changed every 96 hours.
3. 15 mg by SC or IM injection every 4 hours and thereafter titrated up or down as appropriate (approximately one-third of the 24-hour dose of oral morphine divided in equal 4-hourly doses).
4. 25 mg by SC or IM injection or PR (no dose equivalence available) every 4 hours and thereafter titrated up or down as appropriate (parenteral dose is approximately half of the 24-hour dose of oral morphine divided in equal 4-hourly doses).

Question 24

A. Drug choice

1. Tetracosactide (30-minute Synacthen® test) (4 marks). Mr Stratford is likely to have presented with an Addisonian crisis (hyponatraemia, hyperkalaemia, hypercalcaemia, hypoglycaemia, hypotension, leucocytosis, hyperpigmentation of buccal mucosa, nausea, vomiting, weight loss, lethargy, depression and dehydration). A 30-minute (or 'short') Synacthen® test utilises tetracosactide (an analogue of ACTH) to diagnose adrenal insufficiency, such as Addison's disease. The basal plasma cortisol concentration of <170 nmol/L and 30-minute concentration of <600 nmol/L are often diagnostic. Further tests (plasma ACTH and long Synacthen® test) are then used to establish the type and cause of adrenal insufficiency.
2. Tetracosactide (5-hour Synacthen® test) (2 marks). As for previous option; however, is usually only used if the 'short' Synacthen® test suggests adrenal insufficiency. Not very convenient for the patient.[17]

B. Appropriate dose and route (2 marks for each)

1. 250 micrograms by IM or IV injection STAT
2. 1 mg by IM injection STAT[17]

Question 25

A. Drug choice

1. Piperacillin/tazobactam (4 marks). First-line BNF treatment for suspected hospital-acquired pneumonia (HAP) where other antibacterials have been used in the last 3 months (an antipseudomonal penicillin). Since Emily has had a recent course of amoxicillin, the early-onset infection (<5 days after admission to hospital) should be treated as the late-onset one.
2. Ticarcillin/clavulanic acid (3 marks). As for piperacillin/tazobactam. However, piperacillin/tazobactam has activity against a wider range of Gram-negative organisms than ticarcillin/clavulanic acid and is more active against *Pseudomonas aeruginosa*.
3. Ceftazidime (3 marks). One of the first-line BNF treatments for suspected HAP where other antibacterials have been used in the last 3 months (a broad-spectrum cephalosporin with good activity against pseudomonas and other Gram-negative bacteria). Less commonly used for the treatment of HAP than piperacillin/tazobactam – reserved for patients allergic to penicillins.

4. Ceftriaxone (2 marks). As for ceftazidime. However, lower activity against pseudomonas. Also, usually reserved for severe infections, such as meningitis, and patients allergic to penicillin.
5. Cefotaxime (2 marks). As for ceftriaxone.

NB quinolones, such as ciprofloxacin, may also be considered as a valid option for the treatment of late-onset HAP in certain patients. However, Emily's age (elderly) should discourage the prescriber from using quinolones as the first-line treatment (risk of antibiotic-associated colitis and Clostridium difficile *infection) unless the patient has a severe allergy to beta-lactams.*

B. Appropriate dose, route/pharmaceutical form, frequency of administration and duration of treatment (1 mark for each)

1. 4.5 g every 8 hours (TDS) by IV infusion

NB review within 48 hours, duration up to 7 days – applicable to all treatment options shown here. 'IV' or 'IM' (without words 'infusion' or 'injection') are considered to be a sufficient answer for the purpose of this exercise.

2. 3.2 g every 6–8 hours (QDS–TDS) by IV infusion
3. 1 g every 8 hours (TDS), i.e. maximum 3 g/day in elderly patients, by IM injection or IV injection or infusion
4. 1 g daily (OD) by deep IM injection or by IV injection or infusion
5. 1 g every 12 hours (BD) by IM injection or IV injection or infusion

Question 26

A. Drug choice

Adrenaline mg/mL (1 in 1000) nebulised solution (4 marks). The likely diagnosis is severe croup unresponsive to corticosteroid (dexamethasone) treatment. The classic symptoms of 'seal-like barking' and wheeze are reported together with persistent fever. Daniel has been misleadingly administered ceftriaxone to cover any possible bacterial pathogens.[18–20]

B. Appropriate dose and route (2 marks for each)

5 mg (the total dose is calculated as 400 micrograms/kg = 5.6 mg; however, a maximum dose should not exceed 5 mg) via the nebuliser.

Question 27

A. Drug choice

1. Clopidogrel (4 marks). A first-line antiplatelet used in combination with aspirin for patients who have undergone PCI.
2. Prasugrel (2 marks). Normally reserved for patients undergoing primary rather than elective percutaneous coronary intervention (for NSTEMI, STEMI or unstable angina) who have experienced a stent thrombosis during the treatment with clopidogrel. It can be used as a first-line antiplatelet in patients with diabetes mellitus undergoing elective PCI; however, the relatively high-cost (compared with clopidogrel) often makes it an alternative option.
3. Ticagrelor (1 mark). Normally reserved for patients undergoing primary rather than elective percutaneous coronary intervention (for NSTEMI, STEMI or unstable angina) in whom clopidogrel cannot be used. The associated cost is even higher than that of prasugrel and it has to be taken twice daily, thus increasing the risk of non-adherence. It is also a black triangle drug.[21,22]

B. Appropriate dose, route/pharmaceutical form, frequency of administration and duration of treatment (1 mark for each)

1. 75 mg OD PO for 12 months
2. 10 mg OD PO for up to 12 months
3. 90 mg BD PO for up to 12 months

This exercise assumes that the loading dose of a relevant medicine has already been administered before the interventional procedure.

Question 28

A. Drug choice

1. Mirena® (levonorgestrel) intra-uterine system (4 marks). A long-acting progestogen-only contraceptive that is unaffected by enzyme-inducing drugs such as nevirapine (Viramune®).
2. Depo-Provera® (medroxyprogesterone acetate) (3 marks). A long-acting parenteral progestogen-only contraceptive not affected by enzyme-inducing drugs could be used as one of the options for Miss MN. However, her fear of needles is a factor which prevents this type of contraception making Mirena® the first-line option.

3. Noristerat® (norethisterone enantate) (3 marks). As for Depo-Provera®.

B. Appropriate dose, route/pharmaceutical form, frequency of administration and additional instructions (1 mark for each)

1. 20 micrograms/24 hours inserted into uterine cavity within 7 days of onset of menstruation or any time if reasonably certain that the woman is not pregnant and there is no risk of conception. Replaced every 5 years.
2. 150 mg by deep IM injection within first 5 days of cycle. Repeated every 12 weeks.
3. 200 mg by deep IM injection given very slowly into gluteal muscle within first 5 days of cycle. Repeated every 8 weeks.

NB Nexplanon® should not be recommended for Miss MN because the effectiveness of this etonogestrel-releasing implant may be lowered by enzyme-inducing drugs. Miss MN has a reported copper allergy, which makes copper-based intra-uterine devices less suitable.[23]

Question 29

A. Drug choice

1. Beractant (bovine lung extract) (4 marks). The pulmonary surfactant prophylaxis should generally be given within 15 minutes of life for selected extremely preterm babies (28 weeks or less of gestation) and for the majority of those who are <26 weeks of gestation. Such babies are often deficient in their own natural pulmonary surfactant due to poorly developed lungs. In this case, urgent administration of the pulmonary surfactant is essential because it appears that the consultant/registrar probably considered baby Stevens to be at a high risk of neonatal respiratory distress syndrome (hence, the insertion of the endotracheal tube). However, the surfactant was by accident not prescribed by the registrar before she left the ward.[24–28]
2. Poractant alfa (4 marks). As for beractant.

B. Appropriate dose and route (2 marks for each)

1. 74 (or 75) mg of phospholipid (equivalent to a volume of 3 mL) by endotracheal tube
2. 74 (or 75)–150 mg by endotracheal tube

Question 30

A. Drug choice

1. Spironolactone (4 marks). A first-line aldosterone antagonist for patients with moderate to severe chronic heart failure (New York Heart Association (NYHA) Class III to IV). Low doses of spironolactone reduce symptoms and mortality in such patients[29]. The aldosterone antagonist (spironolactone or eplerenone – *see* following points) may also help by increasing the plasma concentration of K^+, which is reduced by furosemide therapy in Kevin's case.

2. Eplerenone (3 marks). A second-line aldosterone antagonist usually reserved for patients in whom spironolactone cannot be used or in those with acute myocardial infarction and evidence of left ventricular systolic dysfunction (started 3–14 days after MI). It has a positive effect on both mortality and morbidity in patients with NYHA Class II (mild–moderate) CHF and LVEF of 35% or less[30]. However, Kevin has likely presented with moderate to severe disease and LVF, which makes spironolactone a more favourable option. Eplerenone is also significantly more expensive than spironolactone.

3. Hydralazine in combination with a nitrate (2 marks). Likely to be of some benefit in moderate to severe CHF; however, it is rarely used and normally reserved for patients of African and/or Caribbean origin. It also adds a burden of two extra medicines compared with only one with aldosterone antagonists above. Finally, only one medicine is required to be prescribed as part of this exercise.

4. Candesartan (1 mark). May be of limited benefit, but is only recommended for patients with mild to moderate heart failure (NYHA Class II or III). Combination of an ACE inhibitor and an angiotensin-II receptor blocker may also increase the long-term risk of hyperkalaemia.

5. Losartan (1 mark). As for candesartan.

6. Valsartan (1 mark). As for candesartan.[8,9,31,32]

B. Appropriate dose (2 marks), route/pharmaceutical form and frequency of administration (1 mark for each)

1. 25 mg PO OM

2. 25 mg PO OM

3. Hydralazine 25 mg PO TDS QDS

Isosorbide dinitrate 40–160 mg daily in divided doses (or any preparation of isosorbide mononitrate providing an equivalent dose).

NB the clinical evidence for the use of nitrates other than isosorbide dinitrate in combination with hydralazine for patients with CHF is lacking.

4. 4 mg PO OM
5. 12.5 mg PO OM
6. 40 mg PO BD

Question 31

A. Drug choice

Olanzapine (4 marks). A first-line option for the management of acute manic episodes of bipolar disorder in patients already receiving optimised lithium (Camcolit®) and valproic acid therapies.

NB olanzapine orodispersible tablets or risperidone orodispersible tablets/liquid or quetiapine could generally be used as alternative options for the management of acute manic episodes; however, Mrs VB is refusing to take any medicines by mouth, which makes parenteral olanzapine the only viable option in this case.[33,34]

B. Appropriate dose and route (2 marks for each)

5–10 mg IM STAT; this may be followed by 5–10 mg after 2 hours if necessary.

Question 32

A. Drug choice

Doxycycline (4 marks). The main differential diagnoses, which have not yet been ruled out for Miss TY, include bacterial vaginosis, genital chlamydia and gonorrhoea (both ± pelvic inflammatory disease). Miss TY has already had a 7/7 course of PO metronidazole, which did not appear to be effective (perhaps excluding the diagnosis of bacterial vaginosis). You have given her a STAT dose of ceftriaxone to cover for possible gonorrhoeal infection. However, she also requires an appropriate treatment for suspected chlamydial infection, such as azithromycin or doxycycline. Macrolides (azithromycin or erythromycin) may aggravate myasthenia gravis and therefore doxycycline is the first-line choice for this lady.[35–37]

B. Appropriate dose, route/pharmaceutical form, frequency of administration and duration of treatment (1 mark for each)

100 mg PO BD for 7 days

Question 33

A. Drug choice

Malarone® (proguanil and atovaquone) (4 marks). The state of Maranhao in Brazil carries a high risk of malaria and is associated with marked chloroquine resistance. The recommended antimalarial chemoprophylaxis for travellers going to this area (according to the antimalarial prophylaxis table in the BNF) include mefloquine, doxycycline or Malarone®. Mefloquine is contraindicated for Mrs Williams due to her history of epilepsy. It should also preferably be started at least 2.5 weeks before entering the endemic area. The history states Mrs Williams will be travelling to Brazil in a week's time. Doxycycline is contraindicated for Mrs Williams because of her history of acute porphyria (see acute porphyria table in the BNF).

B. Appropriate dose, route/pharmaceutical form, frequency of administration and duration of treatment (1 mark for each)

One tablet (proguanil 100 mg/atovaquone 250 mg) PO OD started 1–2 days before entering endemic area and continued for 1 week after leaving.

Question 34

A. Drug choice

1. Indapamide (4 marks). Mr LK presents with uncontrolled stage 2 hypertension and end organ damage (i.e. previous NSTEMI with residual heart failure). He is a gentleman of Caribbean origin and therefore calcium channel blockers would be indicated as the first-line treatment option for hypertension. However, these medicines should be avoided in the presence of heart failure leaving thiazide-like diuretics, such as indapamide or chlortalidone, as the best available choice. These diuretics may also help counteract the hyperkalaemic effects of eplerenone and candesartan.
2. Chlortalidone (4 marks). As for indapamide.

B. Appropriate dose (2 marks), route/pharmaceutical form and frequency of administration (1 mark for each)

1. 2.5 mg PO OM or 1.5 mg of MR tablets PO OM
2. 25 mg PO OM

Question 35

A. Drug choice

Phytomenadione (vitamin K) (4 marks). Almost all neonates are relatively defi-cient in vitamin K and some of them are at a risk of serious bleeding including intracranial haemorrhage. The chief medical officer and the chief nursing officer have recommended that all newborn babies should receive vitamin K to prevent vitamin K deficiency bleeding. The operative delivery itself has been reported as one of the risk factors for vitamin K deficiency bleeding in neonates. Mrs Brown's PMH of deep vein thrombosis should not prevent her baby from receiving a STAT dose of vitamin K unless agreed otherwise by the parents.[38,39]

B. Appropriate dose and route (2 marks for each)

1. 1 mg IM STAT
2. 2 mg of colloidal preparation PO STAT – this would be followed by the second 2 mg dose at 4–7 days post partum
3. 1 mg capsule PO STAT

NB the regimen should be chosen after discussion with parents in the antenatal period.

Question 36

A. Drug choice

Colchicine (4 marks). The likely diagnosis is an acute attack of gout. Colchicine is the first-line treatment option in patients who cannot tolerate NSAIDs or in whom they should be avoided. In this case, the history of ischaemic heart disease and duodenal ulcer helps to rule out NSAIDs as the best option for the management of the acute attack. These medicines carry an increased risk of thrombotic events (e.g. myocardial infarction or stroke). NSAIDs are also linked to serious gastro-intestinal events (including peptic ulcers), particularly in the elderly. Ibuprofen is associated with the lowest cardiovascular and gas-trointestinal risks, however it is not used in the treatment of gout. Naproxen is also associated with a lower risk of thrombotic events and may be used as an alternative to colchicine. The fact that this lady was prescribed ezetimibe instead of a statin (the latter usually recommended for secondary prophylaxis following ischaemic heart disease), should have triggered a thought that the answer to the question may have involved colchicine, which could interact with statins. Similarly to NSAIDs, systemic corticosteroids (e.g. prednisolone) are associated with peptic ulceration and perforation making colchicine a more suitable option for Mrs VM. Systemic corticosteroids should only be prescribed for the treatment of acute gout where NSAIDs and colchicine are not tolerated or are both contraindicated (intra-articular corticosteroids are usually reserved for more severe gout and initiated under the care of a specialist).[40–42]

B. Appropriate dose, route/pharmaceutical form, frequency of administration and duration of treatment/max. cumulative dose per course (1 mark for each)

500 micrograms PO BD–QDS until symptoms relieved (maximum 6 mg per course).

Question 37

A. Drug choice

1. Cyclizine (4 marks). The likely diagnosis is hyperemesis gravidarum. Antihistamines, such as cyclizine and promethazine, are recommended as the first-line option for the management of nausea and vomiting in pregnancy. They may also help fight the vertigo/dizziness which is accompanying Christine's nausea.
2. Promethazine (3 marks). As for cyclizine. However, promethazine is not available in a parenteral form and, although recommended, it is not licensed for use during pregnancy.
3. Prochlorperazine IM (1 mark). A second-line treatment option for nausea and vomiting in pregnancy; however, Christine has already tried prochlorperazine (Buccastem®), which did not appear to be effective thus reducing the likelihood that IM prochlorperazine would be effective. It should also be prescribed on a 'once-only' rather than 'regular medicines' chart.
4. Ondansetron IM/IV (1 mark). Likely to be effective; however, it is not licensed for this indication, and the safety in pregnancy has not been studied extensively.

NB metoclopramide is the second-line treatment option for nausea and vomiting in pregnancy, however it should be avoided in patients under 20 years of age (Christine is 19) due to a higher risk of extrapyramidal side effects in this population. In such circumstances, the use of metoclopramide should be reserved for intractable vomiting of known cause, vomiting due to radiotherapy/cytotoxics, for use as an aid to gastrointestinal intubation and for premedication.

B. Appropriate dose (2 marks), route/pharmaceutical form and frequency of administration (1 mark for each)

1. 50 mg by IM or IV injection TDS
2. 25 mg PO ON (up to a maximum of 100 mg/day) (unlicensed)
3. 12.5 mg IM STAT, followed if necessary after 6 hours by an oral dose
4. 4–8 mg IM/IV TDS (unlicensed)

Question 38

A. Drug choice

1. Chloramphenicol 1% eye ointment (4 marks). The likely diagnosis is blepharitis. The first-line treatment for blepharitis often includes hygiene measures that have already been tried by this gentleman prior to his presentation at the clinic. Where hygiene measures fail, topical antibiotics may be used. Chloramphenicol eye ointment is usually the first-line option. The recommendation that topical chloramphenicol should be avoided because of an increased risk of aplastic anaemia is not well founded (even though the manufacturer advises avoiding it in patients with a family or personal history of blood dyscrasia including aplastic anaemia).[43,44]
2. Ciprofloxacin 0.3% eye ointment (2 marks). Not included among the treatments recommended by NICE Clinical Knowledge Summaries, but licensed for the treatment of blepharitis (see product SPC).[45]
3. Brimonidine 0.15% eye ointment (2 marks). As for ciprofloxacin answer.[46]

B. Appropriate dose/directions for application, route/pharmaceutical form, frequency of administration and duration of treatment (1 mark for each)

1. Apply three to four times a day to the conjunctival sac or to the lid margins of both eyes for 5–7 days (for up to 6 weeks) or until infection has resolved
2. Apply 1.25 cm of eye ointment to the conjunctival sac or to the lid margins of both eyes TDS for 2 days, then BD for 5 days
3. Apply to the conjunctival sac or to the lid margins of both eyes OD BD for 5–7 days (up to 6 weeks) or until infection has resolved

Question 39

A. Drug choice

Erythromycin (4 marks). The first-line antibacterial for the prevention of pneumococcal infection in patients with sickle-cell disease and allergy to penicillin (note the blood-tinged sputum in keeping with likely pneumococcal infection).[47]

B. Appropriate dose, route/pharmaceutical form, frequency of administration and duration of treatment (1 mark for each)

500 mg PO BD long-term

Question 40

A. Drug choice

Dexamethasone (4 marks). May help to temporarily relieve dysphagia and may reduce the extent of anorexia experienced by Mr Barnett.

B. Appropriate dose (2 marks), route/pharmaceutical form and frequency of administration (1 mark for each)

4–8 mg by IM injection, slow IV injection or IV infusion OD (in practice often administered BD).

Question 41

A. Drug choice

Dinoprostone controlled-release pessary, vaginal gel or vaginal tablets (4 marks). Dinoprostone vaginal tablet, gel or pessary are the first-line preparations used for the induction of labour at term.

NB oxytocin is not recommended for use without a vaginal prostaglandin (dinoprostone). Misoprostol is not licensed for this indication and its use is not recommended as routine practice. It needs to be given every few hours, rather than as a one-off dose. Usually only offered if there is an intra-uterine foetal death or as part of a clinical trial.[48–51]

B. Appropriate dose and route (2 marks for each)

Pessaries: 1 pessary (10 mg over 24 hours) by vaginal delivery STAT
Vaginal gel: 1 mg by vaginal delivery STAT
Vaginal tablets: 3 mg by vaginal delivery STAT

Question 42

A. Drug choice

Duloxetine (4 marks). The first-line choice of medicine for Mrs Bedford because it may help with both bereavement-associated major depressive episodes and stress incontinence.

NB amitriptyline or imipramine may help fight depression (tricyclic antidepressants) and reduce incontinence due to their antimuscarinic effects. They are sometimes used to treat nocturnal enuresis in children but they are not used for stress incontinence in adults, leaving duloxetine as the main choice of treatment.[52]

B. Appropriate dose (2 marks), route/pharmaceutical form and frequency of administration (1 mark for each)

20–40 mg PO BD or

60 mg PO OD

Question 43

A. Drug choice

Gentamicin (4 marks). The first-line antibacterial option for Mrs Khan. Her allergy to penicillin rules out the choice of co-amoxiclav. The fact that her eGFR is less than 60 mL/min/1.73 m² (creatinine clearance based on the ideal body weight of 52.4 kg = 32 mL/min), makes nitrofurantoin unsuitable/ineffective because of inadequate urine concentration and risk of peripheral neuropathy. Therefore, the once-daily regimen of gentamicin appears to be the most logical choice. Careful monitoring of the 'trough' (pre-dose) levels will be required considering Mrs Khan's poor kidney function. The first level is usually taken 16–24 hours after the first dose (ideally 1 hour before the second dose). If it is <1 mg/L, gentamicin can be continued safely at the same dosing regimen. The multiple daily dose regimen is inconvenient and rarely used other than in the treatment of infective endocarditis.[16,53]

B. Appropriate dose, route/pharmaceutical form, frequency of administration and duration of treatment (1 mark for each)

Dose is 3–5 mg/kg of adjusted body weight (the patient is obese) every 24 hours IV. This translates into 190–310 mg every 24 hours. To be reviewed prior to the second dose, i.e. within 24 hours.

Ideal body weight = 45.5 + 2.3 × number of inches over 5 feet =
45.5 + 2.3 × 3 = 52.4 kg

Adjusted body weight = ideal body weight + 0.4 × (actual body
weight – ideal body weight) = 62.6 kg

*NB the definition of 'obese' in this case complies with both BMI ≥30 kg/m² and >20%
above the ideal body weight. A 'renal impairment' dose of 3 mg/kg every 24 hours is
acceptable for the purpose of this exercise as per dosages recommended in the* Renal
Drug Handbook *(for CrCl of 30–70 mL/min).*[54,55]

Question 44

A. Drug choice

1. Codeine (4 marks). Loperamide and codeine are the two opioids of choice
   used to reduce the volume of stoma output. However, in contrast to loperamide, codeine may also provide an additional benefit of pain relief for
   Mr Robinson. Once Mr Robinson's pain subsides, codeine can be switched
   to an adequate dose of loperamide to reduce the risk of opioid addiction.
2. Loperamide (2 marks). *See* codeine answer.
3. Co-phenotrope (1 mark). It is likely to reduce the volume of stoma output,
   however is rarely used primarily due to its atropine content, which may
   predispose the patient to antimuscarinic adverse side effects.

B. Appropriate dose (2 marks), route/pharmaceutical form and frequency of administration (1 mark for each)

1. 15–60 mg PO every 4 hours (TDS–QDS) PRN (up to a maximum of
   240 mg/day)
2. 4–8 mg PO daily in divided doses up to a maximum of 16 mg daily in
   divided doses (higher unlicensed doses are sometimes needed)
3. Initially four tablets of 2.5 mg/0.025 mg strength PO, followed by two tablets every 6 hours PRN

Question 45

A. Fluid choice

1. Isotonic albumin solution (4.5% or 5%) (4 marks). The most suitable colloidal solution to help expand the circulatory volume for Mr BW after acute surgical blood loss. The use of albumin also appears to be associated with lower mortality after CABG surgery compared with non-protein colloids.[56] Note that the BNF advises that 'the use of albumin solutions in acute blood loss may be wasteful'; however, taking into account individual patient factors (such as kidney impairment), albumin would be the most appropriate option for the initial management of blood loss until blood transfusion is available.
2. Etherified starch (3 marks). Etherified starch solutions should be used with adequate caution in renal impairment, and therefore albumin may be preferred in Mr BW's case.
3. Dextran 70 (2 marks). Dextrans have been reported to carry an increased risk of bleeding as well as higher (than with other colloids) risk of hypersensitivity reactions. They are rarely used. The administration of hypertonic dextran 70 needs to be immediately followed by the administration of isotonic fluids.

NB gelatin is also likely to be effective and is widely used for volume expansion. However, Mr BW is vegan, which automatically rules out the choice of gelatin solutions. The benefits of crystalloid solutions (e.g. normal saline or Hartmann's solution) are also limited in patients with such significant volume of blood loss as in Mr BW's case. Yet larger volumes of crystalloid solutions may be required to restore the circulating volume (e.g. 2 L or more) because crystalloids can quickly redistribute into the interstitial fluid. The excess of fluid in the interstitial space may then add to pulmonary oedema causing further complications.

B. Appropriate dose/volume (2 marks), type of infusion/route and duration of administration (1 mark for each)

1. 250–1000 mL by IV infusion at a maximum rate of 5 mL/min
2. Tetrastarch, pentastarch or hetastarch 500–1000 mL by IV infusion at a rate not exceeding 30 mL/hr

NB for the purpose of this exercise, the test dose of non-protein colloids is not required.

3. 250 mL over 2–5 min, followed immediately by administration of isotonic fluids[6,56–61]

Question 46

A. Drug choice

1. Rivaroxaban (4 marks). The most suitable choice of pharmacological venous thromboembolism (VTE) prophylaxis for Mrs ME (*see* other options).

NB considering Mrs ME's PMH of non-valvular AF and hypertension together with her unsuitability for warfarin, she may be a candidate for long-term newer anticoagulants such as rivaroxaban or apixaban. Following 5 weeks of 10 mg OD, the dose of rivaroxaban may be titrated up to 15 mg OD for stroke and systemic embolism prophylaxis in AF (see the renal impairment section for rivaroxaban in BNF/ SPC). Aspirin would then most likely be discontinued (lack of convincing evidence for adequate stroke prevention in AF patients).

2. Apixaban (3 marks). *See* rivaroxaban answer. The second most suitable choice of VTE prophylaxis for Mrs ME. More expensive than rivaroxaban and has to be taken twice daily.
3. Dabigatran (2 marks). The third most suitable choice of VTE prophylaxis for Mrs ME. However, Mrs ME is receiving both concomitant verapamil (Securon SR®) and amiodarone (two P-glycoprotein inhibitors), which may increase the plasma concentration of dabigatran. This may in turn increase the risk of bleeding. In addition, following 27–34 days of post-surgical VTE prophylaxis with dabigatran, Mrs ME would have to be switched to alternative long-term AF thromboprophylaxis (e.g. rivaroxaban or apixaban). While she has a PMH of non-valvular AF and hypertension, her age (under 65) makes dabigatran unsuitable for this indication.

NB parenteral anticoagulants, such as LMWHs and fondaparinux, are unsuitable for Mrs ME because of her needle phobia.

B. Appropriate dose, route/pharmaceutical form, frequency of administration and duration of treatment (1 mark for each)

1. 10 mg PO OD for 5 weeks starting 6–10 hours after surgery
2. 2.5 mg PO BD for 32–38 days starting 12–24 hours after surgery

3. 75 mg PO OD for 27–34 days starting 1–4 hours after surgery (the dose adjusted for eGFR 30–50 mL/min/1.73 m^2 and concomitant verapamil + amiodarone)[5,62]

Question 47

A. Drug choice

Tobramycin (4 marks). The first-line option for eradication of chronic *P. aeruginosa* infection in patients who cannot tolerate ciprofloxacin or colistin. In addition, the fact that *Pseudomonas* culture was sensitive to tobramycin should have prompted the prescriber to choose this antimicrobial over colistin.

B. Appropriate dose, route/pharmaceutical form, frequency of administration and duration of treatment (1 mark for each)

300 mg via the nebuliser every 12 hours for 28 days (the course of up to 3 months may sometimes be required for complete eradication)[63,64]

Question 48

A. Drug choice

1. Mirtazapine (4 marks). Usually considered to be the second-line choice of antidepressant in patients who fail to respond to selective serotonin re-uptake inhibitors (SSRIs). However, Molly's PMH of epilepsy and concomitant use of ritonavir (as part of Kaletra®) makes SSRIs and tricyclic antidepressants (TCAs) less suitable. SSRIs and TCAs may antagonise the anticonvulsant effect of valproate increasing the risk of seizures. Ritonavir can 'boost' the plasma concentration of SSRIs or TCAs predisposing patients to their toxicity, such as the serotonin syndrome. Mirtazapine, venlafaxine and reboxetine are not known to exhibit any significant interactions with anticonvulsant or antiretroviral medicines. Adequate caution is necessary when initiating mirtazapine, venlafaxine (and to a lesser extent) reboxetine in an epileptic patient, however seizures with these antidepressants are less common than with SSRIs and TCAs.
2. Reboxetine (3 marks). *See* mirtazapine answer. More expensive and used less frequently than mirtazapine. Has to be taken twice daily (compared to once at night for mirtazapine) which may predispose the patient to non-adherence.
3. Venlafaxine (2 marks). *See* mirtazapine answer. Usually reserved for more severe forms of depression unresponsive to mirtazapine or reboxetine.

NB other antidepressant agents, such as agomelatine or duloxetine, are available but are used further down the line in the management of depression, unless the patient has individual factors which may suggest treatment with these agents, e.g. stress incontinence may suggest the use of duloxetine.

B. Appropriate dose (2 marks), route/pharmaceutical form and frequency of administration (1 mark for each)

1. 15–30 mg PO ON
2. 4 mg PO BD
3. 37.5 mg PO BD; alternatively, modified-release preparation can be used at an initial dose of 75 mg OD[65–67]

References

1. National Institute for Health and Clinical Excellence. *Type 2 Diabetes: NICE guideline 87 – quick reference guide*. London: NICE; 2010. Available at: www.nice.org. uk/nicemedia/live/12165/44322/44322.pdf

2. National Institute for Health and Clinical Excellence. *Chronic Obstructive Pulmonary Disease: NICE guideline 101 – quick reference guide*. London: NICE; 2010. Available at: www.nice.org.uk/nicemedia/live/13029/49399/49399.pdf

3. Jenkins CR, Beasley R. Tiotropium Respimat increases the risk of mortality. *Thorax*. 2013; **68**(1): 5–7.

4. National Institute for Health and Clinical Excellence. *Atrial Fibrillation: NICE guideline 36 – quick reference guide*. London: NICE; 2006. Available at: www.nice. org.uk/nicemedia/live/10982/30054/30054.pdf

5. National Institute for Health and Clinical Excellence. *Venous Thromboembolism – Reducing the Risk: NICE guideline 92 – quick reference guide*. London: NICE; 2011. Available at: www.nice.org.uk/nicemedia/live/12695/47197/47197.pdf

6. Medusa Injectable Medicines Guide Online: National Health Service. Available at: www.injguide.nhs.uk

7. Ballinger A, Patchett S. Heart failure. In: Kumar P, Clark M, editors. *Pocket Essentials of Clinical Medicine*. 4th ed. London: Saunders Elsevier; 2007. pp. 423–34.

8. National Institute for Health and Clinical Excellence. Chronic Heart Failure: NICE guideline 108 – quick reference guide. London: NICE; 2010. Available at: www.nice.org.uk/nicemedia/live/13099/50526/50526.pdf

9. McAnaw J, Hudson SA. Chronic heart failure. In: Walker R, Whittlesea C, editors. *Clinical Pharmacy and Therapeutics*. 4th ed. London: Churchill Livingstone Elsevier; 2007. pp. 298–318.

10. National Institute for Health and Clinical Excellence. *Osteoarthritis: NICE guideline 59 – quick reference guide*. London: NICE; 2008. Available at: www.nice.org. uk/nicemedia/live/11926/39554/39554.pdf

11. National Institute for Health and Clinical Excellence. *Alendronate, etidronate, risedronate, raloxifene, strontium ranelate and teriparatide for the secondary prevention of osteoporotic fragility fractures in postmenopausal women: NICE guideline 161 – quick reference guide*. London: NICE; 2008. Available at: www.nice.org.uk/nicemedia/live/11748/42508/42508.pdf

12. National Institute for Health and Clinical Excellence. *Denosumab for the Prevention of Osteoporotic Fractures in Postmenopausal Women: NICE guideline 204 – quick reference guide*. London: NICE; 2010. Available at: http://guidance.nice.org.uk/TA204/QuickRefGuide/pdf/English

13. Trissel LA. *Handbook on Injectable Drugs* [Online] 2013. Available at: www.medicinescomplete.com

14. Watson M, Lucas C, Hoy A, *et al*. Palliative Care Guidelines Plus [Online]; 2011. Available at: http://book.pallcare.info/index.php?wpage=3.

15. *How do I manage nausea and vomiting in people with Parkinson's disease?* [Online]. Clinical Knowledge Summaries; 2009 [cited 30 November 2013]. Available at: http://cks.nice.org.uk/parkinsons-disease#!scenariorecommendation:13

16. *Antimicrobial Policies and Guidelines*. Redhill: Surrey and Sussex Healthcare NHS Trust; 2012.

17. Ballinger A, Patchett S. Addison's disease – primary hypoadrenalism. In: Kumar P, Clark M, editors. *Pocket Essentials of Clinical Medicine*. 4th ed. London: Saunders Elsevier; 2007. pp. 621–3.

18. *Croup* [Online]. Clinical Knowledge Summaries; 2012 [cited 30 November 2013]. Available at: http://cks.nice.org.uk/croup

19. National Institute for Health and Care Excellence. *Feverish illness in children: NICE guideline 160*. London: NICE; 2013. Available at: www.nice.org.uk/nicemedia/live/14171/63908/63908.pdf

20. *Diagnosing Croup* [Online]. London: NHS Choices; 2012 [cited 15 November 2012]. Available at: www.nhs.uk/Conditions/Croup/Pages/Diagnosis.aspx

21. Wykrzykowska JJ, Arbab-Zadeh A, Godoy G, *et al*. Assessment of in-stent restenosis using 64-MDCT: analysis of the CORE-64 Multicenter International Trial. *AJR Am J Roentgenol*. 2010; **194**(1): 85–92.

22. *Guidelines for Percutaneous Coronary Intervention* [Online]. European Society of Cardiology; 2005 [cited 18 November 2012]. Available at: www.bcis.org.uk/resources/documents/esc_pci2005.pdf

23. *Summary of Product Characteristics Nexplanon 68 mg Implant for Subdermal Use* [Online]. Electronic Medicines Compendium; 2012 [cited 18 November 2012]. Available at: www.medicines.org.uk/EMC/medicine/23824/SPC/Nexplanon+68+mg+implant+for+subdermal+use/#INTERACTIONS

24. Sweet DG, Carnielli V, Greisen G, *et al*.; European Association of Perinatal Medicine. European consensus guidelines on the management of neonatal respiratory distress syndrome in preterm infants – 2010 update. *Neonatology*. 2010; **97**(4): 402–17.

25. *Neonatal Respiratory Distress Syndrome* [Online]. PubMed Health; 2011 [cited 21 November 2012]. Available at: www.ncbi.nlm.nih.gov/pubmedhealth/PMH0002530/

26. *Assessments for Newborn Babies* [Online]. Lucile Packard Children's Hospital at Stanford; 2012 [cited 21 November 2012]. Available at: www.lpch.org/DiseaseHealthInfo/HealthLibrary/hrnewborn/assess.html

27. *Neonatal Handbook: Blood Pressure* [Online]. The Royal Children's Hospital (Australia); 2012 [cited 21 November 2012]. Available at: www.netsvic.org.au/nets/handbook/index.cfm?doc_id=450

28. Tinnion R, Vasey N. Neonatal care: the sick neonate. *Clin Pharm.* 2012; **4**: 165–9.

29. Pitt B, Zannad F, Remme WJ, *et al.* The effect of spironolactone on morbidity and mortality in patients with severe heart failure. Randomized Aldactone Evaluation Study Investigators. *N Engl J Med.* 1999; **341**(10): 709–17.

30. Zannad F, McMurray JJ, Krum H, *et al.* Eplerenone in patients with systolic heart failure and mild symptoms. *N Engl J Med.* 2011; **364**(1): 11–21.

31. McMurray JJ, Adamopoulos S, Anker SD, *et al.*; ESC Committee for Practice Guidelines. ESC Guidelines for the diagnosis and treatment of acute and chronic heart failure 2012: the Task Force for the Diagnosis and Treatment of Acute and Chronic Heart Failure 2012 of the European Society of Cardiology. *Eur Heart J.* 2012; **33**(14): 847–1787.

32. Ballinger A, Patchett S. Investigations in cardiac disease. In: Kumar P, Clark M, editors. *Pocket Essentials of Clinical Medicine.* 4th ed. London: Saunders Elsevier; 2007. pp. 397–408.

33. National Institute for Health and Clinical Excellence. *Bipolar Disorder: NICE guideline 38 – quick reference guide.* London: NICE; 2006. Available at: www.nice.org.uk/nicemedia/live/10990/30191/30191.pdf

34. Pratt JP. Affective disorders. In: Walker R, Whittlesea C, editors. *Clinical Pharmacy and Therapeutics.* 4th ed. London: Churchill Livingstone Elsevier; 2007. pp. 424–37.

35. *Chlamydia – Uncomplicated Genital* [Online]. Clinical Knowledge Summaries; 2009 [cited 30 November 2013]. Available at: http://cks.nice.org.uk/chlamydia-uncomplicated-genital

36. *Gonorrhoea* [Online]. Clinical Knowledge Summaries; 2011 [cited 30 November 2013]. Available at: http://cks.nice.org.uk/gonorrhoea

37. *Acute Pelvic Inflammatory Disease: tests and treatment* [Online]. Royal College of Obstetricians and Gynaecologists; 2010 [cited 24 November 2012]. Available at: www.rcog.org.uk/files/rcog-corp/Acute%20Pelvic%20Inflammatory%20Disease%20%28PID%29_0.pdf

38. *Vitamin K and Vitamin K Deficiency Bleeding of the Newborn* [Online]. Royal Free Hampstead NHS Trust; 2008 [cited 25 November 2012]. Available at: www.royalfree.nhs.uk/pip_admin/docs/vitamin_K_1057.pdf

39. Hey E. Vitamin K: what, why, and when. *Arch Dis Child Fetal Neonatal Ed.* 2003; **88**(2): F80–3.

40. *Gout* [Online]. Clinical Knowledge Summaries; 2012 [cited 30 November 2013]. Available at: http://cks.nice.org.uk/gout

41. Jordan KM, Cameron JS, Snaith M, *et al.* British Society for Rheumatology and British Health Professionals in Rheumatology guideline for the management of gout. *Rheumatology (Oxford).* 2007; **46**(8): 1372–4.

42. Roddy E. Gout: presentation and management in primary care. *Reports on the Rheumatic Diseases (Hands On).* 2011; **6**(9): 1–8.

43. *Blepharitis* [Online]. Clinical Knowledge Summaries; 2012 [cited 30 November 2013]. Available at: http://cks.nice.org.uk/blepharitis

44. *Summary of Product Characteristics Boots Infected Eyes 1% w/w Eye Ointment* [Online]. Electronic Medicines Compendium; 2011 [cited 27 March 2013]. Available at: www.medicines.org.uk/EMC/medicine/26610/SPC/Boots+Infected +Eyes+1++w+w+Eye+Ointment/#CONTRAINDICATIONS

45. *Summary of Product Characteristics Ciloxan 3mg/g Eye Ointment* [Online]. Electronic Medicines Compendium; 2013 [cited 19 September 2013]. Available at: www. medicines.org.uk/emc/medicine/17044/SPC/Ciloxan+3mg+g+Eye+Ointment/

46. *Summary of Product Characteristics Brolene Eye Ointment* [Online]. Electronic Medicines Compendium; 2012 [cited 19 September 2013]. Available at: www. medicines.org.uk/emc/medicine/9938/SPC/Brolene+Eye+Ointment/#INDICA TIONS

47. Rees DC, Olujohungbe AD, Parker NE, *et al.* Guidelines for the management of the acute painful crisis in sickle cell disease. *Br J Haematol.* 2003; **120**(5): 744–52.

48. National Institute for Health and Clinical Excellence. *Induction of Labour: NICE guideline 70 – quick reference guide.* London: NICE; 2008. Available at: www.nice. org.uk/nicemedia/live/12012/41266/41266.pdf

49. *Summary of Product Characteristics Prostin E2 Vaginal Gel 1mg, 2mg* [Online]. Electronic Medicines Compendium; 2011 [cited 8 December 2012]. Available at: www.medicines.org.uk/EMC/medicine/1562/SPC/Prostin+E2+Vaginal+Gel+1m g%2c+2mg/

50. *Martindale: the complete drug reference* [Online]. Available at: www.medicines complete.com/

51. Tenore JL. Methods for cervical ripening and induction of labor. *Am Fam Physician.* 2003; **67**(10): 2123–8.

52. *Incontinence – Urinary, In Women* [Online]. Clinical Knowledge Summaries; 2009 [cited 30 November 2013]. Available at: http://cks.nice.org.uk/ incontinence-urinary-in-women

53. *Urinary Tract Infection (Lower) – Women* [Online]. Clinical Knowledge Summaries; 2009 [cited 30 November 2013]. Available at: http://cks.nice.org.uk/urinary-tract-infection-lower-women

54. Ashley C, Currie A; UK Renal Pharmacy Group. *The Renal Drug Handbook.* 3rd ed. Oxford: Radcliffe Publishing; 2009.

55. Pai MP, Paloucek FP. The origin of the 'ideal' body weight equations. *Ann Pharmacother.* 2000; **34**(9): 1066–9.

56. Sedrakyan A, Gondek K, Paltiel D, *et al.* Volume expansion with albumin decreases mortality after coronary artery bypass graft surgery. *Chest.* 2003; **123**(6): 1853–7.

57. Ballinger A, Patchett S. Acute disturbances of haemodynamic function (shock). In: Kumar P, Clark M, editors. *Pocket Essentials of Clinical Medicine.* 4th ed. London: Saunders Elsevier; 2007. pp. 552–62.

58. Schumacher J, Klotz KF. Fluid therapy in cardiac surgery patients. *Cardiopulmonary Pathophysiology.* 2009; **13**: 138–42.

59. Magder S, Potter BJ, Varennes BD, *et al.* Fluids after cardiac surgery: a pilot study of the use of colloids versus crystalloids. *Crit Care Med.* 2010; **38**(11): 2117–24.

60. Floss K, Borthwick M, Clark C. Intravenous fluids – principles of treatment. *Clin Pharm.* 2011; **3**(9): 274–83.

61. Staples A, Dade J, Acomb C. Intravenous fluids – practical aspects of therapy. *Clin Pharm.* 2011; **3**(9): 285–91.

62. *Summary of Product Characteristics Eliquis 2.5 mg Film-Coated Tablets* [Online]. Electronic Medicines Compendium; 2011 [cited 16 December 2012]. Available at: www.medicines.org.uk/EMC/medicine/24988/SPC/Eliquis+2.5+mg+film-coated+tablets/#INDICATIONS

63. British Medical Association; Royal Pharmaceutical Society. *British National Formulary for Children* [Online]. London: Pharmaceutical Press; 2012. Available at: www.medicinescomplete.com

64. *Antibiotic Treatment for Cystic Fibrosis* [Online]. UK Cystic Fibrosis Trust; 2009 [cited 30 November 2013]. Available at: https://www.cysticfibrosis.org.uk/media/82010/CD_Antibiotic_treatment_for_CF_May_09.pdf

65. *Summary of Product Characteristics Edronax 4mg Tablets* [Online]. Electronic Medicines Compendium; 2011 [cited 27 March 2013]. Available at: www.medicines.org.uk/EMC/medicine/8386/SPC/Edronax+4mg+Tablets/

66. National Institute for Health and Clinical Excellence. *Depression in Adults: NICE guideline 90 – quick reference guide.* London: NICE; 2009. Available at: www.nice.org.uk/nicemedia/live/12329/45890/45890.pdf

67. *Stockley's Drug Interactions* [Online]. Available at: www.medicinescomplete.com/

CHAPTER 2: PRESCRIPTION REVIEW

Question 1

Question A

ACE inhibitors, such as lisinopril, have been reported to cause (acute) renal impairment. 'Renal effects' are described in a distinct paragraph under the ACE inhibitor section of the BNF (section 2.5.5.1). Acute renal failure is reported as a very rare adverse drug reaction for aciclovir, however the likelihood that aciclovir is implicated in this case is increased by the fact that the AKI appeared soon after the patient was initiated on aciclovir treatment.

Question B

Metformin should be avoided if the eGFR is <30 mL/min/1.73 m^2 because of an increased risk of lactic acidosis. Sitagliptin is primarily eliminated via the renal route and requires a dose reduction to 25 mg once daily if the eGFR is <30 mL/min/1.73 m^2.

Question 2

Question A

Citalopram, amitriptyline and tramadol can all increase serotonergic transmission and place the patient at risk of serotonin syndrome, which presents with signs/symptoms reported in this case (indicated as the CNS toxicity in the Interactions section of the BNF). The CNS toxicity was most likely precipitated by tramadol, which was newly initiated during admission.

Question B

Rifampicin (a rifamycin antibiotic) is an inducer of the P450 isoenzyme system(s) that metabolise(s) warfarin. The increase in warfarin metabolism leads to a reduced anticoagulant effect as indicated by the drop in the INR (from 2.2 to 1.6).[1]

Question 3

Question A

Glibenclamide (a long-acting sulfonylurea) is associated with a higher risk of hypoglycaemia and should be avoided in the elderly (Mrs Roberts was hypoglycaemic on admission). Prochlorperazine (phenothiazine antipsychotic) should be avoided in elderly patients with dementia because it may increase the risk of mortality/stroke/TIA in this population of patients (Mrs Roberts has already had a stroke). The elderly are also more susceptible to postural hypotension and temperature fluctuations induced by antipsychotics. Lorazepam (benzodiazepine) should be avoided in the elderly as it may increase the risk of confusion (due to postural hypotension) and ataxia, leading to falls (Mrs Roberts was admitted following a fall).

Question B

Trimethoprim is not an appropriate choice of treatment since the urine dip was negative for nitrites ruling out a UTI. Trimethoprim may also contribute to the development of hyperkalaemia (note that the most recent K^+ level was 4.9).

Question 4

Question A

Carbamazepine is contraindicated in patients with a history of acute porphyria. Safer options, such as levetiracetam, are available. Quinolones (moxifloxacin) should be used with caution in patients with a history of epilepsy (they may increase the risk of convulsions) and in children (because of the risk of arthropathy in weight-bearing joints). If the patient does not respond to flucloxacillin, safer (than moxifloxacin) alternatives include clindamycin or vancomycin (unless Gram-negative organisms are suspected in which case broad-spectrum antibacterials, such as cephalosporins, may be appropriate until the culture sensitivity data becomes available). Convulsions have been reported in patients receiving methylphenidate therapy, however such reports are very rare and the benefits of continuing methylphenidate therapy probably outweigh the risks (unless there is an increase in seizure frequency). Alternatives, including atomoxetine and dexamfetamine, also carry a small risk of convulsions.

Question B

The maximum recommended dose of lamotrigine as the adjunctive therapy of seizures (with enzyme inducing drugs, such as carbamazepine) without valproate for children aged 2–12 years is 400 mg daily (300 mg BD is equivalent to 600 mg daily, which exceeds this recommendation). The maximum recommended dose of methylphenidate for the treatment of ADHD in children aged 6–18 years is 90 mg daily (50 mg BD is equivalent to 100 mg daily, which exceeds this recommendation).

Question 5

Question A

Mr BT presented with typical symptoms of lithium toxicity/poisoning as indicated in the Emergency Treatment of Poisoning section of the BNF.

Question B

Lithium toxicity can be aggravated by hyponatraemia (the body retains lithium which is an ion similar to sodium). ACE inhibitors (perindopril) and loop diuretics (bumetanide) increase the loss of sodium from the body, therefore increasing the retention of lithium. NSAIDs (diclofenac) can increase the risk of lithium toxicity by reducing the excretion of lithium due to fluid retention.

Question 6

Question A

Sulfonylureas (gliclazide) are only indicated in T2DM and are only effective if there is some residual beta-cell activity present (Mrs YG is a type 1 diabetic). Sulfonylureas (with an exception of glibenclamide) should also generally be avoided in pregnancy. Warfarin is teratogenic and should be avoided in pregnancy – low-molecular-weight heparins (e.g. enoxaparin) are a safer alternative. Finally, Mrs YG should have only taken folic acid until week 12 of pregnancy.

Question B

The correct dose of enoxaparin for the treatment of venous thromboembolism in pregnancy (unlicensed indication) is 80 mg twice daily for women with an early pregnancy weight of 70–90 kg.

Question 7

Question A

Sulfasalazine can cause yellow-orange discolouration of the skin. Amiodarone is associated with a slate-grey skin discolouration.

Question B

Beta blockers, particularly the lipid-soluble ones (such as propranolol) can cause sleep disturbances with nightmares. Corticosteroids (such as hydrocortisone) may induce insomnia and nightmares, especially if given later in the day (after 3 p.m.). While sleep disturbances have also been reported with amiodarone, sulfasalazine and lansoprazole, amitriptyline is the third medicine that is most likely to have caused them for Victor. Tricyclic antidepressants (such as amitriptyline) commonly induce CNS effects, including sleep disturbances, irritability and agitation. These effects are particularly common in the elderly (Victor is 75 years old).

Question 8

Question A

Two potential drug-related adverse reactions can be identified in this case. The antiepileptic hypersensitivity syndrome (complicated by possible erythema multiforme or Stevens–Johnson syndrome) may be associated with phenytoin. Strontium ranelate has also been reported to cause severe allergic reactions – drug rash with eosinophilia and systemic symptoms (DRESS). With both reactions, systemic features may be present, and multiple organs, including the liver, kidneys and lungs may be affected.

Question B

Prednisolone, omeprazole, phenytoin and letrozole are all bound to plasma albumin to a certain extent. However, reduced protein binding of prednisolone and phenytoin (particularly in the presence of concurrent liver impairment) is most likely to cause problems due to an increase in the concentration of a free drug (narrow therapeutic range of phenytoin and a wide spectrum of serious adverse corticosteroid effects with prednisolone, e.g. Cushing's syndrome and immunosuppression).[2,3]

Question 9

Question A

Clopidogrel is not licensed for use in patients who have suffered a TIA (as opposed to a 'full' ischaemic stroke). However, it may be used 'off-label' in cases where both aspirin and dipyridamole are not suitable for the patient. According to NICE and BNF guidance on the long-term management of patients following a TIA, Mr Chiew should ideally have been prescribed a combination of aspirin 75 mg OM and dipyridamole 200 mg MR BD after the course of aspirin 300 mg OD was complete. In practice however clopidogrel is often preferred over dipyridamole for both TIA and ischaemic stroke patients due to its once daily administration, better side effect profile and lower cost, i.e. it is commonly prescribed 'off-label' in TIA patients. Considering his medical history of a NSTEMI and TIA, Mr Chiew is at a high risk of future cardiovascular events. Therefore, he would require an adequate lipid-regulating therapy, which according to NICE guidance, should be equivalent to 40 mg of simvastatin/day (20–40 mg/day adjusted thereafter according to the BNF). Hence, the current dose of simvastatin requires further titration or a switch to a higher-intensity statin, e.g. atorvastatin (40–80 mg OD).[4–6]

Question B

Both omeprazole and fluoxetine may reduce the antiplatelet effect of clopidogrel and, whenever possible, their concomitant use should be either kept to a minimum or completely avoided. Omeprazole possibly inhibits the CYP2C19 system which converts clopidogrel into its active metabolite. There has been a debate as to whether or not the interaction between clopidogrel and some PPIs (omeprazole and esomeprazole) is clinically significant. However, in the presence of safer alternatives, such as ranitidine or other PPIs (e.g. lansoprazole), it is advisable to use them instead whenever possible. The mechanism by which fluoxetine may reduce the antiplatelet effect of clopidogrel is unknown, but may be similar to that of omeprazole.[7,8]

Question 10

Question A

According to the G6PD-deficiency table in the BNF, aspirin, gliclazide, nitrofurantoin and quinine all carry a risk of haemolysis in G6PD-deficient individuals. The risk is definite (i.e. significantly greater) with nitrofurantoin and possible with aspirin, gliclazide and quinine. However, the use of aspirin is generally acceptable in such individuals provided the dose does not exceed 1 g/day. Therefore, nitrofurantoin, quinine and gliclazide is the correct answer.

Question B

Calcium-channel blockers, such as amlodipine, increase the risk of simvastatin-related myopathy, e.g. rhabdomyolysis. The mechanism by which amlodipine increases the plasma concentration of simvastatin is currently unknown. The maximum recommended dose of simvastatin with concurrent amlodipine is 20 mg ON.[3,9,10]

Question 11

Question A

Furosemide and vancomycin have both been reported to cause ototoxicity. Therefore, the administration rate of IV furosemide infusions should not exceed 4 mg/min. Note that the initial 240 mg infusion was incorrectly given at a rate of 8 mg/min followed by rather aggressive 80 mg BD treatment IV. Vancomycin should also be used with caution, particularly in patients with renal impairment. Plasma concentrations should be carefully monitored to avoid renotoxic and ototoxic adverse effects.

Question B

Buscopan® (hyoscine butylbromide) is an antimuscarinic agent, which may be associated with all common antimuscarnic adverse effects, including urinary retention, dry mouth and constipation. Ferrous fumarate (oral iron replacement) also commonly causes constipation.

Question 12

Question A

It is common practice to withhold angiotensin-II receptor antagonists (olmesartan) 12–24 hours (24 hours recommended in the BNF) before a major surgical procedure (such as a TURP) to avoid potentially dangerous hypotension after induction of anaesthesia. Amlodipine can be continued safely and may suffice in BP control prior to surgery. Lithium should also be stopped 24 hours prior to major surgery to reduce the risk of toxicity which may arise as a result of any fluid and/or electrolyte disturbances.[11–13]

Question B

Both tamsulosin and tolterodine may be considered for discontinuation following TURP. Mr Rees is likely to have suffered from an overactive bladder, which sometimes co-exists with bladder outlet obstruction induced by BPH. Therefore, he received both antimuscarinic and alpha-1 blocker therapies. With careful monitoring, these may be stopped post TURP, which in itself will provide long-term symptomatic relief.[13,14]

Question 13

Question A

Clozapine, amitriptyline and hyoscine can all cause antimuscarinic adverse effects, one of which is constipation, possibly complicating paralytic ileus. Clozapine and hyoscine are both contraindicated in paralytic ileus whilst amitriptyline should be used with extreme caution.[15]

Question B

Considering the severity of Mrs Gomez's intra-abdominal sepsis and her 'nil by mouth' status, it might be more reasonable to prescribe ciprofloxacin 400 mg BD or TDS IV rather than BD via the NG tube. Note that ciprofloxacin may also interact with calcium and iron in the enteral feeds. Enteral feeds may reduce its absorption by up to 50%.[16]

Question 14

Question A

In light of the venous thromboembolism risk associated with major surgery under general anaesthesia, hormone replacement therapy (HRT), such as FemSeven Conti®, should generally be withheld 4–6 weeks before the procedure. It should only be restarted once the patient is fully mobile.[11,17]

Question B

Diazepam, baclofen and hydrocortisone should not be stopped abruptly prior to major surgery. Abrupt discontinuation of diazepam and baclofen may lead to a hyperactive state, may exacerbate spasticity and precipitate psychiatric reactions or convulsions. Stopping hydrocortisone may worsen the adrenocortical insufficiency – an increase in the corticosteroid dose is often required prior to major surgery to avoid such effects.[11,17]

Question 15

Question A

Mr YR suffered an episode of VT with a significantly prolonged QT interval (likely, torsades de pointes). Escitalopram, domperidone and ondansetron can all prolong the QT interval and carry a recognised arrhythmogenic potential. In addition, they seem to all have been started during hospital admission and therefore (together with hypomagnesaemia) are the most likely precipitants of this episode.[18,19]

Question B

Selective serotonin re-uptake inhibitors (SSRIs; escitalopram) can increase the aspirin-associated risk of bleeding. Serotonin released from platelets potentiates their aggregation. SSRIs block the uptake of serotonin into platelets thus impairing their haemostatic effect.[7] However, note the opposite clinical effect resulting from fluoxetine-clopidogrel interaction (*see* Chapter 2, Question 9).

Question 16

Question A

Loop diuretics, such as furosemide, may cause hyperuricaemia and may exacerbate gout or precipitate an acute attack. Hyperuricaemia may also be observed with thiazide diuretics, such as bendroflumethiazide.

Question B

The dose of alfacalcidol has been prescribed incorrectly and should read 'nanograms' rather than 'micrograms' – see the NPSA signal on the safer use of alfacalcidol.[20] The concentration of oxygen is too high for a patient at risk of hypercapnic respiratory failure (COPD and rising P_aCO_2). The recommended concentrations of oxygen for such patients are 24%–28%.[21] The doses of isosorbide mononitrate are prescribed too far apart from each other (12 hours), which may eventually lead to the development of tolerance to nitrates. In order to reduce such a risk, doses should be given not more than 8 hours apart (e.g. 8 a.m. and 4 p.m.).

Question 17

Question A

Because of its nature as a precursor of dopamine in the CNS, levodopa (co-careldopa or Sinemet Plus®) is well known to cause psychiatric symptoms, including hallucinations. Tricyclic antidepressants (nortriptyline) are commonly associated with CNS side effects, particularly in the elderly. These may include, anxiety, dizziness, agitation, confusion, hallucinations, delusions and others.[22]

Question B

Tricyclic antidepressants and some antipsychotics (risperidone) are a common cause of antimuscarinic adverse effects, such as dry mouth.

NB some antipsychotics, such as clozapine, cause hypersalivation instead.

Question 18

Question A

Betnovate-RD® cream (betamethasone 0.025%), which is usually applied by the patient, is prescribed as Betnovate® cream (betamethasone 0.1%). Tears Naturale® preservative-free 0.4 mL single-use eye drops are prescribed as Tears Naturale® eye drops. The ward staff may get confused and administer multiple-use Tears Naturale® eye drops, which contain benzalkonium chloride as one of the preservatives (Lucas is allergic to this substance). Topical treatment of acute otitis media using gentamicin ear drops is often ineffective and is not recommended. Patients with systemic features may need to receive oral or IV antibacterial treatment as appropriate.

Question B

While OTC Night Nurse® may be given to children over the age of 12, the OTC codeine-containing liquid medicines should not be used in children for cough suppression until they are 18 years old (see MHRA/CHM advice in the BNF). In addition, note that both dextromethorphan and codeine are opioid-based cough suppressants. The mother should be educated to avoid using such a combination in the future in order to minimise any risk of opioid-related adverse effects, such as constipation or respiratory depression.[23,24]

Question 19

Question A

Clozapine is known to cause neutropenia and potentially fatal agranulocytosis. Therefore, regular blood counts are requested throughout the treatment. Permanent discontinuation of treatment may be required if a significant fall in white blood cell or neutrophil count is observed. Mirtazapine has also been reported to cause blood disorders, including granulocytopenia, agranulocytosis, thrombocytopenia and aplastic anaemia. The frequency of such reactions is not known and routine monitoring of blood counts is not recommended.[3,25]

Question B

Methadone is known to cause QT prolongation, particularly in at-risk patients, such as those with electrolyte abnormalities or those receiving concomitant QT interval-prolonging drugs. Quinolones (ciprofloxacin) may also prolong the QT interval. It may be reasonable to replace methadone with another opioid (e.g. morphine sulphate or oxycodone) until the patient completes the course of ciprofloxacin. Alternatively, microbiology advice may need to be sought as to which antimicrobial (other than ciprofloxacin) is suitable for use in this case.

Question 20

Question A

Selective serotonin re-uptake inhibitors (SSRIs), such as citalopram, and tricyclic antidepressants, such as amitriptyline, are known to antagonise the anticonvulsant effects and may lower the seizure threshold. Tramadol also affects the serotonergic and adrenergic pathways, and may lower seizure threshold in susceptible epileptic patients. It is therefore contraindicated in uncontrolled epilepsy. Tramadol would probably have been stopped in Mrs BC's case (at least temporarily). The doses of citalopram and amitriptyline may need to be reduced slowly or these medicines may need to be substituted for alternatives.

Question B

Owing to the risk of dose-dependent QT interval prolongation, the maximum daily dose of citalopram recommended for use in patients over 65 years of age by the MHRA is 20 mg.[26]

Question 21

Question A

Similar to ACE inhibitors, angiotensin II receptor blockers (losartan) should be avoided in pregnancy as far as possible because of the risk of adverse effects on fetal/neonatal blood pressure control and renal function; skull defects and oligohydramnios have also been reported. Alternatives that could be used to control blood pressure during pregnancy include labetalol (avoid if history of asthma), methyldopa and nifedipine. Halibut liver oil capsules are a rich source of vitamin A, which is a known teratogenic substance. Pregnant women are therefore advised not to take vitamin A supplements and not to eat liver products, such as liver paté or liver sausage.

Question B

Taste disturbances are common with both metformin and zopiclone. Patients taking zopiclone often report a mild-bitter or metallic aftertaste. Zopiclone should not be used regularly and/or long-term in pregnancy, and taste disturbances generally cease once the drug is withdrawn. If such effects are intolerable with metformin, alternatives, such as insulin or glibenclamide (from 11 weeks of gestation), may be appropriate.[27]

Question 22

Question A

Quinolones (ciprofloxacin) are known to trigger seizures or to lower seizure threshold and should be used with caution in patients with a history of epilepsy – alternatives may need to be used. Although the amount of ciprofloxacin which appears in breast milk is probably too small to be harmful, its use should be avoided due to a potential risk of articular damage in an infant. A broad-spectrum cephalosporin (e.g. cefuroxime) may be used as an alternative in this case. Because of a large variation in composition and unpredictable metabolic effects, St John's wort should be avoided in patients receiving anticonvulsant medicines. The use of herbal medicines, including St John's wort, is also generally discouraged in pregnancy and breastfeeding.[28]

Question B

Carbamazepine (Tegretol® Prolonged Release) is an enzyme inducer, which accelerates the metabolism of oestrogens present in Norinyl-1® tablets and may therefore reduce its effectiveness. Considering long-term concomitant use, a COC with a higher oestrogen content (50 micrograms) has been chosen and is taken as a 'tricyclic' regimen (i.e. taking three packets of tablets without a break followed by a shortened tablet-free interval of 4 days). St John's wort also contains some enzyme-inducing substances and therefore may reduce the effectiveness of COCs. Concomitant use should generally be avoided if possible.[29–31]

Question 23

Question A

As many as one-third of all patients taking vigabatrin experience visual field defects. Any signs and symptoms suggestive of such defects should be referred for an urgent ophthalmology opinion, and gradual withdrawal of vigabatrin should be considered. Isotretinoin commonly causes dryness of the eyes, which may be accompanied by blepharitis and/or conjunctivitis. This may or may not require the withdrawal of treatment.[32]

Question B

Antihistamines (such as chlorphenamine) may reduce the blink rate and lacrimation, which may introduce discomfort for patients wearing contact lenses. Isotretinoin can affect the contact lens wearer by causing conjunctival inflammation.[32]

Question 24

Question A

Corticosteroids (prednisolone) and NSAIDs, such as naproxen, may lead to fluid accumulation (precipitating a component of heart failure) and a rise in blood pressure. The patient is not receiving regular paracetamol, which may reduce the need for an NSAID to manage his osteoarthritis. Long-term prednisolone is not generally indicated for the management of COPD. Mr JH is not on a regular long-acting antimuscarinic agent (e.g. tiotropium) or theophylline, which should be tried before the long-term corticosteroid is initiated. Pseudoephedrine is a vasoconstrictor and may induce hypertension. It should be withdrawn since there is no clear indication for its use in this patient.[33,34]

Question B

Amiodarone commonly causes the development of reversible corneal microdeposits which sometimes presents with night glare and may affect the patient's ability to drive in the dark.[35]

References

1. *SSRIs (Selective Serotonin Reuptake Inhibitors) – Side Effects* [Online]. London: NHS Choices; 2012 [cited 27 March 2013]. Available at: www.nhs.uk/Conditions/ SSRIs-%28selective-serotonin-reuptake-inhibitors%29/Pages/Side-effects.aspx

2. *Erythema Multiforme* [Online]. PubMed Health; 2012 [cited 1 January 2013]. Available at: www.ncbi.nlm.nih.gov/pubmedhealth/PMH0001854/

3. *Martindale: the complete drug reference* [Online]. Available at: www.medicines complete.com/

4. National Institute for Health and Clinical Excellence. *Clopidogrel and Modified-Release Dipyridamole for the Prevention of Occlusive Vascular Events (Review of Technology Appraisal Guidance 90): quick reference guide.* London: NICE; 2010. Available at: www.nice.org.uk/nicemedia/live/13285/52189/52189.pdf

5. National Institute for Health and Clinical Excellence. *Lipid Modification: NICE guideline 67 – quick reference guide.* London: NICE; 2010. Available at: www.nice. org.uk/nicemedia/live/11982/40675/40675.pdf

6. Schwartz GG, Olsson AG, Ezekowitz MD, *et al*. Effects of atorvastatin on early recurrent ischemic events in acute coronary syndromes: the MIRACL study: a randomized controlled trial. *JAMA*. 2001; **285**(13): 1711–18.

7. *Stockley's Drug Interactions* [Online]. Available at: www.medicinescomplete.com/

8. *Clopidogrel and Proton Pump Inhibitors: interaction – updated advice* [Online]. Medicines and Healthcare Products Regulatory Agency; 2010 [cited 21 September 2013]. Available at: www.mhra.gov.uk/Safetyinformation/DrugSafetyUpdate/CON087711

9. *Rhabdomyolysis* [Online]. PubMed Health; 2011 [cited 4 January 203]. Available at: www.ncbi.nlm.nih.gov/pubmedhealth/PMH0001505/

10. *Simvastatin: updated advice on drug interactions – updated contraindications* [Online]. Medicines and Healthcare Products Regulatory Agency; 2012 [cited 4 January 2013]. Available at: www.mhra.gov.uk/Safetyinformation/DrugSafetyUpdate/CON180637

11. Blood S. Medication considerations before surgery. *Pharm J*. 2012; **288**: 179.

12. Rahman MH, Beattie J. Peri-operative medication in patients with cardiovascular disease. *Pharm J*. 2004; **272**: 352–4.

13. Smith I, Jackson I. Beta-blockers, calcium channel blockers, angiotensin converting enzyme inhibitors and angiotensin receptor blockers: should they be stopped or not before ambulatory anaesthesia? *Curr Opin Anaesthesiol*. 2010; **23**(6): 687–90.

14. Wu ZL, Geng H. Combination of tolterodine and tamsulosin for benign prostatic hyperplasia [Chinese]. *Zhonghua Nan Ke Xue*. 2009; **15**(7): 639–41.

15. Cagir B. Ileus [Online]. *Medscape*; 2013 [cited 27 March 2013]. Available at: http://emedicine.medscape.com/article/178948-overview#a0199

16. White R, Bradnam V. *Handbook of Drug Administration via Enteral Feeding Tubes* [Online] 2013. Available at: www.medicinescomplete.com

17. Rahman MH, Beattie J. Medication in the peri-operative period. *Pharm J*. 2004; **272**: 287–9.

18. *Domperidone: small risk of serious ventricular arrhythmia and sudden cardiac death* [Online]. Medicines and Healthcare Products Regulatory Agency; 2012 [cited 6 January 2013]. Available at: www.mhra.gov.uk/Safetyinformation/DrugSafety Update/CON152725

19. *Intravenous Ondansetron: important new dose restriction* [Online]. Medicines and Healthcare Products Regulatory Agency; 2012 [cited 6 January 2013]. Available at: www.mhra.gov.uk/Safetyinformation/Safetywarningsalertsandrecalls/Safetywarningsandmessagesformedicines/CON178189

20. National Patient Safety Agency. *Prevention of Harm with Alfacalcidol Preparations* [Online]; 2011 [cited 22 September 2013]. Available at: www.nrls.npsa.nhs.uk/signals/?entryid45=132827

21. O'Driscoll BR, Howard LS, Davison AG; British Thoracic Society. BTS guideline for emergency oxygen use in adult patients. *Thorax*. 2008; **63**(6): vi1–68. Available at: www.brit-thoracic.org.uk/portals/0/guidelines/emergency%20oxygen%20guideline/appendix%201%20summary%20of%20recommendations.pdf

22. Lee A. Mental health disorders. In: *Adverse Drug Reactions*. 2nd ed. London: Pharmaceutical Press; 2006. pp. 352–5.

23. Proprietary Association of Great Britain. *OTC Directory 2010/2011*. London: Communications International Group; 2010.

24. Summary of Product Characteristics Night Nurse [Online]. Electronic Medicines Compendium; 2012 [cited 22 September 2013]. Available at: www.medicines.org.uk/emc/medicine/19915/SPC/Night+Nurse/#INDICATIONS

25. *Summary of Product Characteristics Mirtazapine 15mg Tablets* [Online]. Electronic Medicines Compendium; 2010 [cited 26 January 2013]. Available at: www.medicines.org.uk/EMC/medicine/23038/SPC/Mirtazapine+15mg+Tablets/#MACHINE OPS

26. *Citalopram and escitalopram: QT interval prolongation – new maximum daily dose restrictions (including in elderly patients), contraindications, and warnings* [Online]. Medicines and Healthcare Products Regulatory Agency; 2011 [cited 10 February 2013]. Available at: www.mhra.gov.uk/Safetyinformation/DrugSafetyUpdate/CON137769

27. *Summary of Product Characteristics Zopiclone 3.75mg Tablets* [Online]. Electronic Medicines Compendium; 2009 [cited 10 February 2013]. Available at: www.medicines.org.uk/EMC/medicine/24285/SPC/Zopiclone+3.75mg+Tablets./

28. Burgess A. *Is It Safe for Breast Feeding Women to Take Herbal Medicines?* [Online]. NHS Evidence; 2012 [cited 30 November 2013]. Available at: www.evidence.nhs.uk/search?q=%22Is+it+safe+for+breastfeeding+women+to+take+herbal+medicines%22

29. *Summary of Product Characteristics Tegretol Prolonged Release 200mg and 400mg Tablets (Formerly Tegretol Retard)* [Online]. Electronic Medicines Compendium; 2012 [cited 10 February 2013]. Available at: www.medicines.org.uk/EMC/medicine/24201/SPC/Tegretol+Prolonged+Release+200mg+nd+400mg+Tablets+%28formerly+Tegretol+retard%29/

30. *Summary of Product Characteristics Ciprofloxacin 500mg Film-Coated Tablets* [Online]. Electronic Medicines Compendium; 2012 [cited 10 February 2013]. Available at: www.medicines.org.uk/EMC/medicine/25756/SPC/Ciprofloxacin+500mg++Film-Coated+Tablets/#PREGNANCY

31. *Summary of Product Characteristics Norinyl-1 Tablets* [Online]. Electronic Medicines Compendium; 2007 [cited 10 February 2013]. Available at: www.medicines.org. uk/EMC/medicine/1920/SPC/Norinyl-1+Tablets/#INTERACTIONS

32. *Summary of Product Characteristics Isotretinoin 20mg Capsules* [Online]. Electronic Medicines Compendium; 2012 [cited 10 February 2013]. Available at: www.medicines. org.uk/EMC/medicine/15655/SPC/Isotretinoin+20mg+capsules/

33. *Summary of Product Characteristics Prednisolone 1mg Tablets* [Online]. Electronic Medicines Compendium; 2012 [cited 10 February 2013]. Available at: www.medicines. org.uk/EMC/medicine/24113/SPC/Prednisolone+1mg+Tablets/

34. *Summary of Product Characteristics Day Nurse Capsules* [Online]. Electronic Medicines Compendium; 2012 [cited 10 February 2013]. Available at: www. medicines.org.uk/EMC/medicine/20671/SPC/Day+Nurse+Capsules/

35. *Summary of Product Characteristics Amiodarone 100mg Tablets* [Online]. Electronic Medicines Compendium; 2012 [cited 10 February 2013]. Available at: www.medicines. org.uk/EMC/medicine/25743/SPC/Amiodarone+100mg+Tablets/

CHAPTER 3: PLANNING MANAGEMENT

Question 1

Correct answers: A and C

Amoxicillin is indicated as part of the triple eradication regimen for *H. pylori*. A is the correct dose as per the *H. pylori* eradication table in the BNF for this regimen. Option B contains an incorrect dose of amoxicillin. Metronidazole is indicated as part of the *H. pylori* eradication regimen together with amoxicillin. Clarithromycin is not indicated for *H. pylori* eradication because the patient has recently received a course of erythromycin (a macrolide).

Question 2

Correct answers: C and D

The likely diagnosis is an overdose of aspirin in view of the tinnitus and metabolic acidosis. Activated charcoal is not indicated in this case because it has been more than 1 hour after the patient has had an overdose of aspirin. The patient's Ca^{2+} is just below the normal range and is not a priority. Correcting a low K^+ and pH are significantly more important in the presence of a metabolic acidosis. Moreover, concomitant administration of Ca^{2+} and bicarbonate should be avoided as it can result in precipitation. Option C is correct because plasma K^+ should be corrected before administration of bicarbonate as hypokalaemia may complicate alkalinisation of the urine. Sodium bicarbonate would enhance the excretion of salicylates and would help to correct severe metabolic acidosis experienced in this case. Correcting PO_4^{3-} is not a priority because it is just outside the normal range and therefore Option E is incorrect.

Question 3

Correct answers: C and E

Co-amoxiclav is indicated as antibiotic prophylaxis in colectomy, however it should be administered as a monotherapy. Teicoplanin is only added to prophylactic antibiotic regimens in colectomy where there is a high risk of MRSA. Metronidazole is indicated as antibiotic prophylaxis in colectomy (up to three further doses of 500 mg may be given if needed) when used together with gentamicin (1.5 mg/kg). Cefuroxime is indicated as antibiotic prophylaxis in colectomy when used together with metronidazole, nevertheless it should be given at a dose of 1.5 g 30 minutes before the procedure (with up to three further doses of 750 mg given if required).

Question 4

Correct answers: A and E

The likely diagnosis is sympathetic block induced by epidural anaesthesia (bupivacaine). Ephedrine is a preferred pressor drug used to treat hypotension/bradycardia resulting from this block. Noradrenaline or phenylephrine can be used to treat acute hypotension; however, ephedrine is a preferred choice of drug for the reversal of hypotension from epidural anaesthesia. In practice, the general rule would be to instigate more oxygen than less as the following step. This is especially important in pregnant patients who are at risk of PEs. In the majority of cases it would be reasonable to start at an O_2 concentration of 40% aiming for a saturation of >95%. A saturation level of 88%–92% is usually reserved for COPD patients at risk of hypercapnic respiratory failure.

Question 5

Correct answers: B and C

Glyceryl trinitrate (GTN) is not licensed to control BP following a haemorrhagic stroke. It is used to control BP and myocardial ischaemia in cardiac surgery, congestive heart failure and unstable angina. Nimodipine, a calcium-channel blocker, is given to reduce cerebral artery spasm and further neurological deterioration following an aneurysmal subarachnoid haemorrhage. It is also likely to help cautiously control the hypertension experienced by Mr GH. Mr GH has suffered major bleeding (potentially due to excessive anticoagulation secondary to newly started amiodarone, which increases the effect of warfarin). He should be treated as per 'major bleeding' guidance for warfarin patients in the BNF. Phenindione (an oral anticoagulant) should not be confused with phytomenadione (or vitamin K), which is a natural coagulant. The regimen outlined in Option E relates to the management of 'minor bleeding' as opposed to the 'major bleeding' that was experienced by Mr GH in this case.

Question 6

Correct answers: A and E

The likely diagnosis is suspected pelvic inflammatory disease (PID). Ceftriaxone is indicated for the treatment of suspected PID; however, the patient has a severe allergy to beta-lactams (ceftriaxone). Therefore, the regimen comprising doxycycline + metronidazole + ceftriaxone can be ruled out.

The alternative regimen comprises ofloxacin + metronidazole. Azithromycin is not indicated for the treatment of PID.[1]

Question 7

Correct answers: B and D

The likely diagnosis is severe acute asthma, and therefore both oral prednisolone (at a dose of 40 mg rather than 50 mg OD for a 7-year-old) and salbutamol nebules are indicated. Ipratropium should only be used for severe acute asthma (as per BNF table for the Management of Acute Asthma) if initial response to short-acting beta$_2$ agonist (e.g. salbutamol) is inadequate after 15–30 minutes. Terbutaline is indicated as part of the management of severe acute asthma, however this administration interval is more appropriate for life-threatening rather than severe acute asthma.

Question 8

Correct answers: C and E

The likely diagnosis is DKA. Calcium gluconate is used to treat hyperkalaemia, however the patient only has a marginally raised potassium and hence treatment is not required. The Levemir® treatment should be continued as it is generally not recommended to stop the established subcutaneous therapy with long-acting insulin analogues during the treatment of DKA. An infusion of soluble insulin should be initiated alongside the regular established long-acting insulin therapy. Glucose 10% infusion should only be initiated when the BM falls below <14 mmol/L. NaCl 0.9% infusion replaces fluids lost during a DKA episode. Potassium replacement is necessary to maintain the plasma K$^+$ within normal range once the action of insulin becomes apparent.[2]

Question 9

Correct answers: A and C

It is likely that Mrs O'Neill exhibits the signs of methotrexate-induced neutropenia with a tendency to progress to pancytopenia. The risk factors for bone marrow suppression with methotrexate include old age, renal impairment (methotrexate is cleared renally) and concomitant use with other anti-folate drugs, such as trimethoprim. Acute diarrhoea may act as another indicator of methotrexate toxicity. Note that methotrexate itself may also induce renal failure and acute tubular necrosis. Such effects may have precipitated the accumulation of the drug and may have predisposed Mrs O'Neill to toxicity. In addition, it should not be forgotten that dementia and allied confusion may have led to an unintentional overdose of methotrexate by the patient herself. Both methotrexate and trimethoprim should be stopped. Alternative management options should be sought once the patient recovers from this episode. Donepezil can be safely used and does not need to be stopped. The administration of calcium folinate (folinic acid) is a common 'rescue' therapy in suspected methotrexate toxicity. In contrast to folic acid, folinic acid does not require activation by dihydrofolate reductase and therefore is unaffected by methotrexate, which inhibits this enzyme. The initial dose of folinic acid should generally be equal to or exceed the dose of methotrexate implicated in the toxicity. Afterwards, advice from the poisons information service should be sought. Despite the fact that the patient is still neutropenic, she is also apyrexic, and low inflammatory markers make neutropenic sepsis a rather unlikely diagnosis. There is no sensitivity data available to suggest a switch to an alternative antimicrobial therapy (i.e. Option D is incorrect). The underlying cause of pancytopenia should be treated as appropriate. Current antimicrobials should be stopped once infection is completely ruled out. It may be reasonable to continue lenograstim for a few more days with careful monitoring of the WBC and neutrophil count. Once folinic acid starts working, a marked increase in these counts may be expected making further administration of lenograstim unnecessary, i.e. a total treatment duration of 10 days may be excessive.[3]

Question 10

Correct answers: B and D

While Mr McKee is known to the palliative care team, he does not appear to be permanently nil by mouth or critically unwell in order to be considered for continuous subcutaneous infusions. Oxycodone is an alternative strong opioid in patients who cannot tolerate morphine. In this case intolerance presented as gastrointestinal upset and hypotension. According to the dose equivalence chart for morphine salts (oral) and oxycodone (oral), a 10 mg dose of morphine is equal to a 6.6 mg dose of oxycodone. This may be administered as OxyContin® 5 mg BD. The 4- to 6-hourly 'breakthrough pain' dose of oxycodone (OxyNorm®) is equal to one-tenth to one-sixth of the regular 24-hour total daily dose, i.e. 10 mg × 1/10 or 10 mg × 1/6 = 1.0–1.5 mg every 4–6 hours. Transdermal opioid preparations (e.g. fentanyl) are generally initiated when the patient's opioid requirements are stable over time. Note that opioid preparations for Mr McKee were only started about a week before hospital admission, and their doses are still likely to change considerably. Diamorphine by SC or IM injection would be a 'breakthrough pain' option if Mr McKee's nausea and vomiting were prolonged and/or if he was to be initiated on a continuous subcutaneous diamorphine infusion.

Question 11

Correct answers: B and E

Mrs King is likely to have presented with primary angle-closure glaucoma (PACG), which may have been precipitated by amitriptyline and/or chlorphenamine (the two medicines which possess antimuscarinic activity). PACG is managed by surgical interventions, i.e. iridectomy or iridotomy. Following surgery, amitriptyline may either be re-started (if iridectomy/iridotomy remains patent) or (more realistically) be switched to a safer alternative, such as pregabalin. Chlorphenamine should also be withheld before the procedure and may either be re-started following surgery or switched to alternatives with lower antimuscarinic activity, such as loratadine or cetirizine. Beta-blockers, such as betaxolol, are of great benefit in primary open-angle glaucoma, however they are inappropriate for use in PACG where an urgent reduction in intra-ocular pressure and surgical intervention is required. A beta-blocker is sometimes prescribed as a supplementary treatment following surgery for PACG. Mannitol helps to urgently reduce the intra-ocular pressure in PACG and is often prescribed prior to surgery. Where necessary, this may be accompanied by an IV injection of acetazolamide, a carbonic anhydrase inhibitor, which also lowers intra-ocular pressure.[4-8]

Question 12

Correct answers: A and B

Four drops (8 mg) of citalopram liquid are equivalent to the therapeutic effect of a 10 mg tablet. Therefore, a 20 mg dose of citalopram is equivalent to approximately eight oral drops. Ninety-two milligrams of phenytoin base (contained in Epanutin® Infatabs®) is equivalent to approximately 100 mg of phenytoin sodium (contained in Epanutin® capsules). Therefore, a 150 mg dose of Epanutin® Infatabs® is equivalent to 150 mg × 100 mg/92 mg, or 163 mg, of Epanutin® capsules. The powder in Epanutin® capsules (175 mg) should be mixed with 10 mL of water and 9.3 mL of the dispersion (10 mL × 163 mg/175 mg) should be administered via the NG tube. Note that Epanutin®

suspension is thixotropic and cannot be administered via the NG tube. No such information regarding NG administration is available for Epanutin® Infatabs®. IV vancomycin does not significantly permeate the intestinal wall and therefore is not effective in the treatment of *C. difficile*. Nevertheless, it may still predispose the patient to adverse effects, such as nephro- and oto-toxicity. In this case, the IV vancomycin powder may have to be given orally because the contents of vancomycin capsules are gel-formed and are not suitable for administration via the NG tube. IV metronidazole is an option; however, Mr Landgren has already completed at least 4 days of oral vanco-mycin and therefore it may be more appropriate for him to finish a 10- to 14-day course of vancomycin before IV metronidazole is tried (the dose of vancomycin may be increased to 250–500 mg QDS if deemed appropriate fol-lowing a discussion with the Microbiologist). Although the dose equivalence is correct (100 mg of Tegretol® tablets = 125 mg of Tegretol® suppositories), the administration of carbamazepine PR is normally reserved for patients in whom this medicine is used to manage epilepsy. Whilst this may partially be the case for Mr Landgren, it is more likely that carbamazepine is prescribed to help his trigeminal neuralgia (TDS dosing). Considering the fact that he is to have an NG tube inserted, it may be more appropriate to switch Tegretol® tablets to Tegretol® liquid (100 mg/5 mL). The unnecessary three times daily administration of suppositories may also be rather inconvenient for nursing staff and unpleasant for the patient.[9–11]

Question 13

Correct answers: C and E

Alpha$_1$-selective alpha blockers, such as tamsulosin, are generally indicated by NICE as the first-line treatment option in men with moderate to severe lower urinary tract symptoms resembling benign prostatic hyperplasia (BPH). However, Mr PO's history of postural hypotension and previous/upcoming cataract surgeries makes tamsulosin a less suitable choice for the management of suspected BPH. NICE recommends 5-alpha reductase inhibitors, such as finasteride, as a treatment option in men with lower urinary tract symptoms and a prostate that is estimated to be larger than 30 g (or prostate-specific antigen greater than 1.4 ng/mL and high risk of progression). Since an alpha blocker is not a suitable option in this case, finasteride should be considered as the second-line most effective therapy for Mr PO. Levodopa has been reported to cause urinary retention, however this effect is rather rare. It is necessary to maintain an effective control of Parkinson's disease, hence the dose reduction of Stalevo® is not a reasonable option. As a mineralocorticoid, fludrocortisone has an intrinsic effect of fluid retention. However, the importance of preventing postural hypotension (and any consequences, such as accidental falls) is likely to outweigh the risks associated with fluid retention, particularly at a dose as low as 50 micrograms a day. Mr PO does not have any past medical history of urinary incontinence. It is therefore likely that oxybutynin, an antimuscarinic agent, was prescribed to manage the urgency experienced by Mr PO in the past, which may have been an early symptom of BPH. Oxybutynin may cause urinary retention as an antimuscarinic adverse effect and should be avoided in Mr PO's case as far as possible.[12]

References

1. *Pelvic Inflammatory Disease* [Online]. London: Clinical Knowledge Summaries; 2013 [cited 2 December 2013]. Available at: http://cks.nice.org.uk/pelvic-inflammatory-disease

1. *The Management of Diabetic Ketoacidosis in Adults* [Online]. Joint British Diabetes Societies Inpatient Care Group; 2010 [cited 22 September 2013]. Available at: www.bsped.org.uk/clinical/docs/DKAManagementOfDKAinAdultsMarch20101.pdf

2. *Summary of Product Characteristics Methotrexate 2.5 mg Tablets* [Online]. Electronic Medicines Compendium; 2012 [cited 28 March 2013]. Available at: www.medicines.org.uk/EMC/medicine/12033/SPC/Methotrexate+2.5+mg+Tablets/#PHARMACOKINETIC_PROPS

3. Titcomb LC, Andrew SD. Glaucoma. In: Walker R, Whittlesea C, editors. *Clinical Pharmacy and Therapeutics*. 4th ed. London: Churchill Livingstone Elsevier; 2007. pp. 789–806.

4. National Institute for Health and Clinical Excellence. *Neuropathic Pain – pharmacological management: NICE guideline 96 – quick reference guide*. London: NICE; 2010. Available at: www.nice.org.uk/nicemedia/pdf/CG96QuickRefGuide.pdf

5. *Summary of Product Characteristics Lyrica Capsules* [Online]. Electronic Medicines Compendium; 2009 [cited 29 March 2013]. Available at: www.medicines.org.uk/EMC/medicine/14651/SPC/Lyrica+Capsules/

6. *Summary of Product Characteristics Amitriptyline 10mg Film-coated Tablets* [Online]. Electronic Medicines Compendium; 2005 [cited 29 March 2013]. Available at: www.medicines.org.uk/EMC/medicine/25741/SPC/Amitriptyline+10mg+Film-coated+Tablets/

7. *Summary of Product Characteristics Piriton Allergy Tablets* [Online]. Electronic Medicines Compendium; 1997 [cited 29 March 2013]. Available at: www.medicines.org.uk/EMC/medicine/16103/SPC/Piriton+Allergy+Tablets/

8. *Summary of Product Characteristics Vancomycin 1g Powder for Solution for Infusion* [Online]. Electronic Medicines Compendium; 2008 [cited 29 March 2013]. Available at: www.medicines.org.uk/EMC/medicine/20835/SPC/Vancomycin+1 g+Powder+for+Solution+for+Infusion+%28Wockhardt+UK+Ltd%29/#PHARM ACOKINETIC_PROPS

9. White R, Bradnam V. *Handbook of Drug Administration via Enteral Feeding Tubes* [Online] 2013. Available at: www.medicinescomplete.com

10. *Antimicrobial Policies and Guidelines*. Redhill: Surrey and Sussex Healthcare NHS Trust; 2012.

11. Gower RL. Benign prostatic hyperplasia. In: Walker R, Whittlesea C, editors. *Clinical Pharmacy and Therapeutics*. 4th ed. London: Churchill Livingstone Elsevier; 2007. pp. 691–8.

12. National Institute for Health and Clinical Excellence. *The Management of Lower Urinary Tract Symptoms in Men: NICE guideline 97 – quick reference guide*. London: NICE; 2010. Available at: www.nice.org.uk/nicemedia/live/12984/48575/48575. pdf

CHAPTER 4: COMMUNICATING INFORMATION

Question 1

Correct answers: B and E

There is no need to avoid alcohol while being treated with pioglitazone. However, pioglitazone should be discontinued if jaundice develops because of rare reports of liver toxicity. The incidence of heart failure is increased when pioglitazone is combined with insulin (not metformin). Pioglitazone carries a small increased risk of bladder (not prostate) cancer. Therefore, haematuria, dysuria or urinary urgency should be reported during treatment.[1]

Question 2

Correct answers: D and E

Although NSAIDs can potentially reduce the excretion of methotrexate, there is no need to stop taking diclofenac since it had been initiated before methotrexate was started. The patient should be monitored for any signs/symptoms of methotrexate toxicity. Paracetamol does not increase the risk of methotrexate toxicity. Folic acid should be taken once weekly on a *different* day from methotrexate (to provide a time interval for the therapeutic effect of methotrexate). Methotrexate has been reported to cause pulmonary toxicity, e.g. pneumonitis (hence, the symptoms of dyspnoea or cough) and liver toxicity, e.g. cirrhosis (hence the symptoms of nausea or abdominal discomfort).

Question 3

Correct answers: B and E

Both heparin (and low-molecular-weight heparins, such as enoxaparin) and losartan may induce hyperkalaemia (the risk is higher in renal impairment). Withhold heparin and losartan until potassium is within normal range. A STAT dose of NeoRecormon® (epoetin beta) is unlikely to be of any benefit in this situation. In fact it may make hyperkalaemia worse (hyperkalaemia is reported among the side effects of epoetin beta). The patient is not suffering from significant metabolic acidosis – and hence there is no need for bicarbonate. Calcium gluconate and insulin are given for the management of acute hyperkalaemia.

Question 4

Correct answers: C and E

In order to complete a 90-day cycle, she should take 1 *white* tablet (etidronate) for 14 days, followed by 1 *pink* tablet (calcium carbonate) for 76 days. She should avoid food for at least 2 hours before and *2 hours after* taking the white tablet (disodium etidronate). The absorption of bisphosphonates may also be reduced by oral iron (ferrous sulphate). Leaving a 2- to 3-hour gap between the administration of these medicines may reduce the risk of such an interaction. The warning presented in Option B applies to other bisphosphonates, including alendronic acid and risedronate. It is not applicable to etidronate. Following the advice set out in Option C may help to reduce the risk of developing serious osteonecrosis of the jaw that may be induced by bisphosphonate treatment.[2]

Question 5

Correct answers: A and D

Pancreatin is inactivated by gastric acid and therefore is best taken with food (or immediately before or after food). Creon® should be taken immediately after being mixed with fluids/food, otherwise dissolution of the enteric coating might occur. While she should avoid mixing Creon® with hot fluids or foods (pancreatin is inactivated by heat), using antacids with Creon® would not do any harm. In fact, it may help by reducing the acidity of the gastric environment. Option C is incorrect because Creon® 10000 is not a higher-strength preparation of pancreatin. While the mum should be aware of the possibility that Creon® may cause lower bowel strictures, this has been mainly reported for higher-strength preparations of pancreatin (excluding higher-strength preparations of Creon®).[3]

Question 6

Correct answers: B and C

Although a theoretical interaction between temazepam (benzodiazepine) and paroxetine (SSRI) does exist, it may not be clinically significant and it is best for Debbie to continue temazepam until the effects of paroxetine kick in. Temazepam can then be reviewed for discontinuation (provided her insomnia was depression-induced). She should stop taking OTC sumatriptan (5HT$_1$ agonist) because its concomitant use with paroxetine may increase the risk of CNS toxicity. It is important to review the aetiology of her headaches and to ensure the most appropriate treatment is prescribed by the GP or by the specialist. Similarly to other SSRIs, paroxetine has been associated with suicidal behaviour, particularly in children and young adults, and at the beginning of the treatment (Option C). While the symptoms presented in Option D may warrant a medical consultation, Debbie should not stop the treatment abruptly as that may cause an antidepressant withdrawal reaction. In fact, all the symptoms in Option D can be implicated as part of the withdrawal reaction. The angle-closure glaucoma may very rarely be precipitated by SSRIs; however, it is not a common side effect.

Question 7

Correct answers: D and E

As a hepatic enzyme inhibitor, erythromycin *increases* the plasma concentration and hence the effect of ethinylestradiol contained in Microgynon 30®. However, Miss AP should still resume taking her 'pill' as soon as possible and then abstain from intercourse or use an additional method of contraception such as condoms for the next 7 days because she missed two 'pills' in a row due to nausea and vomiting. 'Tricycling' (unlicensed regimen) is only recommended for cases where hormonal contraceptives are used with enzyme-inducing medicines (except rifampicin and rifabutin), e.g. ritonavir or St John's wort. The symptoms presented in Option E may indicate venous thromboembolism (deep vein thrombosis or pulmonary embolism) and may warrant a prompt discontinuation of the 'pill' followed by appropriate treatment.

Question 8

Correct answers: C and D

While peripheral neuropathy has been reported as a side effect of amiodarone therapy, the stiffness and coldness of Paul's legs are more likely to be caused by a beta blocker (carvedilol). Myopathy is a well-known side effect of statin therapy; however, the stiffness and coldness of Paul's legs are more likely to be a result of a beta-blocker therapy. Acebutolol, a beta blocker with intrinsic sympathomimetic activity (partial agonist), is an alternative to carvedilol and may cause less coldness of the extremities. Beta blockers are known to cause fluctuations in T2DM control (both hyper- and hypoglycaemia). Cardio-selective beta blockers, such as bisoprolol, may be an alternative option in such cases. Even though water-soluble beta blockers are less likely to cause sleep disturbances, they are not necessarily a better choice in T2DM (with an exception of atenolol, which is cardioselective).

Question 9

Correct answers: A and E

The 'colour-dose' guidance in Option A is correct: 1 mg (brown) tablet + 3 mg (blue) tablet = 4 mg. It is important that the patient does not misinterpret the caution with vitamin K-containing products. She should be advised to not introduce major changes to her diet while on warfarin rather than be asked to stop taking one class of food, because cutting out the vitamin K products from her diet may destabilise the patient further and increase her risk of bleeding. She should avoid introducing major changes to the consumption of alcohol (e.g. binge drinking), which may affect the anticoagulant control. A few glasses of wine a week taken at regular intervals should not be harmful. Grapefruit juice should not be confused with cranberry juice, which can enhance the anticoagulant effect of warfarin (but be careful about using grapefruit juice and statins!). Aspirin and NSAIDs (e.g. ibuprofen or diclofenac) can enhance the anticoagulant effects of warfarin, and in order to avoid that, the patient should be advised not to self-medicate with these products unless recommended to do so by her doctor or another competent healthcare professional.

Question 10

Correct answers: B and C

Baby Thomas is due for the first dose of pneumococcal polysaccharide conjugate vaccine; however, Prevenar 13®, a 13-valent conjugate vaccine, rather than Synflorix®, a 10-valent conjugate vaccine, is recommended as part of the childhood immunisation schedule. The 'high dose' diphtheria toxoid-containing vaccines, such as Pediacel®, are used in primary immunisation of children under 10 years of age. Option C is correct and reflects the advice set out in the BNF under 'Post-immunisation pyrexia in infants'. If pyrexia persists, parents should be advised to seek medical advice. The dose of ibuprofen recommended for post-immunisation fever under 'Post-immunisation pyrexia in infants' is 50 mg (only given under doctor's advice). The actual dose that baby Thomas may have (according to the Children's BNF) is 5 mg/kg or about 25 mg three to four times daily. Option E would be correct for any live attenuated vaccines. In contrast, baby Thomas is to receive an inactivated vaccine of poliomyelitis (as part of Pediacel®) rather than the live attenuated one. The live (oral) poliomyelitis vaccine is reserved for use during infection outbreaks.[4]

Question 11

Correct answers: A and E

Isotretinoin therapy should be started at 500 micrograms/kg/day, i.e. 0.5 mg × 56 kg = 28 mg in Janette's case. This rounds up to 30 mg, or one 10 mg and one 20 mg capsule taken once daily in total. If needed, the dose can be increased to 1 mg/kg/day after a further review. Women receiving isotretinoin should avoid blood donations during the treatment and for at least *one* month after stopping isotretinoin. Isotretinoin is teratogenic and this requires the use of at least *one* method of contraception (two methods are preferred). However, POCs are not considered effective, and women of childbearing potential should seek alternatives, such as COCs. Women of childbearing potential receiving isotretinoin should be tested for pregnancy *every month* during the treatment (unless there are reasons to suggest that there is no risk of pregnancy) and 5 weeks after stopping the treatment. The pregnancy test should be performed in the first 3 days of the menstrual cycle. Both doxycycline and isotretinoin have been reported to cause photosensitivity reactions. Women receiving isotretinoin should avoid exposure to UV light (including sunlight), and should use sunscreen and emollientS from the start of the treatment.[5]

Question 12

Correct answers: C and D

Qvar® contains extra-fine particles and is approximately twice as potent as Clenil Modulite® inhaler, suggesting an equivalent dose of 100 micrograms BD. This answer would therefore be correct for a patient with well-controlled asthma. However, Layla was admitted to hospital with an acute exacerbation, suggesting poorly controlled chronic asthma. As a result, she should receive a dose of 200 micrograms BD until further review (see BNF guidance under the Qvar® monograph). Inhaled corticosteroid inhalers should be used regularly as 'preventers'; however, it takes approximately 3–7 days to achieve alleviation of symptoms. Inhaled beclometasone is not known to pose any significant risks to the baby during pregnancy and breastfeeding. Poorly controlled asthma may itself threaten pregnancy, and therefore the benefits of using asthma medicines during pregnancy often outweigh the risks. It is probable that beclometasone is excreted in mothers' milk; however, considering the inhaled route of administration and relatively low doses, the risk to the baby is minimal. For Option D, see BNF guidance under 'Candidiasis' for inhaled corticosteroids. Spacer devices (AeroChamber Plus®) reduce the impact of the drug on the oropharynx, hence the larger proportion of particles is deposited in the lungs. Spacer devices should be cleaned as stated in Option E. However, cleaning the spacer once a month is sufficient, i.e. daily washing is not required. More frequent cleaning may induce electrostatic charges that may in turn affect drug delivery.[6]

Question 13

Correct answers: A and C

For Option A, see the side effects of 'Prostaglandin analogues and prostamides' in the BNF. Prostaglandin analogues, such as latanoprost, may cause brown rather than blue pigmentation of the eyes, particularly in those with mixed-colour irides. Applying pressure on the lacrimal punctum of the eye for at least 1 minute after instilling the eye drops reduces the nasolacrimal drainage. This may also decrease the systemic absorption of the eye drops from the nasal mucosa. One drop of latanoprost should generally be applied to each eye in the evening. Instillation of more than one drop may not provide any benefit but instead may increase the risk of systemic side effects. An interval of at least 5 (not 15) minutes should be left between the application of two different eye drop preparations. In case of eye gels or suspensions, this interval may be extended further. See the 'Administration of drugs to the eye' in the BNF.[7,8]

References

1. National Institute for Health and Clinical Excellence. *Type 2 Diabetes: NICE guideline 87 – quick reference guide*. London: NICE; 2010. Available at: www.nice.org. uk/nicemedia/live/12165/44322/44322.pdf

2. *Stockley's Drug Interactions* [Online] 2013. Available at: www.medicinescom plete.com/mc/stockley/current/x07-3726.htm?q=diltiazem%20phenytoin& t=search&ss=text&p=1#_hit

3. *Summary of Product Characteristics Creon 10000 Capsules* [Online]. Electronic Medicines Compendium; 2013 [cited 29 March 2013]. Available at: www.medicines. org.uk/EMC/medicine/2068/SPC/Creon+10000+Capsules/#POSOLOGY

4. British Medical Association; Royal Pharmaceutical Society. *British National Formulary for Children* [Online]. London: Pharmaceutical Press; 2012. Available at: www.medicinescomplete.com

5. *Summary of Product Characteristics Isotretinoin 20mg Capsules* [Online]. Electronic Medicines Compendium; 2012 [cited 10 February 2013]. Available at: www.medicines. org.uk/EMC/medicine/15655/SPC/Isotretinoin+20mg+capsules/

6. *Summary of Product Characteristics Qvar MDI 100 micrograms* [Online]. Electronic Medicines Compendium; 2012 [cited 28 October 2012]. Available at: www.medicines. org.uk/EMC/medicine/23274/SPC/Qvar+MDI+100+micrograms

7. *Patient Information Leaflet Latanoprost 50mcg/ml Eye Drops* [Online]. Electronic Medicines Compendium; 2012 [cited 28 October 2012]. Available at: www.medicines.org.uk/EMC/medicine/25680/PIL/Latanoprost+50mcg+ml+eye+drops/

8. *Patient Information Leaflet Tears Naturale* [Online]. Electronic Medicines Compendium; 2010 [cited 28 October 2012]. Available at: www.medicines.org.uk/EMC/medicine/17865/PIL/Tears+Naturale/

CHAPTER 5: CALCULATION SKILLS

Question 1

Correct answer: 130 mg

    Working:

1. Weight (kg) = 6.35 kg × 10 = 63.5 kg
2. Height (cm) = (5 × 12 + 8) × 2.54 cm = 172.7 cm
3. BSA (m^2) = (63.5 kg × 172.7 cm / 3600)$^{1/2}$ m^2 ≈ 1.75 m^2
4. Dose (mg) = 75 mg/m^2 × 1.75 m^2 = 131.25 mg ≈ 130 mg.

Question 2

Correct answer: 9.4 mL/hr

    Working:

1. Dose (mg/min) = 3 µg/kg/min × 83 kg = 249 µg = 0.249 mg/min ≈ 0.25 mg/min
2. Dose (mg/hr) = 0.25 mg/min × 60 min = 15 mg/hr
3. Dose (mL/hr) = 15 mg/hr × 1 mL / 1.6 mg = 9.375 mL/hr ≈ 9.4 mL/hr.

NB the height of the patient, the strength of glucose solution and the size of the dopamine bag are irrelevant to the calculation.

Question 3

Correct answer: 2 mL

    Working:

1. Bioavailable fraction of digoxin tablets = 125 µg × 63 / 100 = 78.75 µg
2. Dose of digoxin elixir (micrograms) = 78.75 µg × 100 / 75 = 105 µg
3. Dose of digoxin elixir (mL) = 105 µg × 1 mL / 50 µg = 2.1 mL ≈ 2 mL.

Question 4

Correct answer: 800 mL

    Working:

1. The amount required for 1 week (mL) = 200 mL + 200 mL = 400 mL
2. The amount required for 2 weeks (mL) = 400 mL × 2 = 800 mL (200 mL × 4).

NB see the table of 'Suitable quantities of dermatological preparations to be prescribed for specific areas of the body' in the BNF, section 13.1.12.

Question 5

Correct answer: 0.4 mL

Working:

1. Dose (mg) = 5 mg/kg × 3.5 kg = 17.5 mg
2. Volume to be withdrawn from the vial (mL) = 17.5 mg × 1 mL / 40 mg = 0.4375 mL ≈ 0.4 mL.

NB the strength of sodium chloride infusion, the total volume of the final solution and the administration time are irrelevant to the calculation.

Question 6

Correct answer: 150 mg

Working:

1. Total daily dose of chlorpromazine = 100 mg × 3 = 300 mg
2. Total daily dose of clozapine = 300 mg × 50 / 100 = 150 mg.

NB see the table of 'Equivalent doses of oral antipsychotics' in the BNF, section 4.2.1.

Question 7

Correct answer: 192 mL

Working:

1. The number of millimoles to be infused over 24 hours = 4 mmol × 24 hours = 96 mmol
2. The volume of 50% magnesium sulphate solution required to provide 96 mmol = 96 mmol × 1 mL / 2 mmol = 48 mL
3. The total volume of the infusion = 10 mL/hr × 24 hours = 240 mL
4. The volume of glucose 5% required to produce the infusion = 240 mL – 48 mL = 192 mL.

NB the details of initial injection are irrelevant to the calculation.

Question 8

Correct answer: 40 hours

Working:

1. $T_{1/2}$ = 0.693/k = 0.693 / 0.03 h^{-1} = 23.1 hours ≈ 23 hours
2. A minimal fall in concentration required = 52 mg/L / 15 mg/L = 3.467 times ≈ 3.5 times

3. Time required to achieve a 3.5 times fall in concentration = 3.5 × 23 hours / 2 = 40.25 hours ≈ 40 hours.

NB the dose of phenytoin, the Vd and clearance equations are irrelevant to the calculation.[1,2]

Question 9

Correct answer: 30 mg
   Working:
1. The amount of morphine sulphate Mrs LM received as part of her background infusion in 24 hours = 2 mg × 24 h = 48 mg
2. The amount of morphine sulphate Mrs LM received as part of her PCA in 24 hours = 1 mg × 10 = 10 mg
3. The total amount of morphine sulphate Mrs LM received in 24 hours = 48 mg + 10 mg = 58 mg
4. The 12-hourly dose of MST Continus® required = 58 mg / 2 = 29 mg ≈ 30 mg.[3]

Question 10

Correct answer: 140 mg
   Working:
1. Weight (kg) = 7 × 6.35 kg + 5 × 0.45 kg = 46.7 kg
2. GFR (mL/min) = (140 – 87) × 46.7 kg × 1.04 / 145 μmol/L = 17.75 mL/min ≈ 18 mL/min
3. Dose (mg) = 3 mg/kg daily = 3 mg/kg × 46.7 kg = 140.1 mg ≈ 140 mg.

NB height is irrelevant to this calculation as ideal body weight is not required.

Question 11

Correct answer: 0.6%
   Working:
1. Background incidence of breast cancer over 10 years per 1000 women in Europe not using HRT (age range 50–59 years) = 20 (from the HRT Risk table in the BNF)
2. HRT-free 10-year risk of breast cancer expressed as % = 20 / 1000 × 100% = 2%

3. Additional cases over 10 years per 1000 women using oestrogen only HRT (age range 50–59 years) = 6
4. Total incidence over 10 years per 1000 women using oestrogen only HRT = 20 + 6 = 26
5. Total 10-year risk of breast cancer in women using oestrogen only HRT expressed as % = 26 / 1000 × 100% = 2.6%
6. Percentage difference in the risk of breast cancer with Evorel® '50' compared with HRT-free life = 2.6% – 2.0% = 0.6%.

NB see the table of 'HRT Risk' in the BNF, section 6.4.1.1.

Question 12

Correct answer: 690 mg
   Working:
1. Mean weight for a 7-year-old (kg) = 23 kg (see the table at the back of the BNF)
2. Loading dose (mg) = 20 mg/kg = 20 mg × 23 kg = 460 mg
3. Maintenance dose (mg) = 5 mg/kg = 5 mg × 23 kg = 115 mg
4. Total 24-hour dose (mg) = 460 mg + 115 mg × 2 = 690 mg.

Question 13

Correct answer: 21%. Yes, lipid-regulating therapy is indicated in Arjan's case.
   Working:
1. According to Joint British Societies' charts (at the back of the BNF), the 'baseline' 10-year risk of CVD for a non-diabetic, non-smoker male under 50 years of age with a systolic BP of 140 mmHg and a TC:HDL-C ratio of 4.7 mmol/L is approximately 10% (the upper range of the green zone). Where the HDL value is not available, one should assume it is equal to 1 mmol/L (see further guidance in the BNF).
2. However, the 'actual' CVD risk, which considers patients' ethnic background (originating from Indian subcontinent) and family history (first-degree relative had a CVD before the age of 65 years for a female), is approximately: 10% × 1.4 × 1.5 = 21%.
3. Lipid-regulating therapy for primary CVD prevention is likely to be of benefit in all patients with a 10-year CVD risk of 20% or more (i.e. high risk of CVD). This applies to Arjan's case, and he may benefit from lipid-regulating therapy, such as simvastatin 20–40 mg ON.[4]

References

1. Fitzpatrick R. Practical pharmacokinetics. In: Walker R, Whittlesea C, editors. *Clinical Pharmacy and Therapeutics*. 4th ed. London: Churchill Livingstone Elsevier; 2007. pp. 24–39.

2. *Summary of Product Characteristics Epanutin Capsules 25, 50 and 100mg* [Online]. Electronic Medicines Compendium; 2012 [cited 2 December 2013]. Available at: www.medicines.org.uk/emc/medicine/25070/SPC/Epanutin+capsules+25%2c+50+and+100mg/

3. Rahman MH, Beattie J. Managing post-operative pain. *Pharm J*. 2005; **275**: 145–8.

4. National Institute for Health and Clinical Excellence. *Lipid modification: NICE guidance 67 – quick reference guide*. London: NICE; 2010. Available at: www.nice.org.uk/nicemedia/live/11982/40675/40675.pdf

CHAPTER 6: ADVERSE DRUG REACTIONS

Question 1

Correct answers: A and D

Weight gain is a common adverse effect of sodium valproate treatment. Liver toxicity is a known adverse drug reaction (ADR) of sodium valproate therapy; however, it is relatively rare compared with weight gain or hair loss. Blood and hepatic disorders have been reported in patients receiving sodium valproate, but they are also rare. Transient hair loss is a rather common side effect of sodium valproate treatment. Pancreatitis has also been reported in patients taking sodium valproate; however, it is a very rare ADR of this medicine.

Question 2

Correct answers: C and D

A deterioration in renal function due to aspirin therapy (most likely as a result of afferent arteriolar constriction) has been reported; however, it is relatively uncommon. Clopidogrel does not appear to cause any detectable renal impairment. Metformin itself does not cause renal impairment. Nevertheless, it may lead to lactic acidosis in the presence of renal failure induced by iodine-containing contrast media, which causes renal medullary ischaemia because of renal vasoconstriction. Similarly, ciclosporin (Neoral®) can induce ischaemic acute tubular necrosis. While prednisolone should be used with caution in patients with renal impairment, it has not been reported to cause deterioration in kidney function.[1–5]

Question 3

Correct answers: D and E

ACE inhibitors (ramipril) have been reported to cause myalgia on rare occasions; however, there is no significant interaction between ramipril and other medicines in the question that may predispose Mrs BU to this effect. Furosemide may indirectly interact with digoxin causing hypokalaemia, which increases the risk of digoxin toxicity. On the other hand, this interaction is irrelevant to the current clinical situation (likely rhabdomyolysis). Allopurinol does not exhibit any significant interactions with medicines listed in the question. Concomitant administration of digoxin and colchicine may increase the risk of myopathy (probably due to the competition for P-glycoprotein). The likelihood of this interaction causing myopathy is increased by the fact that colchicine was acutely started during the previous admission about a week ago. In studies where such an interaction was suspected, colchicine was stopped with a resolution of the adverse effect.[6]

Question 4

Correct answers: C and E

Desferrioxamine is a preferred agent of choice in the treatment of acute iron overload, unless contraindicated or previously not tolerated. Deferiprone is only licensed to treat iron overload in patients in whom desferrioxamine is contraindicated or inadequate. In this situation there is no evidence to suggest that it may be the case. Venesection may be considered for the treatment of iron overload associated with haemochromatosis; however, desferrioxamine would be preferred in acute iron overload associated with thalassaemia.[7] Metoclopramide should be avoided in patients under 20 years of age. Cyclizine may help to temporarily reduce the nausea and vomiting associated with iron overload.

Question 5

Correct answers: C and D

Oculogyric crisis and the neuroleptic malignant syndrome have been reported as rare ADRs of levodopa treatment, and are less common than postural hypotension or discolouration of the urine. Henoch–Schönlein purpura is very rare with levodopa treatment.

Question 6

Correct answers: B and C

Pulmonary oedema has been reported with methotrexate, but it has not been associated with ankle swelling (peripheral oedema). Calcium-channel blockers (felodipine) commonly induce peripheral oedema. NSAIDs may sometimes cause fluid retention (rarely precipitating congestive heart failure). This may lead to peripheral oedema. Unless renal dysfunction occurs, sulfasalazine is unlikely to cause peripheral oedema. Angioedema has been reported in patients taking angiotensin-II receptor antagonists (irbesartan); however, such an effect may be ruled out in this case because Mrs Nathan has not presented with any signs/symptoms of an allergic reaction. While irbesartan is not normally associated with ankle swelling, peripheral oedema has been reported for some other medicines of the same class, such as olmesartan.[8,9]

Question 7

Correct answers: C and E

Ethinylestradiol (an oestrogen) contained in Yasmin® may have reduced the plasma concentration of lamotrigine, thus predisposing this lady to an increased risk of seizures. This interaction is made even more likely because Miss GT takes a high dose of ethinylestradiol (60 micrograms) as a 'tricyclic' regimen, i.e. continuously for three cycles, then followed by a tablet-free interval of 4 days. Phenytoin reduces the plasma concentration of lamotrigine; however, considering the fact that phenytoin was started before lamotrigine (10 years ago), it is unlikely that this interaction had contributed to the seizures experienced by Miss GT. Paracetamol and amoxicillin have not been reported to possess any significant interaction with other medicines included in the question.

Question 8

Correct answers: A and D

It is not known how long ago the overdose of diazepam occured, and therefore the administration of activated charcoal may be reasonable. On the other hand, since the patient is already demonstrating symptoms of systemic toxicity (confusion), this measure is less suitable than flumazenil, a benzodiazepine antagonist used to manage benzodiazepine toxicity [unlicensed indication]. Benzodiazepines are sometimes used to treat SSRI poisoning-induced seizures. However, since benzodiazepine overdose is suspected, lorazepam is not a suitable agent because it may contribute to diazepam toxicity. Naloxone is used to manage opioid rather than benzodiazepine toxicity.[8]

Question 9

Correct answers: A and E

Bradypnoea, or respiratory depression, is a well-known, dose-related ADR of opioid therapy. Abnormal pain sensitivity (hyperalgesia) and adrenal insufficiency have been reported in patients on opioid therapy; however, they are more common with long-term use. *Urinary retention* rather than incontinence is among the common side effects of opioid therapy, probably due to their anticholinergic properties. Both bradycardia and (paradoxical) tachycardia are reported as common ADRs of opioid therapy.

Question 10

Correct answers: B and D

Cholestatic jaundice and hepatitis have been reported in patients on flucloxacillin therapy; however, these effects are very rare. Hepatobiliary disorders have been reported in patients on sodium fusidate. According to the manufacturer, the frequency of such effects is unknown but the BNF reports reversible jaundice (especially after high dosage) as a 'less common' ADR (i.e. higher incidence than 'very rare' with flucloxacillin). Paracetamol-induced liver damage occurs primarily in an overdose and is rare within the safe dose range. Biliary spasm, which in certain cases causes an increase in liver enzymes, has been reported among the common side effects in patients on opioid therapy, including codeine. Antihistamines, such as cyclizine, have been reported to cause hepatic dysfunction, but such effects are rare.[8,10–13]

Question 11

Correct answers: B and D

Amiodarone, which has most likely been started for Mrs Thompson to manage the newly diagnosed AF (note the loading regimen of 200 mg TDS), may have doubled the plasma concentration of digoxin leading to a higher risk of digoxin toxicity. Mrs Thompson exhibited nausea and vomiting, the early signs of digoxin toxicity, which were accompanied by another 'classic' sign of yellow vision. This was then followed by severe bradycardia possibly leading to a circulatory collapse. The patient may require atropine and if necessary the digoxin-binding Fab antibody fragments to reverse the toxicity. A blood sample should be taken to measure the plasma digoxin level and serum U&Es (the risk of digoxin toxicity is increased in the presence of hypokalaemia, hypomagnesaemia and hypercalcaemia). Digoxin, bisoprolol and amiodarone should be withheld, and the patient should be monitored closely, preferably with specialist cardiology input. The concomitant use of digoxin and beta blockers (such as bisoprolol) may increase the risk of atrioventricular block and bradycardia. However, this interaction is irrelevant in this case because Mrs Thompson was already taking digoxin and bisoprolol prior to hospital admission. Some ACE inhibitors, e.g. captopril, have been reported to possibly increase the plasma concentration of digoxin; however, the clinical significance of such an interaction is doubtful.[14]

Question 12

Correct answers: C and D

Mrs GJ is actively vomiting, which may make oral PPI treatment (oral pantoprazole) unsuitable. IV omeprazole by injection or short IV infusion (Option B) may be a reasonable option if OGD results were not known. Endoscopy-confirmed active major peptic ulcer bleeding requires a continuous IV omeprazole infusion (preceded by a short 40- to 60-minute initial infusion). Indometacin should be discontinued because NSAIDs are contraindicated in patients with a previous or active peptic ulcer. Vitamin K (phytomenadione or menadiol) is generally not required unless the patient is on regular anticoagulant (warfarin) therapy or has severe liver disease.

Question 13

Correct answers: A and E

Ciclosporin (Neoral®) carries an increased risk of hyperkalaemia, particularly in patients with renal dysfunction. In fact, it can itself cause intrarenal vasoconstriction, which may lead to ischaemic acute tubular necrosis. However, in this case the acute rise in the concentration of nitrogenous products is probably related to urosepsis rather than ciclosporin therapy. Co-amoxiclav (Augmentin®) 1.2 g vials contain about 1 mmol of K^+/vial. Even though this is a relatively minute amount, it may predispose the patient to high plasma potassium when used with other 'hyperkalaemic' medicines, such as ciclosporin, especially in the presence of an acute kidney injury. Note that the usual recommended dose of IV co-amoxiclav to be used in a patient with such a degree of renal impairment (eGFR of 21 mL/min/1.73 m^2) is 1.2 g IV STAT, followed by 600 mg BD; however, the patient was prescribed 1.2 g IV TDS, thus further increasing the risk of co-amoxiclav-related hyperkalaemia. Prednisolone may cause hypo- rather than hyperkalaemia. The risk of hypokalaemia is rather low because of a relatively weak mineralocorticoid effect possessed by this corticosteroid. Salbutamol nebules can cause hypo- rather than hyperkalaemia, especially when used with concomitant theophylline and corticosteroids. Nevertheless, Lynn uses them on a PRN basis, and therefore salbutamol is unlikely to have influenced the blood test results significantly. Similarly to salbutamol, theophylline (Slo-Phyllin®) may cause hypo- rather than hyperkalaemia.[15,16]

References

1. *Summary of Product Characteristics Aspirin Tablets BP 300mg* [Online]. Electronic Medicines Compendium; 2010 [cited 29 March 2013]. Available at: www.medicines.org.uk/EMC/medicine/23776/SPC/Aspirin+Tablets+BP+300mg/#UNDESIRABLE_EFFECTS

2. Thomsen HS, Morcos SK. Contrast media and the kidney: European Society of Urogenital Radiology (ESUR) guidelines. *Br J Radiol*. 2003; **76**(908): 513–18.

3. *Summary of Product Characteristics Prednisolone Tablets BP 5 mg* [Online]. Electronic Medicines Compendium; 2013 [cited 29 March 2013]. Available at: www.medicines.org.uk/EMC/medicine/26657/SPC/Prednisolone+Tablets+BP+5+mg/#UNDESIRABLE_EFFECTS

4. Mathew R, Haque K, Woothipoom W. Acute renal failure induced by contrast medium: steps towards prevention. *BMJ*. 2006; **333**(7567): 539–40.

5. Stegall MD, Everson GT, Schroter G, *et al*. Prednisone withdrawal late after adult liver transplantation reduces diabetes, hypertension, and hypercholesterolemia without causing graft loss. *Hepatology*. 1997; **25**(1): 173–7.

6. *Stockley's Drug Interactions* [Online]. Available at: www.medicinescomplete.com/

7. *BNF for Children September 2013: iron overload* [Online]. Medicines Complete; 2013 [cited 25 September 2013]. Available at: www.medicinescomplete.com/mc/bnfc/current/PHP13936-iron-overload.htm?q=thalassaemia&t=search&ss=text&p=1#_hit

8. *Martindale: the complete drug reference* [Online]. Available at: www.medicinescomplete.com/

9. *Summary of Product Characteristics Methotrexate 2.5 mg Tablets* [Online]. Electronic Medicines Compendium; 2012 [cited 28 March 2013]. Available at: www.medicines.org.uk/EMC/medicine/12033/SPC/Methotrexate+2.5+mg+Tablets/#PHARMACOKINETIC_PROPS

10. *Summary of Product Characteristics Fucidin Tablets* [Online]. Electronic Medicines Compendium; 2012 [cited 29 March 2013]. Available at: www.medicines.org.uk/EMC/medicine/2448/SPC/Fucidin+Tablets/#UNDESIRABLE_EFFECTS

11. *Summary of Product Characteristics Cyclizine 50mg Tablets* [Online]. Electronic Medicines Compendium; 2012 [cited 30 March 2013]. Available at: www.medicines.org.uk/EMC/medicine/27036/SPC/Cyclizine+50mg+Tablets/

12. *Summary of Product Characteristics Codeine Phosphate Tablets 30mg* [Online]. Electronic Medicines Compendium; 2010 [cited 16 September 2012]. Available at: www.medicines.org.uk/EMC/medicine/23910/SPC/Codeine+Phosphate+Tablets+30mg/#UNDESIRABLE_EFFECTS

13. Kennedy P, O'Grady J. Liver disease. In: Walker R, Whittlesea C, editors. *Clinical Pharmacy and Therapeutics*. 4th ed. London: Churchill Livingstone Elsevier; 2007. pp. 215–31.

14. *Summary of Product Characteristics Digoxin Tablets BP 125 micrograms* [Online]. Electronic Medicines Compendium; 2012 [cited 30 March 2013]. Available at:

www.medicines.org.uk/EMC/medicine/23943/SPC/Digoxin+Tablets+BP+125+
micrograms/#UNDESIRABLE_EFFECTS

15. Ballinger A, Patchett S. Hyperkalaemia. In: Kumar P, Clark M, editors. *Pocket Essentials of Clinical Medicine*. 4th ed. London: Saunders Elsevier; 2007. pp. 324–5.

16. *Summary of Product Characteristics Neoral Soft Gelatin Capsules, Neoral Oral Solution* [Online]. Electronic Medicines Compendium; 2012 [cited 27 October 2012]. Available at: www.medicines.org.uk/EMC/medicine/1307/SPC/Neoral+Soft+G elatin+Capsules%2c+Neoral+Oral+Solution/#CLINICAL_PRECAUTIONS

CHAPTER 7: DRUG MONITORING

Question 1

Correct answers: C and E

A rather 'old-fashioned' approach of using the Hartford nomogram is normally restricted to once-daily dosing of gentamicin and is unsuitable for 12-hourly dosing in the treatment of endocarditis. Option B presents a non-existent approach to monitoring. Both 'peak' (1 hour post dose) and 'trough' (immediate pre-dose) levels of gentamicin should be obtained at around the third or fourth dose for multiple-dose regimens (used in endocarditis). Thereafter, where 'peak' concentration is high, the dose must be decreased. Where 'trough' concentration is high, the dosing interval should be increased. The target 'peak' concentration in the treatment of endocarditis should be 3–5 mg/L, while the target 'trough' serum concentration should be <1 mg/L.

Question 2

Correct answers: C and D

It is likely that one of the causes of Mrs Jones' exacerbation was her re-initiated smoking and drinking habits, which in the long-term induced the metabolism and reduced the effective plasma concentration of theophylline therapy (see the monograph on theophylline in the BNF). This may require an increase in the dose from 250 to 500 mg BD. Slo-Phyllin® contains theophylline rather than aminophylline. Aminophylline levels are not usually measured. Instead, a theophylline level should be requested 4–6 hours after the dose (post dose) at least 5 days after increasing the dose to 500 mg BD (aim for a post-dose theophylline plasma level of 10–20 mg/L). Owing to the irreversible nature of COPD, the ideal clinical monitoring targets may not always be achievable. Therefore, it is reasonable to aim for pre-exacerbation spirometry results as a goal, i.e. FEV_1 predicted ≈40% and FEV_1/FVC 0.65. Considering the previous blood gas measurements, the targets of a P_aO_2 of 12 kPa and P_aCO_2 of 5 kPa may not be easily achievable in Mrs Jones' case. As long as she maintains her P_aO_2 over 8 kPa and P_aCO_2 at the pre-exacerbation level, she may avoid the need for long-term oxygen therapy.[1]

Question 3

Correct answers: B and C

FBC, U+Es and LFTs should generally be measured before initiating olanzapine treatment and annually thereafter. No measurement is required at 6 months post treatment initiation (see the BNF, 'Monitoring', section 4.2.1 on antipsychotic drugs). Patients taking olanzapine or clozapine require more frequent monitoring of blood lipids and weight than patients taking other antipsychotic medicines: every 3 months for the first year, then yearly. ECG monitoring is not generally required unless pre-treatment physical examination identifies cardiovascular risk factors, the patient has a history of cardiovascular disease, the patient is admitted as an inpatient or the patient is prescribed haloperidol or pimozide. Physical health monitoring should be undertaken annually rather than 3- or 6-monthly. DSM-IV and ICD-10 tools are used to diagnose mental health disorders and are not generally used for reassessment of symptomatic improvement.

Question 4

Correct answers: A and E

COCs should be avoided in females with a BMI of, or higher than, 35 kg/m^2 due to a high risk of venous thromboembolism (Miss Thompson's BMI is about 32 kg/m^2). Moreover, the efficacy of contraceptive patches is reduced in women with a body weight of, or more than, 90 kg. A sudden occurrence of severe back pain may warrant a clinical examination and review but is rather unlikely to be related to Evra® patches. This is not to be confused with a sudden occurrence of severe chest or unilateral calf pain. Unless it is severe and requiring clinical examination, diarrhoea and vomiting are only a concern in patients taking oral contraceptives (not in those using contraceptive patches). COCs should be used with caution in patients who suffer from hyperprolactinaemia; however, there is nothing to suggest that this is the case for Miss Thompson. Therefore, there is no need to monitor prolactin levels as such. The increase in headache frequency or onset of focal symptoms may indicate a stroke or a transient ischaemic attack and may require an immediate discontinuation of therapy followed by a neurological review.

Question 5

Correct answers: B and D

Erythromycin inhibits the metabolism of warfarin and therefore, increases the anticoagulant effect (INR) with a consequent increase in the risk of haemorrhage. Erythromycin also inhibits the metabolism of simvastatin, and therefore increases the risk of statin-related myopathy. The usual practice is to withhold simvastatin during treatment with erythromycin. This generally does not cause any harm to the patient since statin therapy is a long-term preventative measure against cardiovascular events.

Question 6

Correct answers: C and D

Amiodarone is a class III rather than class II antiarrhythmic agent according to Vaughan-Williams classification. It has a minor effect on reducing the sinus rate and does not generally have a significant effect on the amplitude of the QRS complex. However, amiodarone can significantly prolong the QT interval and increase the risk of torsades de pointes, especially in patients with hypokalaemia. It has been associated with hepatotoxicity (hence, the monitoring requirements), and treatment should be stopped if severe liver function abnormalities or clinical signs of liver disease develop. Amiodarone has also been reported to cause pneumonitis and therefore a baseline chest X-ray is required at the beginning of treatment, irrespective of whether or not the signs/symptoms are present.[2-4]

Question 7

Correct answers: B and C

Visual acuity testing should be undertaken prior to treatment; however, the concerning medicine that may cause ophthalmic effects is ethambutol rather than isoniazid. The degree of renal impairment may guide further adjustments to the regimen. For instance, the dose of ethambutol may need to be reduced as appropriate. Diabetes is one of the risk factors for isoniazid-induced peripheral neuropathy. Therefore, Juliet was prescribed pyridoxine as a prophylactic measure. Liver function should be checked before initiating treatment. Two-monthly checks are only required in patients with pre-existing liver disease or chronic alcohol use. Option E is applicable; however, rifampicin changes the colour of the urine to orange-red rather than brown.

Question 8

Correct answers: B and E

Concomitant use of nebulised salbutamol, IV aminophylline and IV hydrocortisone increases the risk of serious hypokalaemia, which may in turn result in the development of cardiac arrhythmias. Therefore, it is essential to maintain plasma K^+ at or above 3.5 if possible. Salbutamol, aminophylline and hydrocortisone do not have a significant direct effect on the acid-base balance, although in exceptional circumstances they may impair this balance by causing hypokalaemia. Plasma theophylline concentration should be measured 4–6 hours after the start of an IV aminophylline infusion. The target O_2 saturation and PEF, which are at or above those used to diagnose moderate acute asthma, are reasonable at the beginning of the treatment for life-threatening acute asthma.[5,6]

Question 9

Correct answers: D and E

The level of rivaroxaban-induced anticoagulation does not correlate with the INR or APTT. Therefore, INR or APTT are not reliable measures of the bleeding risk or thromboprophylactic effect associated with this oral anticoagulant. The pharmacodynamic effects of rivaroxaban may be assessed using the anti-factor Xa tests; however, such tests are very expensive and time-consuming. They are not routinely undertaken in practice. A fall in Hb may help to diagnose the active bleeding caused by rivaroxaban and/or naproxen, whereas a stable Hb may indicate cessation of bleeding. Together with a fall in Hb, repeated episodes of coffee ground vomiting (haematemesis) may indicate continuation of active bleeding due to a possible NSAID-induced peptic ulcer.[7]

Question 10

Correct answers: B and D

Hartmann's is a 'balanced solution' with electrolyte composition that closely resembles that of blood plasma. It reduces the risk of hyperchloraemic acidosis, which exists with isotonic sodium chloride solution. Haemodilution is a known complication of fluid overload. Although the blood loss experienced by Mr Teddington was modest, he was prescribed a comparatively large volume of crystalloid fluids, which may cause a drop in haemoglobin. This should ideally be discussed prior to fluid administration. Alternatively, where the patient has already received the fluids, the Hb should be monitored carefully. Renal function should be monitored as appropriate; however, Hartmann's solution is unlikely to cause hyperoncotic acute renal failure, which has been reported with colloids, such as starch solutions. Crystalloids, such as Hartmann's solution or glucose 5%, can leak into the interstitial space causing significant tissue oedema, which may lead to an increase in nausea and vomiting where the small bowel is affected. The fluctuations in blood sugar are unlikely because at 5% concentration glucose is metabolised rapidly and is mainly used to replace the loss of water.[8,9]

Question 11

Correct answers: B and E

Digoxin toxicity increases progressively through the range of 1.5–3 micrograms/L. A level of <1.5 micrograms/L is unlikely to be associated with digoxin toxicity. An optimum therapeutic range for digoxin is 0.8–2 micrograms/L. The units in Option C are incorrect: micrograms/mL instead of micrograms/L. Spironolactone may increase K^+ and the risk of digoxin toxicity, but the two effects are unrelated. Spironolactone may increase digoxin toxicity by reducing its renal excretion or by reducing its volume of distribution. Furosemide-induced hypokalaemia may increase the risk of digoxin toxicity. Digoxin competes with K^+ for the binding site on Na^+/K^+ ATPase. Therefore, K^+ depletion increases the pharmacodynamic effect of digoxin. However, such an interaction is unlikely in this case because of the co-prescription of spironolactone, which causes a rise in K^+.[10]

Question 12

Correct answers: C and E

The renal protective dose of ramipril should be titrated to a maximum of 5 mg OD even if the BP is below 130/80. Titration should stop if the BP is significantly reduced (risk of organ hypoperfusion) or the patient is otherwise unable to tolerate the increasing dose of ramipril. The use of ramipril at an optimum dose would minimise the progression of microvascular diabetic complications, such as nephropathy. Monitor renal function to ensure the continuing benefit of this therapy and to minimise the likelihood of any problems. Ramipril should be used with caution in renal disease because of a higher risk of complications such as hyperkalaemia; however, problems rarely appear unless eGFR is <30 mL/min/1.73 m² (however, note the recommendation to avoid ACE inhibitors in severe bilateral renal artery stenosis or severe stenosis of the artery supplying a single functioning kidney). In addition to information in Option C, ramipril-induced hypersensitivity can also manifest as a rash which may be associated with pruritus and urticaria. Ramipril induces hyper- as opposed to hypokalaemia (Option D is incorrect).[11,12]

Question 13

Correct answers: C and D

Both ritonavir and lopinavir (Kaletra®) increase the plasma concentration of simvastatin and therefore the risk of the related myopathy. The concomitant use of these protease inhibitors and simvastatin should be avoided. The interaction between them and atorvastatin appears to be less significant, and hence atorvastatin may be used as an alternative option to simvastatin in this case. Once the baseline creatine kinase is confirmed as satisfactory, further tests are not required in patients who remain asymptomatic. All antiretrovirals, particularly protease inhibitors (such as ritonavir (Kaletra®), may lead to the development of the lipodystrophy syndrome, which is a combination of fat redistribution, insulin resistance and dyslipidaemia. Miss NA exhibits a few features of this syndrome (dyslipidaemia and a 'buffalo hump'). The risk is higher in patients receiving combinations of protease inhibitors (Kaletra®) and nucleoside reverse transcriptase inhibitors (Kivexa®). Plasma lipids and blood glucose should normally be measured before starting the therapy, after 3–6 months of treatment and annually thereafter. Since Miss NA was diagnosed with HIV more than 6 months ago, she only needs to be followed up annually. Non-cardioselective beta blockers, such as carvedilol, may lead to the development of hypoglycaemia. It is possible that carvedilol was started for Miss NA 3 weeks ago when her AF was first diagnosed, and therefore it is the most likely cause of hypoglycaemia. Beta blockers may also mask the autonomic response to hypoglycaemia, e.g. tachycardia – Miss NA's HR was 74 beats/min despite profound hypoglycaemia. Her GP should monitor her blood glucose carefully and should consider replacing carvedilol with a trial of a cardioselective beta blocker, such as atenolol or bisoprolol. Blood glucose should be rechecked by the GP at the earliest opportunity; however, thiazides do not normally cause hypoglycaemia. Instead, they may lead to the development of hyperglycaemia. Glipizide is a short-acting sulfonylurea and is unlikely to have induced hypoglycaemia since it has been used for 4 years without any major issues.

References

1. National Institute for Health and Clinical Excellence. *Chronic Obstructive Pulmonary Disease: NICE guideline 101 – quick reference guide*. London: NICE; 2010. Available at: www.nice.org.uk/nicemedia/live/13029/49399/49399.pdf

2. Scott DK. Cardiac arrhythmias. In: Walker R, Whittlesea C, editors. *Clinical Pharmacy and Therapeutics*. 4th ed. London: Churchill Livingstone Elsevier; 2007. pp. 319–33.

3. Ballinger A, Patchett S. Ventricular arrhythmias. In: Kumar P, Clark M, editors. *Pocket Essentials of Clinical Medicine*. 4th ed. London: Saunders Elsevier; 2007. pp. 418–22.

4. *Summary of Product Characteristics Amiodarone Injection Minijet 30mg/ml (International Medication Systems)* [Online]. Electronic Medicines Compendium; 2007 [cited 6 October 2012]. Available at: www.medicines.org.uk/EMC/medicine/14156/SPC/

5. Ballinger A, Patchett S. Disorders of the acid-base balance. In: Kumar P, Clark M, editors. *Pocket Essentials of Clinical Medicine*. 4th ed. London: Saunders Elsevier; 2007. pp. 327–32.

6. Ballinger A, Patchett S. Respiratory failure. In: Kumar P, Clark M, editors. *Pocket Essentials of Clinical Medicine*. 4th ed. London: Saunders Elsevier; 2007. pp. 563–7.

7. *Summary of Product Characteristics Xarelto 20mg Film-Coated Tablets* [Online]. Electronic Medicines Compendium; 2012 [cited 30 March 2013]. Available at: www.medicines.org.uk/EMC/medicine/25586/SPC/Xarelto+20mg+film-coated+tablets/

8. Floss K, Borthwick M, Clark C. Intravenous fluids – principles of treatment. *Clin Pharm*. 2011; 3(9): 274–83.

9. Staples A, Dade J, Acomb C. Intravenous fluids – practical aspects of therapy. *Clin Pharm*. 2011; 3(9): 285–91.

10. *Stockley's Drug Interactions* [Online]. Available at: www.medicinescomplete.com/

11. Hackett EA, Thomas SM. Diabetes mellitus. In: Walker R, Whittlesea C, editors. *Clinical Pharmacy and Therapeutics*. 4th ed. London: Churchill Livingstone Elsevier; 2007. pp. 629–55.

12. Ballinger A, Patchett S. Complications of diabetes. In: Kumar P, Clark M, editors. *Pocket Essentials of Clinical Medicine*. 4th ed. London: Saunders Elsevier; 2007. pp. 663–8.

CHAPTER 8: DATA INTERPRETATION

Question 1

Correct answer: E

Mrs Hopkins is likely to have presented with amiodarone-induced hypo-thyroidism (AIH), which typically appears as fatigue, dry skin, cold intolerance and hormone changes resembling those of primary hypothyroidism. It is commonly related to the Wolff–Chaikoff effect, i.e. the presence of excess iodine and is more prevalent in elderly females living in areas of *adequate* iodine intake. In contrast to amiodarone-induced thyrotoxicosis, the management of AIH involves continuing the medicine and initiating thyroid hormone replacement therapy. The benefits of continuing amiodarone therapy often outweigh the risks of AIH. Amiodarone therapy should be continued (at the same dose and dosage frequency) with careful monitoring and thyroid hormone replacement therapy.[1,2]

Question 2

Correct answer: D

The next dose should be omitted, and subsequent dosing should be adjusted to 500 mg every 48 hours (i.e. decreased by two levels of dosing from 750 mg 24-hourly) as per guidance for 'trough' level of 25–30 mg/L.[3]

Question 3

Correct answer: D

Antibiotic therapy should be discontinued because the likely diagnosis is nitrofurantoin-induced acute pulmonary toxicity, which commonly presents as pulmonary eosinophilia resembling Loeffler's syndrome. Piperacillin/tazo-bactam or AmBisome® is unlikely to help because eosinophilic pneumonia is a hypersensitivity reaction rather than infection. There is no need to consult the microbiology department (no pathogens were isolated in blood/sputum cultures). The resolution of acute pulmonary toxicity is almost always reversible and complete on nitrofurantoin withdrawal. Atenolol (beta blocker) can precipitate bronchospasm; however, the clinical picture of the reaction suggests nitrofurantoin-induced pulmonary toxicity.[1,4] Note that a normal eosinophil count with fine end inspiratory crepitations on chest examination and finger clubbing would imply a diagnosis of pulmonary fibrosis.

Question 4

Correct answer: C

Severe hepatocellular damage has been reported with labetalol. It manifests as acute (often reversible) hepatitis and requires prompt discontinuation of treatment. Re-challenge with labetalol often triggers reoccurrence of acute liver injury and as such should be avoided. In order to minimise hypertension-related foetal risks, Mrs Ivanovic should be prescribed an alternative agent, such as nifedipine. Although nifedipine is metabolised by the liver and requires adequate caution in hepatic disease (e.g. dose reduction), it may be safer than methyldopa which itself has been reported to cause hepatitis and jaundice. UFH is metabolised by the liver (for renal excretion) and therefore is contraindicated in severe hepatic disease. Dalteparin has been reported to cause transient elevations in liver transaminases (it may require dose reduction in liver failure), however the benefits of continuing its use for Mrs Ivanovic may outweigh the risks associated with stopping the treatment, e.g. recurrent venous thromboembolism.[1,5–10]

Question 5

Correct answer: B

Ezetimibe can be used in conjunction with a statin for the management of hypercholesterolaemia, but has a limited benefit in the treatment of hyper-triglyceridaemia (no or little effect on the absorption of TGs). The main pharmacodynamic effect of fibrates, such as fenofibrate, is a reduction in serum TGs. Fenofibrate is recommended as an addition to statin therapy in T2DM patients with well-controlled diabetes whose serum TGs exceed 2.3 mmol/L despite 6 months of treatment with a statin. The use of gemfibrozil in combination with a statin increases the risk of rhabdomyolysis considerably and should be avoided whenever possible. Bile acid sequestrants, such as colestyramine, can be added to a statin to manage hypercholesterolaemia; however, (similarly to ezetimibe) they have little or no effect on serum TGs. Mr Scharpf is already receiving a 'high-intensity' statin (at least simvastatin 40 mg OD or equivalent), and therefore the initiation of rosuvastatin is unlikely to have a major effect on the level of TGs.[11–13]

Question 6

Correct answer: E

Assuming the blood loss has been corrected, Miss Lam's daily fluid requirements include about 2.4 L of total fluids (30 mL/kg/day), 80–112 mmol of Na^+ (1.0–1.4 mmol/kg/day) and 56–72 mmol of K^+ (0.7–0.9 mmol/kg/day). The current fluid prescription provides her with 3.5 L of total fluids, 75 mmol of Na^+ and 50 mmol of K^+. Therefore, she has been receiving an excess of over 1 L fluid with a lack of the two electrolytes. The resulting hyponatraemia caused the retention of lithium (usual range 0.4–1.0 mmol/L) and symptoms of toxicity, such as apathy and restlessness (often confused with symptoms arising from the patient's illness). This situation requires a withdrawal of lithium (Priadel®) until the level is within range (psychiatry advice should normally be sought). It may also require fluid restriction and sodium replacement, which would be best achieved with a low volume of normal saline solution (rather than Hartmann's or potassium chloride in glucose). Hypotonic saline should not be used in this case because it can further exacerbate dilutional hyponatraemia. Hypertonic saline is normally restricted to severe hyponatraemia (Na^+ <110 mmol/L). Advice from the National Poisons Information Service should be sought if necessary.[14–17]

Question 7

Correct answer: D

Jane's asthma is not well controlled (PEFR = 121 L/192 L × 100% = 63% of predicted), which suggests a step up in treatment. The second step in the management of chronic asthma in children over 5 years of age involves the addition of a regular standard-dose corticosteroid. Alternatives, such as montelukast, are considerably less effective. Considering Jane's satisfactory inhaler technique, choosing oral therapy, which may predispose her to systemic adverse effects, is not reasonable. Mometasone is not recommended for use in children. The dose of fluticasone in Option C is correct; however, in children aged 5–15 years, corticosteroid therapy should be routinely delivered via the spacer device. The dose of fluticasone prescribed in Option E is too high (high-dose corticosteroid instead of the recommended standard-dose one).[18,19]

Question 8

Correct answer: C

Mr Thornton is likely to have experienced tumour lysis syndrome (TLS), which is more prevalent in patients with high-grade lymphomas (such as DLBCL). He was on allopurinol 300 mg OM for the prophylaxis of gout prior to starting his chemotherapy; however, this dose did not prevent the rise in plasma urate post chemotherapy, causing a possible urate nephropathy. Rasburicase IV infusion for up to 7 days (until serum urate is controlled) is the cornerstone of TLS treatment. Allopurinol should be stopped during rasburicase administration because it inhibits the production of uric acid, the substrate for rasburicase. Unless symptomatic, the correction of low calcium should usually be avoided because the administration of this electrolyte in the presence of excess phosphate may lead to formation of calcium phosphate precipitates. Where needed, hyperphosphataemia can be treated with adequate hydration and a phosphate binder. Calcium gluconate can also be used to protect the myocardium from hyperkalaemia; however, this has already been managed prior to the scenario. Options D and E contain an incorrect dose of rasburicase.[20–22]

Question 9

Correct answer: B

St John's wort should be stopped because it may have induced the metabolism of carbamazepine thus reducing the therapeutic plasma level and increasing the risk of epileptic seizures. No interaction has been reported between cranberry juice and carbamazepine to date; therefore, it is relatively safe for Miss JK to continue using this supplement. The plasma level of carbamazepine is low (usual range, 4–12 mg/L). This requires an increase in carbamazepine dose followed by careful monitoring. Fluoxetine increases the plasma concentration of carbamazepine. Considering the low current plasma level of carbamazepine, the discontinuation of this antidepressant is unreasonable. It may also exacerbate the patient's depression. Clarithromycin inhibits the metabolism of carbamazepine leading to an increase in plasma level of this anticonvulsant. Considering the current low plasma concentration of carbamazepine, stopping clarithromycin before the 7-day course is finished may be unreasonable because it may precipitate further seizures and/or lead to a relapse of an insufficiently treated chest infection.[23]

Question 10

Correct answer: C

Mr BN is likely to have presented with CKD-related anaemia. However, considering the relatively mild degree of anaemia (Hb only slightly below 10 g/dL, ferritin is >100 µg/L and transferrin saturation (iron/TIBC × 100%) >20%), IV iron (CosmoFer® or MonoFer®) is unlikely to be required and oral preparations (e.g. ferrous sulphate) may be sufficient to replenish iron stores. Epoetin (NeoRecormon® or Eprex®) is unlikely to be indicated in Mr BN's clinical circumstances (uncomplicated anaemia and history of prostate cancer). If epoetin is to be prescribed, the iron stores should be replenished accordingly prior to initiating such treatment. In addition, epoetins should be used with particular caution in cancer patients (increased risk of tumour progression) and are generally restricted to those receiving chemotherapy. Metformin does not need to be withheld (eGFR >30 mL/min/1.73 m²), but may require a dose review and/or reduction in light of the increased risk of lactic acidosis. Exenatide does not need to be stopped (eGFR >30 mL/min/1.73 m²); however, it should be used with caution and BMs should be monitored carefully. Ramipril can be used at the same dose with careful monitoring of BP, urea and electrolytes (eGFR >30 mL/min/1.73 m²).[24–26]

Question 11

Correct answer: D

Joanna has presented with symptomatic hypomagnesaemia, likely secondary to omeprazole therapy (typically occurs 3–12 months after starting treatment). Similar to omeprazole, lansoprazole has been reported to cause hypomagnesaemia and would not be an alternative option. In contrast to proton pump inhibitors, ranitidine has not been reported to possess any effect on plasma magnesium and therefore can be safely used once magnesium deficiency is corrected. Pizotifen or lorazepam have not been reported to cause hypomagnesaemia and therefore does not require discontinuation or a change to an alternative medicine. Lorazepam may need to be temporarily withheld if more severe CNS depression is thought to be implicated (which is not the case in this scenario). Magnesium should be replaced as appropriate. With an exception of more serious cases, magnesium sulphate can usually be given as an IV infusion. Joanna's hypomagnesaemia is not severe enough to require an IV bolus dose of 20 mmol of magnesium sulphate. Intramuscular injections of magnesium sulphate can be painful and IV is generally a preferred route of administration.[16,27–29]

Question 12

Correct answer: C

A bolus of short-acting insulin (such as Actrapid® or NovoRapid®) should usually be given before, rather than after, breakfast. The sliding scale should be stopped 30 minutes later. Since Tim's BMs have been relatively high and unstable, it may be reasonable to increase the first dose of insulin by 10%–20% (13–14 units STAT). In addition, the use of NovoRapid® (Tim's regular type of insulin) would be preferred over Actrapid®. Tim's usual regimen of insulin can be restarted with his lunchtime dose of NovoRapid® (rather than in the evening). Levemir® should not be given as a post-sliding scale bolus dose in the morning. It is a long-acting insulin and should be restarted in the evening with careful BM monitoring. BMs should be monitored closely for the first couple of days and may warrant dose adjustments where appropriate. Metformin can be restarted with breakfast (i.e. at least 48 hours post procedure).[30–32]

Question 13

Correct answer: A

Mouth ulcers, fever and non-specific illness may indicate drug-induced neutropenia or agranulocytosis, and should be treated with adequate caution. Both nitrazepam and carbimazole have been reported to cause blood dyscrasias and should be stopped at least until blood test results exclude such a diagnosis. Difflam® spray can only provide temporary relief and should be prescribed once iatrogenic neutropenia/agranulocytosis is ruled out. If neutropenia/agranulocytosis is confirmed, alternative options to nitrazepam and/or carbimazole may need to be considered. For nitrazepam this may include non-benzodiazepine hypnotics, such as zopiclone. Following a discussion with endocrinologists, surgeons and haematologists, carbimazole may be replaced with propylthiouracil or radioactive iodine. Alternatively, the patient may undergo thyroid surgery. Propranolol is used as an adjunct to other antithyroid drugs or radioactive iodine. Beta blockers can slow the heart rate and improve the tremor, but they have little effect on resolving thyroid overactivity. Therefore, propranolol cannot replace carbimazole or propylthiouracil as a monotherapy. In contrast to some other second-generation antipsychotics, such as clozapine or olanzapine, amisulpride has not been linked to blood dyscrasias and can be safely continued (see the Summary of Product Characteristics).[33] In most cases antipsychotics should not be withdrawn abruptly because of the high risk of relapse. Duloxetine has not been reported to cause blood disorders and can be safely continued.[33–39]

References

1. *Martindale: the complete drug reference* [Online]. Available at: www.medicines complete.com/

2. Martino E, Bartalena L, Bogazzi F, *et al.* The effects of amiodarone on the thyroid. *Endocr Rev.* 2001; **22**(2): 240–54.

3. *Antimicrobial Policies and Guidelines.* Redhill: Surrey and Sussex Healthcare NHS Trust; 2012.

4. Twilla J, Winton J, Self TH. Nitrofurantoin pulmonary toxicity: a rare but serious complication [Online]. *Consultant.* 2010: **50**(6). Available at: www.consultant360. com/content/nitrofurantoin-pulmonary-toxicity-rare-serious-complication

5. National Institute for Health and Clinical Excellence. *Hypertension in Pregnancy: NICE guideline 107 – quick reference guide.* London: NICE; 2010. Available at: www.nice.org.uk/nicemedia/live/13098/50416/50416.pdf

6. *Summary of Product Characteristics Heparin Sodium 1,000 I.U./ml Solution for Injection or Concentrate for Solution for Infusion (Without Preservative)* [Online]. Electronic Medicines Compendium; 2009 [cited 13 October 2012]. Available at: www.medicines.org.uk/EMC/medicine/9793/SPC/Heparin+sodium+1%2c000+ I.U.+ml+Solution+for+injection+or+concentrate+for+solution+for+infusion+%2 8without+preservative%29/

7. *Summary of Product Characteristics Fragmin 10,000 IU/0.4ml Solution for Injection* [Online]. Electronic Medicines Compendium; 2013 [cited 31 March 2013]. Available at: www.medicines.org.uk/EMC/medicine/26894/SPC/Fragmin+10% 2c000+IU+0.4ml+solution+for+injection/

8. *Summary of Product Characteristics Adalat* [Online]. Electronic Medicines Compendium; 2013 [cited 13 October 2012]. Available at: www.medicines.org. uk/EMC/medicine/20901/SPC/Adalat/

9. *Summary of Product Characteristics Methyldopa Tablets BP 125mg* [Online]. Electronic Medicines Compendium; 2007 [cited 13 October 2012]. Available at: www.medicines. org.uk/EMC/medicine/24120/SPC/Methyldopa+Tablets+BP+125mg/

10. *Drug Record: Labetalol* [Online]. US National Library of Medicine; LiverTox; 2013 [cited 31 October 2013]. Available at: http://livertox.nih.gov/Labetalol.htm.

11. *Summary of Product Characteristics Ezetrol 10mg Tablets* [Online]. Electronic Medicines Compendium; 2013 [cited 31 March 2013]. Available at: www.medicines. org.uk/EMC/medicine/12091/SPC/Ezetrol+10mg+Tablets/

12. *Summary of Product Characteristics Questran Light* [Online]. Electronic Medicines Compendium; 2005 [cited 14 October 2012]. Available at: www.medicines.org.uk/ EMC/medicine/348/SPC/Questran+Light

13. *Summary of Product Characteristics Fenofibrate 200mg Capsules* [Online]. Electronic Medicines Compendium; 2012 [cited 14 October 2012]. Available at: www.medicines. org.uk/EMC/medicine/23955/SPC/Fenofibrate+200+mg+capsules/

14. *Summary of Product Characteristics Priadel Liquid* [Online]. Electronic Medicines Compendium; 2012 [cited 14 October 2012]. Available at: www.medicines.org.uk/ emc/medicine/6981/SPC/Priadel+Liquid/

15. *Coronary Artery Bypass Graft – Recovery* [Online]. London: NHS Choices; 2012 [cited 24 November 2012]. Available at: www.nhs.uk/Conditions/Coronary-artery-bypass/Pages/Recovery.aspx

16. Medusa Injectable Medicines Guide Online: National Health Service. Available at: www.injguide.nhs.uk

17. *Hyponatraemia (Emergency Care Guidelines)*. Version 4, Feb 2008 edition. Redhill: Surrey and Sussex Healthcare NHS Trust; 2012.

18. *Predictive Normal Values (Nomogram, EU Scale)* [Online]. Essex: Clement Clarke International; 2004 [cited 15 October 2012]. Available at: www.peakflow.com/top_nav/normal_values/index.html

19. British Guideline on the Management of Asthma. *Thorax*. 2008; **63**(Suppl. 4): iv1–121.

20. *Guidelines for the Management of Tumour Lysis Syndrome* [Online]. Surrey, West Sussex and Hampshire Cancer Network; 2012 [cited 31 March 2013]. Available at: www.royalsurrey.nhs.uk/Default.aspx?DN=45ce893f-8494-413f-9dc6-b3c7a6e21a51

21. Cameron L, Loughran C. Lymphomas. In: Walker R, Whittlesea C, editors. *Clinical Pharmacy and Therapeutics*. 4th ed. London: Churchill Livingstone Elsevier; 2007. pp. 731–45.

22. Ballinger A, Patchett S. Hyperkalaemia. In: Kumar P, Clark M, editors. *Pocket Essentials of Clinical Medicine*. 4th ed. London: Saunders Elsevier; 2007. pp. 324–5.

23. *Stockley's Drug Interactions* [Online]. Available at: www.medicinescomplete.com/

24. National Institute for Health and Clinical Excellence. *Anaemia Management in People with Chronic Kidney Disease: NICE guideline 114* – quick reference guide. London: NICE; 2011. Available at: www.nice.org.uk/nicemedia/live/13329/52857/52857.pdf

25. National Institute for Health and Care Excellence. *Anaemia Management in People with Chronic Kidney Disease: NICE guideline 114*. London: NICE; 2011. Available at: www.nice.org.uk/nicemedia/live/13329/52853/52853.pdf

26. Ballinger A, Patchett S. Anaemia. In: Kumar P, Clark M, editors. *Pocket Essentials of Clinical Medicine*. 4th ed. London: Saunders Elsevier; 2007. pp. 183–96.

27. *Summary of Product Characteristics Pizotifen Tablets 0.5mg* [Online]. Electronic Medicines Compendium; 2012 [cited 18 October 2012]. Available at: www.medicines.org.uk/EMC/medicine/24179/SPC/Pizotifen+Tablets+0.5mg

28. *Summary of Product Characteristics Losec Capsules 10mg* [Online]. Electronic Medicines Compendium; 2012 [cited 18 October 2012]. Available at: www.medicines.org.uk/EMC/medicine/7275/SPC/Losec+Capsules+10mg

29. *Summary of Product Characteristics Ranitidine 150mg Tablets* [Online]. Electronic Medicines Compendium; 2012 [cited 18 October 2012]. Available at: www.medicines.org.uk/EMC/medicine/23245/SPC/Ranitidine+150mg+tablets/

30. Rahman MH, Beattie J. Medication in the peri-operative period. *Pharm J*. 2004; **272**: 287–9.

31. Rahman MH, Beattie J. Peri-operative care and diabetes. *Pharm J*. 2004; **272**: 323–5.

32. Rahman MH, Beattie J. Peri-operative medication in patients with cardiovascular disease. *Pharm J*. 2004; **272**: 352–4.

33. *Summary of Product Characteristics Amisulpride 100 mg Tablets* [Online]. Electronic Medicines Compendium; 2012 [cited 27 October 2012]. Available at: www.medicines. org.uk/EMC/medicine/25318/SPC/Amisulpride+100+mg+Tablets/

34. *Summary of Product Characteristics Carbimazole 20 mg Tablets* [Online]. Electronic Medicines Compendium; 2011 [cited 27 October 2012]. Available at: www.medicines. org.uk/EMC/medicine/26933/SPC/Carbimazole+20+mg+tablets/

35. *Summary of Product Characteristics Zopiclone 3.75mg Tablets* [Online]. Electronic Medicines Compendium; 2009 [cited 10 February 2013]. Available at: www.medicines. org.uk/EMC/medicine/24285/SPC/Zopiclone+3.75mg+Tablets./

36. *Summary of Product Characteristics Cymbalta 30mg Hard Gastro-resistant Capsules, Cymbalta 60mg Hard Gastro-resistant Capsules* [Online]. Electronic Medicines Compendium; 2009 [cited 27 October 2012]. Available at: www.medicines.org. uk/EMC/medicine/15694/SPC/Cymbalta+30mg+hard+gastro-resistant+capsule s%2c+Cymbalta+60mg+hard+gastro-resistant+capsules/

37. *Summary of Product Characteristics Nitrazepam Tablets 5mg* [Online]. Electronic Medicines Compendium; 2012 [cited 28 September 2013]. Available at: www. medicines.org.uk/emc/medicine/24136/SPC/Nitrazepam+Tablets+5mg/#UND ESIRABLE_EFFECTS

38. *Summary of Product Characteristics Propranolol Tablets BP 40mg* [Online]. Electronic Medicines Compendium; 2012 [cited 27 October 2012]. Available at: www.medicines. org.uk/EMC/medicine/24090/SPC/Propranolol+Tablets+BP+40mg/

39. *Hyperthyroidism – Clinical Features and Treatment* [Online]. British Thyroid Association; 2012 [cited 27 October 2012]. Available at: www.british-thyroid-association.org/info-for-patients/Docs/bta_patient_hyperthyroidism.pdf

Appendix 1

Templates of the Prescriptions to be used for Questions in Chapter 1

General practice prescription template:

Pharmacy Stamp	Age	Title, Forename, Surname & Address
Please don't stamp over age box	D.o.B 1.8.1966	*18 Anglesea Road Kingston KT1 4TH*

Number of days' treatment N.B. Ensure dose is stated	

Endorsements

Specimen copy

Signature of Prescriber	Date

For dispenser No. of Prescns on form	Dr Who 163827 16 Station Road Kingston Upon Thames KT2 4BB 0299 1234567	FP10NC0106

NHS PATIENTS – please read the notes overleaf

000055559980

Prescribing Safety Assessment: resources [Online]. Medical Schools Council, British Pharmacological Society; [27 March 2013]. Available at: www.prescribe.ac.uk/psa/?page_id=14

An example of a prescription written on a *General practice prescription template*:

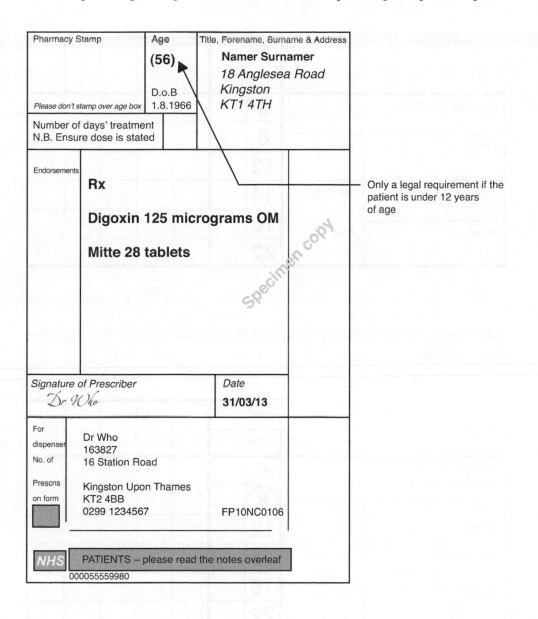

Pharmacy Stamp	Age **(56)** D.o.B 1.8.1966	Title, Forename, Surname & Address **Namer Surnamer** *18 Anglesea Road Kingston KT1 4TH*
Please don't stamp over age box		

Number of days' treatment
N.B. Ensure dose is stated

Endorsements

Rx

Digoxin 125 micrograms OM

Mitte 28 tablets

Only a legal requirement if the patient is under 12 years of age

Specimen copy

Signature of Prescriber *Dr Who*	Date **31/03/13**

For dispenser
No. of
Prescns
on form

Dr Who
163827
16 Station Road

Kingston Upon Thames
KT2 4BB
0299 1234567   FP10NC0106

NHS   PATIENTS – please read the notes overleaf
000055559980

Hospital regular medicines prescription chart template:

	Date					
	Time					
Drug (approved name)	**6**					
Dose / Route	**8**					
	12					
Prescriber – sign + print / Start date	**14**					
Notes / Pharmacy	**18**					
	22					

An example of a prescription written on a *Hospital regular medicines prescription chart template*:

	Date					
	Time					
Drug (approved name) **Lansoprazole**	**6**					
	⑧					
Dose **30 mg** / Route **PO**	**12**					
Prescriber - sign + print *Dr Who* Dr Who / Start date **31/03/13**	**14**					
Notes / Pharmacy	**18**					
	22					

Prescribing Safety Assessment: resources [Online]. Medical Schools Council, British Pharmacological Society; [27 March 2013]. Available at: www.prescribe.ac.uk/psa/?page_id=14

Hospital fluid prescription chart template:

		INFUSION THERAPY						Prescriber's signature	Given by
Date	Start time	Infusion solution				Medicine added			
		Type/strength	Volume	Route	Duration	Approved name	Dose		

Note that the template used during the PSA will contain a column for the 'rate' of the infusion. However, it was deemed unnecessary to include such a column in this publication since the rate of the infusion can be implied from the volume used and the duration over which it is to be administered

An example of a prescription written on a *Hospital fluid prescription chart template*:

		INFUSION THERAPY						Prescriber's signature	Given by
Date	Start time	Infusion solution				Medicine added			
		Type/strength	Volume	Route	Duration	Approved name	Dose		
31/03/13	8:00 am	Sodium chloride 0.9%	100 mL	IV	30 min	Teicoplanin	400 mg	*Dr Who*	

Prescribing Safety Assessment: resources [Online]. Medical Schools Council, British Pharmacological Society; [27 March 2013]. Available at: www.prescribe.ac.uk/psa/?page_id=14

Hospital once-only medicines prescription chart template:

ONCE ONLY MEDICINES

Date	Time	Medicine (approved name)	Dose	Route	Prescriber – sign + print	Time given	Given by

An example of a prescription written on a *Hospital once-only medicines prescription chart template*:

ONCE ONLY MEDICINES

Date	Time	Medicine (approved name)	Dose	Route	Prescriber – sign + print	Time given	Given by
31/03/13	8:00 am	**Benzylpenicillin**	**1.2 g**	**IV**	*Dr Who* **Dr Who**		

Prescribing Safety Assessment: resources [Online]. Medical Schools Council, British Pharmacological Society; [27 March 2013]. Available at: www.prescribe.ac.uk/psa/?page_id=14

Appendix 2

List of Common Abbreviations

A&E	accident and emergency
ACE	angiotensin-converting enzyme
AChEi	acetylcholinesterase inhibitor
ACTH	corticotropin, or adrenocorticotropic hormone
ADHD	attention deficit hyperactivity disorder
ADR	adverse drug reaction
AF	atrial fibrillation
AIH	amiodarone-induced hypothyroidism
AKI	acute kidney injury
ALP	alkaline phosphatase
ALT	alanine transaminase
APTT	activated partial thromboplastin time
B_{12}	vitamin B_{12}
BD	twice daily
BM	randomly taken glucose concentration in blood plasma
BMI	body mass index
BNF	*British National Formulary*
BNP	B-type natriuretic peptide
BP	blood pressure
BPH	benign prostatic hyperplasia
bpm	beats per minute
BPS	British Pharmacological Society
Ca^{2+}	calcium concentration in blood plasma
CABG	coronary artery bypass graft
CCB	calcium-channel blocker

CCF	congestive cardiac failure
CDI	*Clostridium difficile* infection
CHF	chronic heart failure
CHM	Commission on Human Medicines
CHMP	Committee for Medicinal Products for Human Use
CKD	chronic kidney disease
CNS	central nervous system
CO_2	carbon dioxide
COC	combined oral contraceptive(s)
CHCs	combined hormonal contraceptives
COPD	chronic obstructive pulmonary disease
Cr	creatinine concentration in blood plasma
CrCl	creatinine clearance
CRP	C-reactive protein
CSF	cerebrospinal fluid
CT	computed tomography
CVD	cardiovascular disease
CXR	chest X-ray
COX-2	cyclo-oxygenase-2
DH	drug history
DKA	diabetic ketoacidosis
DLBCL	diffuse large B-cell lymphoma
DMARD	disease-modifying anti-rheumatic drug
DRESS	drug rash with eosinophilia and systemic symptoms
DSM-IV	Diagnostic and Statistical Manual of Mental Disorders, 4th Edition
DVT	deep vein thrombosis
DXA	dual energy X-ray absorptiometry
E/C or EC	enteric-coated (tablets)
ECG	electrocardiogram
eGFR	estimated glomerular filtration rate
EU	European Union
Fab	Fragment antigen-binding – a region on an antibody that binds to antigens
FBC	full blood count
FEC	a chemotherapy regimen (5-fluorouracil, epirubicin and cyclophosphamide)

FEV_1	forced expiratory volume in 1 second
FL	femtolitre
FP10	a general practice prescription
FVC	forced vital capacity
FY1	Foundation Year 1
FY2	Foundation Year 2
G6PD	glucose 6-phosphate dehydrogenase
GCS	Glasgow coma score
GFR	glomerular filtration rate
GMC	General Medical Council
GORD	gastro-oesophageal reflux disease
GP	general practitioner/general practice
GPP	good prescribing practice
GTN	glyceryl trinitrate
HAP	hospital-acquired pneumonia
Hb	haemoglobin
HbA_{1c}	glycosylated haemoglobin
HCO_3^-	bicarbonate concentration in blood plasma
HDL-C	high-density lipoprotein cholesterol
HIV	human immunodeficiency virus
HO	house officer (junior doctor)
HR	heart rate
HRCT	high resolution computed tomography
HRT	hormone replacement therapy
$5HT_1$	a subtype of serotonin (5-hydroxytryptamine) receptors
IBS	irritable bowel syndrome
ICD-10	World Health Organization International Statistical Classification of Diseases and Related Health Problems, 10th Revision
ICH	intracerebral haemorrhage
IM	intramuscular
INR	international normalised ratio
INH	inhalation (administration route via an inhaler)
IV	intravenous/intravenously
JVP	jugular venous pressure
K^+	potassium concentration in blood plasma
KCl	potassium chloride

LAD	left anterior descending coronary artery
LD	loading dose
LDL-C	low-density lipoprotein cholesterol
LFT	liver function test
LMWH	low-molecular-weight heparin
LVEF	left ventricular ejection fraction
LVF	left ventricular failure
LVH	left ventricular hypertrophy
MCA	middle cerebral artery
MCV	mean corpuscular volume
MDRD	Modification of Diet in Renal Disease
Mg^{2+}	magnesium concentration in blood plasma
MHRA	Medicines and Healthcare products Regulatory Agency
MI	myocardial infarction
MMSE	mini mental state examination
MR	modified release
MRI	magnetic resonance imaging
MR	modified-release preparation of an oral dosage form
MRSA	methicillin-resistant *Staphylococcus aureus*
MSC	Medical Schools Council
MST	morphine sulphate tablets
ms	millisecond
NB	*nota bene* – an Italian and Latin phrase meaning 'note well'
Na^+	sodium concentration in blood plasma
NaCl	sodium chloride
NAD	no abnormality detected
NPSA	National Patient Safety Agency
NEB	nebulisation (administration route via a nebuliser)
Neut	neutrophil count
NG	nasogastric
NHS	National Health Service
NICE	National Institute for Health and Care Excellence
NKDA	no known drug allergies
NSAID	non-steroidal anti-inflammatory drug
NSTEMI	non-ST-segment elevation myocardial infarction
NYHA	New York Heart Association
O_2	oxygen

O_2 sat	oxygen saturation in arterial blood
OD	every day
OGD	oesophago-gastro-duodenoscopy
OM	every morning
ON	every night
OTC	over the counter
PACG	primary angle-closure glaucoma
P_aCO_2	partial pressure of carbon dioxide in arterial blood
P_aO_2	partial pressure of oxygen in arterial blood
PC	presenting complaint
PCA	patient-controlled analgesia
PCI	percutaneous coronary intervention
PE	pulmonary embolism
PEF	peak expiratory flow
PEFR	peak expiratory flow rate
PEG	percutaneous endoscopic gastrostomy
PDE-5	phosphodiesterase type-5
PID	pelvic inflammatory disease
Plt	platelet count
PMH	past medical history
PO	oral
PO_4^{3-}	phosphate concentration in blood plasma
POC	progestogen-only contraceptive(s)
PPI	proton pump inhibitor
PR	per rectum (rectal or rectally)
PRN	when required
PSA	Prescribing Safety Assessment
PT	prothrombin time
QDS	four times daily
QTc	corrected QT interval
QIPP	Quality, Innovation, Productivity and Prevention
R-CHOP	rituximab, cyclophosphamide, doxorubicin, vincristine and prednisolone
RR	respiratory rate
S_aO_2	arterial oxygen saturation
SC	subcutaneously
SH	social history

SHO	senior house officer (junior doctor)
SMC	Scottish Medicines Consortium
SPC	Summary of Product Characteristics
SpR	specialist registrar (senior doctor)
SR	slow release
SSRI	selective serotonin re-uptake inhibitor
STAT	immediate/immediately
STEMI	ST-segment elevation myocardial infarction
T	one tablet/capsule/sachet/puff/application
T1DM	type 1 diabetes mellitus
T2DM	type 2 diabetes mellitus
T_3	triiodothyronine
T_4	thyroxine
TC	total cholesterol
TCA	tricyclic antidepressant
TDM	therapeutic drug monitoring
TDS	three times daily
TGs	triglycerides
TIA	transient ischaemic attack
TIBC	total iron binding capacity
TLS	tumour lysis syndrome
TOP	topical application (e.g. of cream or ointment)
TSH	thyroid-stimulating hormone
TT	two tablets/capsules/sachets/puffs/applications
TTT	three tablets/capsules/sachets/puffs/applications
TURP	transurethral resection of the prostate
U	urea
U&Es or U+Es	urea and electrolytes
UFH	unfractionated heparin
UK	United Kingdom
UTI	urinary tract infection
UV	ultraviolet
Vd	volume of distribution
VT	ventricular tachycardia
VTE	venous thromboembolism
WBC	white blood cell count

Appendix 3

Introduction to Prescribing and Pharmaceutical Care

The Oxford Dictionaries define prescribing as advising and authorising 'the use of a medicine or treatment for someone, especially in writing'.[1] The prescribing of medicines is the most common type of intervention in the National Health Service (NHS) and accounts for as much as 12% of the total NHS expenditure.[2] The prescribing performance is also one of the key elements of the government's Quality, Innovation, Productivity and Prevention (QIPP) programme whereby NHS organisations are expected to improve the quality of care while achieving a total of £20 billion in savings by 2014–15.[3] Therefore, it is essential that all medical and non-medical prescribers are familiar with the principles of **good prescribing practice** (GPP), which involves the use of medicines and medical devices in the safest, most effective and cost-effective manner.

The clinical significance of GPP may be mapped into the definition of **'pharmaceutical care'** proposed by Hepler and Strand back in early 1990:

> the responsible provision of drug therapy for the purpose of achieving definite outcomes that improve a patient's quality of life. These outcomes are (1) cure of a disease, (2) elimination or reduction of a patient's symptomatology, (3) arresting or slowing of a disease process, or (4) preventing a disease or symptomatology.[4]

Doctors work closely with pharmacists and other healthcare professionals to ensure that these outcomes are met in practice. Indeed, in order to achieve the outcomes of GPP and provide effective pharmaceutical care, the prescriber is required to adapt a structured approach to prescribing practice. The recent guide to *Good Practice in Prescribing and Managing Medicines and Devices* by the GMC outlines the steps to be followed to ensure appropriate prescribing and emphasises the fact that 'serious or persistent failure to follow this guidance will put practitioners' registration at risk'.[5] According to this document, **the main principles** to be adhered to by all prescribers include the following:

- Recognising and working within the limits of practitioners' competence, and keeping their knowledge and skills up to date throughout their working life.
- Utilising electronic and other systems to improve the safety of prescribing.
- Seeking advice from experienced colleagues, including pharmacists, prescribing advisers and clinical pharmacologists.
- Being familiar with the guidance set out in the BNF and the BNF for Children.
- Taking into account the guidelines published by NICE for practitioners in England, the Scottish Medicines Consortium and Health Improvement Scotland (including the Scottish Intercollegiate Guidelines Network) for practitioners in Scotland, the Department of Health, Social Services and Public Safety for practitioners in Northern Ireland, All-Wales Medicines Strategy Group for practitioners in Wales and by the Medical Royal Colleges and other authoritative sources of specialty specific clinical guidelines.
- Avoiding prescribing for himself or herself or anyone with whom the practitioner has a close personal relationship (this particularly applies to medicines governed by the Controlled Drugs legislation).
- Making an assessment of the patient's condition before deciding to prescribe a medicine: any previous adverse reactions to medicines, recent use of other medicines including non-prescription and herbal medicines, illegal drugs and medicines purchased online, adherence to other medicines and other medical conditions.
- Effective shared-care prescribing through liaison with colleagues in other care settings and through ensuring a smooth transition of the patient's pharmaceutical care across the interface.
- Raising concerns about prescribing and administration errors by questioning any decision or action that may be considered unsafe.

- Identifying and reporting suspected adverse drug reactions to the Medicines and Healthcare products Regulatory Agency (MHRA) as appropriate.
- Reviewing medicines' use for any adverse effects, non-adherence or other pharmaceutical problems and arranging monitoring at regular intervals by following the BNF or other authoritative clinical guidance.
- Considering and, if appropriate, acting on any recommendations provided by pharmacists or other healthcare professionals who have reviewed patients' (use of) medicines.
- Ensuring that all repeat prescriptions are safe and appropriate.
- Prescribing unlicensed medicines only where a suitable licensed medicine is not available, commonly in paediatrics, psychiatry or palliative care.[5]

The communication with the patient and/or his or her relative(s)/carer(s) is of paramount importance for safe and effective prescribing. According to the GMC,[5] the prescriber should make an assessment of the patient's condition and reach an agreement with him or her on the treatment options proposed, explaining:

- the likely risks and benefits of treatment, including serious and common adverse effects
- if applicable, the use of an unlicensed medicine or the use of a licensed medicine for an unlicensed indication ('off-label' prescribing)
- what to do in the event of a side effect or reoccurrence of the condition
- how and when to take the medicine
- how to adjust the dose if necessary
- how to use a medical device (e.g. an inhaler)
- the likely duration of treatment
- the arrangements for monitoring, follow-up and review, including further consultation, blood tests or other investigations, processes for adjusting the type or dose of medicine, and for issuing repeat prescriptions.

The prescriber should also check that the patient and/or his or her relative/carer understood the information provided and answer any related questions or address any concerns as appropriate. The special needs of each patient should be taken into account, including any language barrier or disability, and information in other languages or relevant disability aids should be provided.

Any medicines' adherence issues should be investigated and dealt with prior to starting a new medicine.[5]

Considering the time limitations, prescribers are encouraged to liaise with other members of the multidisciplinary healthcare team, such as pharmacists, to carry out medicines reviews and to ensure that patients are appropriately counselled on the above before initiating therapy.

The GMC guide is informative and should be adhered to at all times when prescribing medicines or medical devices,[5] however it may be difficult to follow in day-to-day prescribing practice. The simpler, step-wise approach has been proposed by Webb and colleagues in their 'Clinical Pharmacy Process'.[6]

Step 1: Establishing the Need for Drug Therapy

- Diagnosis
- Risks vs. benefits of treatment
- Patient's health and social circumstances
- Past medical history
- Medication ('drug') history

Step 2: Selecting the Medicine

- Drug–patient interactions (e.g. prescribing warfarin for an elderly, confused patient, prescribing amoxicillin for a patient with a penicillin allergy or prescribing trimethoprim to a pregnant woman)
- Drug–disease interactions (e.g. metformin in renal failure, diltiazem in uncontrolled heart failure, statins in liver impairment, digoxin and hypokalaemia, ciprofloxacin in epilepsy, aspirin in a patient with a history of peptic ulcer bleeding, diclofenac in a patient with a history of myocardial infarction)
- Drug–drug interactions (e.g. simvastatin and clarithromycin, amiodarone and warfarin, methotrexate and non-steroidal anti-inflammatory drugs (NSAIDs), theophylline and smoking, lithium and diuretics, tetracyclines and calcium, alcohol and anticonvulsants)

Step 3: Administering the Medicine

- Calculating the dose (the use of weight/height/body surface area of the patient)
- For parenteral medicines, ensuring appropriate concentrations in compatible fluids and rates of infusion

- Selecting an appropriate regimen (risks associated with parenteral administration, patient's clinical condition, frequency of administration/duration of action/half-life)
- The rate and extent of absorption (oral bioavailability of digoxin liquid vs. digoxin tablets, malabsorption disorders, liver impairment)
- Degree of plasma protein binding (for highly protein-bound drugs, such as phenytoin and prednisolone)
- Volume of distribution (e.g. theophylline and heart failure)

Step 4: Providing the Medicine

- Ensuring the prescription is legal, legible, accurate and unambiguous
- Hospital formulary status (non-formulary or restricted-use) and shared-care guidelines (continuation of supply, monitoring and review in primary or secondary care)

Step 5: Monitoring Therapy

- Effectiveness (e.g. symptomatic improvement of heart failure, forced expiratory volume (FEV_1) in COPD, changes in inflammatory markers with antimicrobial treatment, changes in Disease Activity Score (DAS28) with methotrexate, TDM for narrow therapeutic index drugs, such as vancomycin, digoxin, phenytoin)
- Potential adverse effects (bleeding with anticoagulants/antiplatelets, osteoporosis with long-term corticosteroid use, ciclosporin and acute renal failure, carbamazepine and rash/liver impairment, antidepressants and hyponatraemia)

Step 6: Patient Advice and Education

- Providing accurate and reliable information (e.g. booklets for warfarin or methotrexate, steroid cards for corticosteroids, information booklets produced by Diabetes UK and British Heart Foundation)
- Medicines' reminder charts or medicines' administration charts (e.g. for those patients living in a nursing home)
- Describing the sources of further help and information, encouraging questions

Step 7: Evaluating Effectiveness

- Carrying out regular reviews for each medicine using steps 1–6 presented here
- Taking appropriate action to ensure that healthcare outcomes set at the beginning of treatment (e.g. reduction of a patient's symptomatology) are met as appropriate (e.g. if FEV_1 is more than 50% in a COPD patient who already uses a when-required short-acting beta$_2$ agonist and a long-acting beta$_2$ agonist; however, is still experiencing exacerbations or persistent breathlessness, he or she may require a combination inhaler of a long-acting beta$_2$ agonist plus an inhaled corticosteroid after the inhaler technique and adherence to treatment are reviewed).[6,7]

References

1. Oxford Dictionaries. *Prescribe* [Online]. Oxford: Oxford University Press [cited 10 March 2013]. Available at: www.oxforddictionaries.com/definition/english/prescribe
2. *Medicines and Pharmacy* [Online]. London: Department of Health [cited 10 March 2013]. Available at: http://webarchive.nationalarchives.gov.uk/+/www.dh.gov.uk/en/Healthcare/Medicinespharmacyandindustry/DH_099148
3. Quality, Innovation, Productivity and Prevention (QIPP) [Online]. The Lancet UK Policy Matters [cited 30 November 2013]. Available at: http://ukpolicymatters.thelancet.com/qipp-programme-quality-innovation-productivity-and-prevention/
4. Hepler CD, Strand LM. Opportunities and responsibilities in pharmaceutical care. *Am J Hosp Pharm*. 1990; **47**(3): 533–43.
5. *Good Practice in Prescribing and Managing Medicines and Devices* [Online]. General Medical Council; 2013 [cited 30 November 2013]. Available at: www.gmc-uk.org/Prescribing_Guidance__2013__50955425.pdf
6. Webb DG, Davies JG, McRobbie D. Clinical pharmacy process. In: Walker R WC, editor. Clinical Pharmacy and Therapeutics. 4th ed. London: Churchill Livingstone; 2007. p. 3–11.
7. British Medical Association; Royal Pharmaceutical Society. *British National Formulary 65*. London: Pharmaceutical Press; 2013.

Appendix 4

The Guide to Using and Revising the *British National Formulary*

The BNF is a unique collaboration between numerous organisations, primarily the British Medical Association and the Royal Pharmaceutical Society, which brings together 'authoritative, independent guidance on best practice with clinically validated drug information'.[1] Among other available evidence and information, the BNF considers the available Summaries of Product Characteristics, peer-reviewed articles and systematic reviews/meta analyses, consensus guidelines (e.g. those of NICE), tertiary literature (e.g. Martindale: the Complete Drug Reference), statutory information (e.g. the Medicines Act 1968), expert opinions and comments from industry.

The BNF can be split into three major sections: (1) the introduction (which includes 'Changes for This Edition', 'Guidance on Prescribing' and 'Emergency Treatment of Poisoning'), (2) notes on drugs and preparations (15 chapters arranged broadly according to body systems and types of conditions managed or treated) and (3) appendices/indices.

Each section of the BNF is important in its own right and may be used in different clinical scenarios. Therefore, apart from revising the 15 main chapters, the PSA candidates are reminded to familiarise themselves with the guidance on prescribing (e.g. prescribing in renal impairment, palliative care or pregnancy/breastfeeding), the appendices/indices (e.g. intravenous additives and the use of different diluents for certain intravenous infusions) and the 'back' of the BNF (e.g. the use of Cardiovascular Risk Prediction Charts).

Even though the BNF's index is useful in finding the information needed, the common knowledge of where in the BNF such information is outlined would help the candidate browse to the correct section more efficiently. The following sections outline the main information points for each section/chapter of the BNF that PSA candidates should pay attention to when revising for the assessment and in everyday practice (organised according to the outline of the BNF). This is not an exhaustive list, and there might be questions in the assessment for which you would need to use information in the BNF not highlighted here. You do not need to memorise all the information included in this section or the information in the BNF that this section refers to, but you are advised to familiarise yourself with it to enable you to find it quickly if needed. The most important warnings, tables, guidelines, advice and information points are highlighted here in bold.

How to use the *British National Formulary*

- The symbol that is used to denote preparations that are considered by the Joint Formulary Committee to be less suitable for prescribing
- The symbol that is placed against those preparations that are not prescribable in the NHS (the 'blacklist')
- Selecting a suitable preparation (e.g. the use of 'sugar-free' preparations)

Prescription Writing

- 'Micrograms' and 'nanograms' – no abbreviations
- Avoid decimals unless necessary (e.g. 3 mg, not 3.0 mg)

Controlled Drugs and Drug Dependence

- Prescription requirements for Schedule 2 and 3 drugs (temazepam exemption)

Adverse Reactions to Drugs

- What does the black triangle symbol mean?
- Which ADRs need to be reported for newer drugs and vaccines?
- Which ADRs need to be reported for established drugs and vaccines?
- Which ADRs need to be reported for medical devices?
- Which ADRs need to be reported if they occur in children?
- What are the principles used when listing the side effects in each drug monograph?

- Which drugs can affect the oral mucosa, the teeth and jaw, the periodontium and the salivary glands?
- Which drugs can cause changes in taste or taste disturbances?

Prescribing for Children

- Avoiding intramuscular injections in children
- ADRs in children
- Special prescription requirements (for children under 12 years of age)
- Tablets vs. liquids
- Dose frequency (e.g. giving the night-time dose earlier to avoid waking the child up at night)

Prescribing in Hepatic Impairment

- Which drugs can accumulate in patients with intrahepatic or extrahepatic obstructive jaundice?
- Which drugs are affected by hypoproteinaemia?
- Which drugs can further impair the cerebral function in the presence of severe liver disease?
- Which drugs can exacerbate oedema and ascites in chronic liver disease?

Prescribing in Renal Impairment

- How many half-lives does it take to reach a steady-state plasma concentration?
- **Cockcroft and Gault formula vs. eGFR** and the MDRD formula: which one to use and when?
- Stages of CKD (based on NICE clinical guideline 73)

Prescribing in Pregnancy

- What are the effects of drugs given in different trimesters of pregnancy and around the time of labour?
- What are the late-onset effects that can result from use of drugs during pregnancy?
- Where can you find the information on drugs and pregnancy?

Prescribing in Breastfeeding

- Which drug characteristics may allow them to achieve a concentration in milk that is high enough to expose the infant to adverse effects?

- The main drug example known to inhibit the infant's sucking reflex
- The main drug example to affect lactation

Prescribing in Palliative Care

- The stepwise approach to pain management (i.e. from paracetamol/ NSAIDs to strong opioids)
- **Equivalent single doses of opioid analgesics**
- How to initiate the modified-release opioid analgesics?
- How to calculate the 'breakthrough pain' dose?
- How to convert oral morphine to parenteral morphine?
- How to convert oral morphine to parenteral diamorphine?
- **How to convert oral morphine to transdermal fentanyl or buprenorphine?**
- How to manage gastrointestinal pain?
- How to manage neuropathic pain?
- How to manage excessive respiratory secretions?
- How to manage nausea and vomiting?
- How to manage raised intracranial pressure?
- How to manage restlessness and confusion?
- How to manage a variety of palliative care conditions using continuous infusion devices?
- **Mixing and compatibility of drugs commonly used for continuous subcutaneous infusions**
- **Equivalent doses of morphine and diamorphine (oral vs. subcutaneous infusions)**

Prescribing in the Elderly

- Which drugs are the elderly population more sensitive to?
- Which drugs are affected by changes in renal/hepatic clearance that occurs in the elderly?
- Which drugs commonly cause constipation in the elderly?
- Which drugs commonly lead to hypotension and falls in the elderly?
- What are the main risks associated with the use of hypnotics, diuretics and NSAIDs in the elderly?
- Which other drugs need to be used with caution or should be avoided in the elderly (e.g. co-trimoxazole, glibenclamide, warfarin)?

Prescribing in Dental Practice

- Signs/symptoms and management of hypoglycaemia

Emergency Treatment of Poisoning

- The management of toxicity associated with the following:
  - ‣ aspirin
  - ‣ **paracetamol (be familiar with the plasma concentration against time graph and the use of acetylcysteine)**
  - ‣ opioids
  - ‣ antidepressants
  - ‣ beta blockers
  - ‣ benzodiazepines
  - ‣ iron salts
  - ‣ theophylline
  - ‣ snake bites and animal stings

1: Gastrointestinal System

- How to manage dyspepsia and gastro-oesophageal reflux disease (including special populations, e.g. pregnant women and children)?
- Interactions between antacids and commonly used medicines
- The definition of and significance of 'low Na$^+$' (sodium) and antacid preparations containing 'low Na$^+$'
- The use of antispasmodic (particularly antimuscarinic) drugs in the management of IBS and diverticular disease (including cautions, contraindications and side effects)
- **The testing and eradication of *Helicobacter pylori* infection (including the recommended regimens for adults)**
- The management of NSAID-associated ulcers
- Bezoar formation with sucralfate
- The use of misoprostol in women of childbearing age
- The use of proton pump inhibitors (including cautions and side effects, paying special attention to hyponatraemia, hypomagnesaemia and diarrhoea)
- The management of acute diarrhoea and the use of antimotility drugs (cautions, side effects (e.g. paralytic ileus) and contraindications, such as antibiotic-associated colitis)
- The management of ulcerative colitis vs. the management of Crohn's disease (paying special attention to the use of infliximab)

- The management of *Clostridium difficile* infection
- The management of IBS
- Aminosalicylates and blood disorders, aminosalicylates and 'brand specificity'
- **The 'blue box' for methotrexate (weekly dose, folic acid replacement, blood disorders, liver toxicity, respiratory effects)**
- The use of laxatives (including special populations of children and pregnant women)
- Bowel cleansing preparations (cautions, contraindications and side effects)
- Stoma care (including the use of EC/modified-release preparations, laxatives, antidiarrhoeals, diuretics)
- Colestyramine and absorption of other drugs
- **The administration of pancreatin and higher-strength pancreatin preparations**

2: Cardiovascular System

- Digoxin: the threshold of 60 beats/min, loading in patients with heart failure, renal function and digoxin, toxicity and TDM, hypokalaemia, digoxin-specific antibody fragments
- Diuretics: hypokalaemia and the use of diuretics in the elderly
- Thiazides: cautions, contraindications, renal/hepatic impairment (risk of encephalopathy in alcoholic patients), pregnancy/breastfeeding and main side effects (particularly electrolyte and metabolic disturbances)
- Loop diuretics: as for thiazides, the administration of IV preparations and the risk of ototoxicity (the maximum rate of administration for IV infusion)
- Potassium-sparing diuretics and aldosterone antagonists: indications, cautions, contraindications, side effects, eplerenone vs. spironolactone
- The use of mannitol to treat cerebral oedema and raised intra-ocular pressure
- The management of common arrhythmias, particularly atrial fibrillation (AF) and atrial flutter, arrhythmias after myocardial infarction, ventricular tachycardia
- The Vaughan Williams classification of the anti-arrhythmic drugs
- Anti-arrhythmic drugs which prolong QT interval, e.g. amiodarone
- Dronedarone and hepatic disorders, heart failure, monitoring required
- Amiodarone: cautions, contraindications, side effects, monitoring required

- Beta-adrenoceptor blocking drugs: drugs with intrinsic sympathomimetic activity, water-soluble drugs, sotalol and QT interval, drugs that lower peripheral resistance, cardioselective drugs, common adverse effects, beta blockers and pregnancy/breastfeeding, beta blockers and angina/myocardial infarction, esmolol and supraventricular arrhythmias, beta blockers and heart failure, propranolol and thyrotoxicosis, beta blockers and bronchospasm, **labetalol and liver damage**
- Hypertension: thresholds and targets of treatment (including special populations of elderly, diabetes, renal disease, pregnancy/breastfeeding), the management of hypertension (including special populations as mentioned), hypertensive crises
- Alpha-adrenoceptor blocking drugs: indications, cautions (including drowsiness), side effects
- Heart failure: stepwise approach to heart failure management
- ACE inhibitors: indications, renal effects (note bilateral renal artery stenosis), anaphylactoid reactions, concomitant diuretic use, hepatic impairment and use of prodrugs, other side effects, pregnancy/breastfeeding
- Angiotensin-II receptor blockers: as for ACE inhibitors, drugs licensed for use alone or in a combination with an ACE inhibitor in heart failure
- Nitrates: different preparations of glyceryl trinitrate (GTN) available and their clinical indications, isosorbide dinitrate vs. mononitrate (the variety of dosage forms available), nitrate tolerance, side effects, cautions and contraindications
- Calcium-channel blockers (CCBs): dihydropyridine vs. non-dihydropyridine CCBs, verapamil and negatively inotropic effects, nifedipine and nicardipine vs. amlodipine and felodipine, the use of nimodipine in patients who suffered a subarachnoid haemorrhage, diltiazem and 'brand specificity', side effects, cautions and contraindications
- Other antianginal drugs: clinical indications of nicorandil, **ivabradine (note NICE guidance on the use in CHF)** and ranolazine (caution with QT interval prolongation)
- **Peripheral vasodilators: NICE guidance on the treatment of intermittent claudication, the management of Raynaud's phenomenon**
- The use of sympathomimetics in the treatment of shock
- Cardiopulmonary resuscitation

- Heparin: clinical indications, UFH vs. low-molecular-weight heparins (LMWHs), different routes of administration, APTT monitoring, the use in pregnancy/breastfeeding, the use of protamine sulphate in an event of a haemorrhage, heparin-induced thrombocytopenia, hyperkalaemia, administration around spinal/epidural anaesthesia, renal/hepatic impairment
- LMWHs: *see* 'Heparin' in previous point, monitoring of anti-Factor Xa activity
- Danaparoid, argatroban, bivalirudin, epoprostenol, fondaparinux: clinical indications/uses
- Warfarin: clinical indications, dosing, monitoring (including target INR for different conditions), duration of treatment, the management of haemorrhage/high INR, peri-operative anticoagulation, combined use with antiplatelets, hepatic/renal impairment, pregnancy/breastfeeding, counselling, see interactions in Appendix 1 of the BNF.
- **Dabigatran, apixaban and rivaroxaban: NICE guidance for clinical indications, renal/hepatic impairment and dosing (including special populations, such as elderly or those on interacting medicines), duration of treatment**
- **Antiplatelet drugs: clinical indications, duration of clopidogrel treatment for patients with STEMI/NSTEMI, unstable angina, NICE guidance on clopidogrel and dipyridamole, NICE guidance on the use of prasugrel and ticagrelor, antiplatelet drugs and coronary stents (special attention at durations of treatment)**
- Management of transient ischaemic attack (TIA) and ischaemic stroke: initial management vs. long-term management (antiplatelet drugs, blood pressure control, the use of statins, special populations, such as patients with atrial fibrillation)
- Intracerebral haemorrhage: the use of caval filters, the use of statins
- Management of stable angina vs. acute coronary syndromes (NSTEMI, unstable angina, STEMI): oxygen, pain relief, anti-platelets, beta-blockers and other anti-anginals, ACE inhibitors, statins
- **Fibrinolytic drugs: indications, time frame for thrombolysis, cautions and contraindications to thrombolysis**
- Lipid-regulating drugs: clinical indications and targets (total cholesterol, LDL-C), primary vs. secondary prevention of cardiovascular events, the management of hyperlipidaemias, risks associated with combination

treatment, monitoring, **side effects of statins (especially muscle effects)**, their use in hepatic impairment, pregnancy/breastfeeding, patient counselling, bile acid sequestrants and vitamin supplements, counselling, **NICE guidance on ezetimibe**, fibrates and myotoxicity, nicotinic acid and prostaglandin-mediated symptoms

3: Respiratory System

- The use of inhaled vs. oral vs. parenteral drugs (indications, advantages and risks)
- The control of asthma in pregnancy and breastfeeding
- **Management of chronic asthma and management of acute asthma tables**
- **Chronic obstructive pulmonary disease (COPD) management (including the flow chart of inhaled therapies and the use of oxygen in those at risk of type II respiratory failure)**
- The treatment of croup
- Selective beta$_2$ agonists: **Commission on Human Medicines (CHM) advice on long-acting beta$_2$ agonists**, cautions and side effects (e.g. tremor, QT-interval prolongation, hypokalaemia – note the combined use with theophylline and corticosteroids), counselling for different devices
- Antimuscarinic bronchodilators: clinical indications, ipratropium vs. tiotropium, cautions (especially glaucoma), side effects, counselling for different devices
- Theophylline: indications, variations in plasma theophylline concentration in different populations of patients (note hepatic impairment, smoking, heart failure, enzyme inducing/inhibiting drugs), TDM, theophylline vs. aminophylline, caffeine, 'brand specificity', cautions, side effects, contraindications
- Drug delivery devices: **NICE guidance on inhaler devices**, spacer devices, indications for nebulisation, the use of oxygen vs. air to drive nebulisers for patients at risk of hypercapnia
- Corticosteroids: smoking and corticosteroids, onset of action, cautions (including paradoxical bronchospasm), **MHRA/CHM advice on beclometasone inhalers** (particularly, Qvar® vs. Clenil Modulite®), side effects of inhaled corticosteroids, counselling for different devices
- Leukotriene receptor antagonists: clinical indications, Churg–Strauss syndrome, zafirlukast and hepatic disorders

- Roflumilast: NICE guidance for use in COPD
- Antihistamines: sedating vs. non-sedating antihistamines, clinical indications/uses, cautions and contraindications (e.g. caution in prostatic hypertrophy), hepatic impairment and sedating antihistamines, pregnancy/breastfeeding, side effects
- Omalizumab: **NICE guidance for use in severe persistent allergic asthma,** Churg–Strauss syndrome
- Anaphylaxis: stepwise approach to management, **the table of doses of intramuscular adrenaline,** the use of adrenaline in patients taking beta blockers
- C1-esterase inhibitor: clinical indications
- Pulmonary surfactants: clinical indications
- Oxygen: target oxygen saturation for different populations of patients, including those at risk of hypercapnic respiratory failure, high- vs. low-concentration oxygen therapy (indications), long-term oxygen therapy (indications), oxygen therapy equipment
- Carbocisteine: indications and cautions
- Dornase alfa: indications and dosing
- NICE guidance on mannitol dry powder for inhalation for treating cystic fibrosis
- Hypertonic sodium chloride: indications
- **Cough suppressants: MHRA/CHM advice on over-the-counter (OTC) cough and cold medicines for children, MHRA/CHM advice on OTC codeine-containing liquid medicines for children**
- Systemic nasal decongestants: indications and cautions

4: Central Nervous System

- Benzodiazepines: paradoxical effects, driving, dependence and withdrawal, indications, **approximate equivalent doses,** use in children, elderly and for dental procedures, use in hepatic/renal impairment and pregnancy/breastfeeding, side effects, cautions and contraindications
- Zaleplon, zolpidem and zopiclone vs. benzodiazepines
- Chloral hydrate and clomethiazole: indications
- Melatonin: indications
- Different options in the management of anxiety
- Barbiturates: indications and use in the elderly

- Antipsychotics: **special considerations (the first seven bullet points)**, clinical indications, first- vs. second-generation antipsychotics, cautions, contraindications, **antipsychotic prescribing for the elderly** (particularly those with dementia), driving, withdrawal, hepatic/renal impairment, pregnancy/breastfeeding, side effects (especially extrapyramidal symptoms, cardiovascular risks, neuroleptic malignant syndrome), the choice of antipsychotic (e.g. in patients with diabetes), monitoring requirements, **equivalent doses of oral antipsychotics**, pimozide and ECG monitoring, **clozapine and agranulocytosis, myocarditis/ cardiomyopathy, gastrointestinal obstruction**, CNS and respiratory depression, monitoring, side effects and their management (e.g. the use of hyoscine for hypersalivation), **equivalent doses of depot antipsychotics** and their clinical indications
- Antimanic drugs: the choice of drug/clinical indications, lithium (thyroid disorders, TDM, interactions with ACE inhibitors, NSAIDs, diuretics, etc., signs and symptoms of overdosage/toxicity, withdrawal, 'brand specificity', patient counselling)
- Antidepressant drugs: different classes and choice of antidepressants, St John's wort, **hyponatraemia and antidepressant therapy**, **suicidal behaviour and antidepressant therapy**, the management of depression, antidepressant withdrawal, pregnancy/breastfeeding (for different classes of drugs), tricyclic antidepressants (indications, cautions, especially cardiovascular risks, interactions, contraindications, side effects), monoamine oxidase inhibitors (as for tricyclics, tyramine 'cheese syndrome', advantages of moclobemide), selective serotonin re-uptake inhibitors (**depressive illness in children and adolescents**, cautions (especially epilepsy), interactions, contraindications, side effects (note the cardiovascular risks)), citalopram (QT prolongation, maximum dosage in elderly over 65 years of age, conversion of tablets to oral drops), **mirtazapine** (**blood disorders**, withdrawal), venlafaxine (withdrawal), duloxetine (different indications for different preparations available)
- CNS stimulants: clinical indications, atomoxetine and hepatic disorders, suicidal ideation, dexamfetamine and special cautions in children, methylphenidate and evening dosing, 'brand specificity'
- Orlistat: clinical indications (special criteria), multivitamin use and other cautions, side effects and contraindications, patient counselling, interactions

- Drugs used in nausea and vertigo: clinical indications of different drugs, metoclopramide (dystonic reactions, particularly in the young (aged under 20 years) and very old, also see special restrictions under metoclopramide monograph), domperidone vs. metoclopramide, vomiting during pregnancy (management and supplementation with thiamine), post-operative nausea and vomiting, motion sickness, other vestibular disorders (including Ménière's disease), ondansetron and QT interval prolongation
- Non-opioid analgesics: pain in sickle cell disease, dental and orofacial pain, dysmenorrhoea, clinical indications of drugs available for use, **aspirin (use in children under 16 years of age, hypersensitivity)**, paracetamol (maximum dose of IV preparation)
- Opioid analgesics: cautions, contraindications, hepatic/renal impairment, pregnancy/breastfeeding, major side effects, clinical uses, buprenorphine patches (**fever and external heat**, preparations available, dose adjustment, patient counselling), codeine (variation in metabolism), fentanyl (dose adjustment, duration of action, **patient counselling, fever and external heat, respiratory depression**, special requirements for prescriptions), methadone (indications, **QT interval prolongation**), morphine salts and oxycodone (different preparations available), tramadol (interactions with antidepressants, use in patients with epilepsy)
- Neuropathic pain: drugs available for the treatment of different neuropathies
- Antimigraine drugs: drugs available for use, $5HT_1$-receptor agonists (cautions, especially cardiovascular risks, contraindications, side effects, patient counselling for different preparations), ergotamine and peripheral vasospasm, pizotifen and cautions, treatment of cluster headaches, **NICE guidance on the use of botulinum toxin type A**
- Antiepileptic drugs: considerations when choosing an antiepileptic drug, interactions, withdrawal, **antiepileptic hypersensitivity syndrome**, driving, pregnancy and breastfeeding, carbamazepine (indications/ uses, cautions, **blood, hepatic and skin disorders**, patient counselling, 'brand specificity', routes of administration including switching PO carbamazepine to PR, TDM), oxcarbazepine (**blood, hepatic and skin disorders**), ethosuximide (**blood disorders**), lamotrigine (**blood disorders, skin reactions, counselling**, careful dose titration), phenytoin (indications (not effective in absence seizures), TDM, 'brand and preparation specificity' (phenytoin sodium vs. phenytoin base), protein

binding, signs/symptoms of toxicity, side effects (**blood and skin disorders**), patient counselling, phenytoin vs. fosphenytoin, retigabine (NICE guidance, QT interval prolongation), **topiramate (ocular effects)**, **sodium valproate** (**liver toxicity, blood and hepatic disorders, pancreatitis**, different preparations available, monitoring), **vigabatrin (visual field defects)**, stepwise management of status epilepticus in primary and secondary care (including relevant monitoring), febrile convulsions and paracetamol

- Parkinson's disease: the choice of treatment (consider special populations, such as elderly), dopamine receptor agonists (ergot-derived vs. non-ergot-derived, **impulse control disorders**, withdrawal, **fibrotic reactions, sudden onset of sleep and hypotensive reactions**, apomorphine, use of rotigotine patches (including the dose titration), levodopa (side effects, particularly nausea/vomiting, motor complications, 'end-of-dose' deterioration, reddish discolouration of body fluids, combinations with benserazide and carbidopa, different preparations available, cautions), catechol-O-methyltransferase inbibitors (**tolcapone and hepatotoxicity**, Stalevo®), antimuscarinic drugs (cautions, contraindications, side effects)

- Drugs used in substance dependence: chlordiazepoxide and alcohol withdrawal, treatment of delirium tremens, thiamine and Wernicke's encephalopathy, disulfiram (initiation of treatment and patient counselling), nicotine dependence (bupropion and cautions, choice of nicotine replacement therapy, cautions, side effects, patient counselling, **varenicline and MHRA/CHM advice on suicidal behaviour**), opioid substitution therapy (**missed doses, NICE guidance on buprenorphine and methadone, NICE guidance on naltrexone**)

- Drugs for dementia: clinical indications, **NICE guidance**, donepezil, galantamine, rivastigmine and cardiovascular risks, galantamine and hepatic impairment, memantine and history of convulsions, switching patients from oral to transdermal rivastigmine

5: Infections

- **The table of notifiable diseases**
- Considerations when choosing a suitable antibacterial (e.g. allergies, renal/hepatic function, co-morbidities, ethnic origin, age, pregnancy/breastfeeding)

- Other general principles of antibacterial prescribing (i.e. dose, route, duration)
- **Summary of antibacterial therapy table: be able to navigate within the table according to body systems/different infections**
- **Summary of antibacterial prophylaxis table: be able to navigate within the table according to different surgical procedures and types of infections**
- **NICE guidance on antimicrobial prophylaxis against infective endocarditis in adults and children undergoing interventional procedures**
- Penicillins and beta-lactams: hypersensitivity reactions, encephalopathy, accumulation of sodium/potassium in renal failure, MRSA (know the options available and the general principles of treatment), **flucloxacillin and hepatic disorders**, **co-amoxiclav and cholestatic jaundice**, penicillins vs. cephalosporins vs. carbapenems, aztreonam and specific cautions for inhaled treatment, specific side effects for parenteral treatment
- Tetracyclines: cautions (note myasthenia gravis and systemic lupus), interactions with iron, calcium, aluminium, magnesium, zinc, contraindications (special considerations in children, pregnant and breastfeeding women), renal/hepatic impairment, photosensitivity with doxycycline and demeclocycline, patient counselling
- Aminoglycosides: treatment of endocarditis, once-daily vs. multiple daily dose regimens, **monitoring of serum concentrations**, the use of aminoglycosides in renal impairment, contraindications (myasthenia gravis), **'peak' and 'trough' concentrations for multiple daily dose regimen of gentamicin, amikacin and tobramycin**, using ideal body weight to calculate the dose in obese patients, specific **cautions for inhaled treatment with tobramycin**
- Macrolides: QT interval prolongation, caution in myasthenia gravis, hepatotoxicity **(particularly telithromycin)**, **telithromycin and driving**
- Clindamycin: diarrhoea/colitis, monitoring liver/renal function, injections containing benzyl alcohol in neonates
- Other antibacterials: chloramphenicol **(blood disorders, plasma monitoring in neonates (know the underlying reasons)**, sodium fusidate vs. fusidic acid (bioavailability, **hepatotoxicity**), vancomycin (risk of anaphylactoid reactions with rapid infusion, nephrotoxicity, ototoxicity,

plasma concentration monitoring, oral vancomycin for *Clostridium difficile*), **daptomycin (muscular effects), linezolid (blood disorders, optic neuropathy, interactions), colistin (specific cautions for inhaled treatment and side effects of parenteral/inhaled treatments, monitoring of plasma concentration, preparation of Colomycin® for nebulisation)**

- Sulfonamides and trimethoprim: co-trimoxazole (**restrictions on the use of**, cautions, acute porphyria, use in pregnancy/breastfeeding), **trimethoprim (blood disorders**, folate deficiency, interactions – note methotrexate)
- Antituberculosis drugs: **unsupervised vs. supervised regimens**, monitoring (particularly **hepatic/renal function, visual acuity (ethambutol)**, isoniazid and peripheral neuropathy/pyridoxine, rifampicin and six toxicity syndromes, e.g. thrombocytopenic purpura, interactions, discolouration of body secretions with rifampicin/rifabutin)
- Metronidazole: disulfiram-like reaction, patient counselling
- Quinolones: use in epilepsy, myasthenia gravis, **children/adolescents (see the text box on tendon damage)**, QT interval prolongation, photosensitivity, interactions, drowsiness, patient counselling
- Nitrofurantoin: pulmonary and liver effects, neuropathy, acute porphyria, use in poor renal function (eGFR <60 mL/min/1.73 m^2)
- Antifungal drugs: treatment of different fungal infections (e.g. aspergillosis vs. uncomplicated candidiasis), fluconazole and voriconazole (hepatotoxicity, QT interval prolongation, acute porphyria, interactions), itraconazole (as for fluconazole plus risk of **heart failure**), ketoconazole (hepatotoxicity, interactions), **amphotericin (anaphylaxis**, renal impairment, advantages of lipid formulations over traditional formulations)
- HIV infection: principles of treatment (the commonly used starting regimens), immune reconstitution syndrome, lipodystrophy syndrome, osteonecrosis, drug interactions (particularly ritonavir and other protease inhibitors), lactic acidosis with nucleoside reverse transcriptase inhibitors, **abacavir and hypersensitivity reactions, didanosine and pancreatitis, lamivudine/tenofovir and chronic hepatitis B, darunavir/ fosamprenavir/atazanavir and rash, ritonavir ± lopinavir and pancreatitis, saquinavir and arrhythmias, tipranavir and hepatotoxicity, efavirenz (rash, psychiatric disorders), etravirine and hypersensitivity**

reactions, nevirapine (hepatotoxicity, rash), enfuvirtide and hypersensitivity reactions, raltegravir and rash

- Herpes virus infections: aciclovir vs. famciclovir vs. valaciclovir, aciclovir (renal impairment, hydration, neurological reactions, use of ideal body weight in obese patients)
- Treatment of cytomegalovirus infection: cidofovir and nephrotoxicity, ocular disorders, ganciclovir vs. *valganciclovir* and caution in handling
- Chronic hepatitis B and chronic hepatitis C: **treatment options as endorsed by NICE**
- Influenza: oseltamivir in children, pregnancy/breastfeeding and **NICE guidance on oseltamivir, zanamivir and amantadine**
- The treatment of respiratory syncytial virus: palivizumab (indications), ribavirin (indications, specific cautions for inhaled/oral treatment, contraindications, specific side effects for inhaled/oral treatment)
- Antimalarials: treatment pathway for falciparum malaria vs. benign malaria, **primaquine and glucose-6-phosphate dehydrogenase (G6PD) deficiency**, prophylaxis against malaria (length of prophylaxis, chloroquine/mefloquine and epilepsy, pregnancy/breastfeeding, renal impairment and malarone, anticoagulants, **be familiar with continents, countries, regions outlined in the prophylaxis table**), **mefloquine and driving**, quinine (cardiovascular risks, myasthenia gravis, **equivalent doses of quinine base and different quinine salts**)
- Anthelmintics: be familiar with options available for the treatment of different infections, particularly threadworms, mebendazole and interactions, piperazine and epilepsy, liver/kidney disease

6: Endocrine System

- Insulin: **target glucose and HbA$_{1c}$**, examples of recommended insulin regimens, insulin in pregnancy/breastfeeding, **NICE guidance on continuous subcutaneous insulin infusion**, insulin therapy during peri-operative period, **NICE guidance on insulin detemir and insulin glargine**
- Antidiabetic drugs: **licensed/NICE indications for all commonly used drugs**, the principles of management in pregnancy/breastfeeding, sulfonylureas (hypoglycaemia and glibenclamide vs. gliclazide/tolbutamide, sulfonylureas and surgery, acute porphyria), **metformin (risk factors for lactic acidosis and relevant NICE guidance,**

iodine-containing X-ray contrast media and metformin, anorexia, gastrointestinal side effects, decreased B_{12} absorption), **pioglitazone (NICE guidance on HbA$_{1c}$ changes, MHRA/CHM advice on cardiovascular safety, risk of bladder cancer, liver toxicity**, risk of bone fractures), **dipeptidyl peptidase-4 inhibitors (NICE guidance on HbA$_{1c}$ changes, vildagliptin and liver toxicity**), **glucagon-like peptide-1 activators (NICE guidance on recommended indications, and HbA$_{1c}$ and weight changes, exenatide and pancreatitis, patient counselling**)

- Management of diabetic ketoacidosis (fluids, insulin and relevant monitoring) and hypoglycaemia (oral/IV glucose and glucagon)
- Management of diabetic nephropathy and diabetic neuropathy (use in conjunction with relevant NICE guidance)
- Thyroid hormones: levothyroxine vs. liothyronine, **levothyroxine (initial dosage, baseline ECG and symptomatic monitoring)**
- Anti-thyroid drugs: carbimazole (initiation of therapy and dose adjustment, **neutropenia and agranulocytosis**, rashes and pruritus), treatment of thyrotoxic crisis, drugs during pregnancy/breastfeeding, **propylthiouracil (hepatotoxicity**, leucopenia)
- Corticosteroids: corticosteroid replacement in Addison's disease and acute adrenocortical insufficiency, **equivalent anti-inflammatory doses of corticosteroids**, properties and uses of different corticosteroids, cautions and adverse effects, particularly adrenal suppression (including the use of corticosteroids peri-operatively and recommendations on **withdrawal of treatment**), risk of infections, psychiatric reactions, metabolic disturbances, osteoporosis, **advice to patients/steroid treatment card**, the use in pregnancy/breastfeeding
- Female sex hormones and their modulators: HRT (risk of VTE, stroke, endometrial cancer (but note the reduced risk by progestogen), breast cancer, ovarian cancer, coronary heart disease, **be familiar with the HRT risk table and know how to use it to estimate individual risks**, the choice of HRT, HRT and surgery, contraindications to HRT, **withdrawal bleeding**, counselling on patches), raloxifene (venous thromboembolism, stroke, breast cancer, endometrial cancer), progestogens (fluid retention, history of liver tumours, genital/breast cancer, arterial disease)
- Male sex hormones and antagonists: testosterone (cardiovascular disease, epilepsy, diabetes, skeletal metastases, women and androgenic side effects),

cyproterone (risk of hepatic tumours, **driving**), finasteride (caution in women of childbearing potential, contraception, **male breast cancer**)

- Tetracosactide: different types of Synacthen® tests and how they are undertaken
- Posterior pituitary hormones: vasopressin vs. desmopressin vs. terlipressin, **desmopressin and hyponatraemic convulsions**
- Drugs affecting bone metabolism: **NICE guidance on primary vs. secondary prevention of fractures in postmenopausal women**, options for the management of corticosteroid-induced osteoporosis, bisphosphonates (**osteonecrosis of the jaw, MHRA/CHM advice on atypical femoral fractures, oesophageal reactions, patient counselling for alendronic acid, disodium etidronate, ibandronic acid, risedronate sodium and sodium clodronate, zoledronic acid and renal function**), **NICE guidance on denosumab, strontium ranelate (severe allergic reactions and patient counselling)**

7: Obstetrics, Gynaecology and Urinary Tract Disorders

- Drugs used for the induction of abortion (know different preparations available)
- Drugs used for the induction and augmentation of labour (know different preparations available)
- Drugs used to treat vaginal and vulval candidiasis (different preparations available)
- CHCs: low- vs. high-strength preparations, risk of venous thromboembolism, action to be taken if one or more pills are missed (different requirements for different preparations), delayed application or detached patch, action to be taken if diarrhoea and vomiting occurs after taking the pill, interactions with enzyme inducing drugs (short vs. long courses), special considerations for patients undergoing surgery, **indications for immediate withdrawal of treatment (e.g. sudden chest pain), risk factors for venous thromboembolism and for arterial disease, CHCs and migraines, CHCs and breast/cervical cancers**, changing from one preparation to another, special considerations in secondary amenorrhoea, post-partum, after abortion or miscarriage, know how to find different preparations in the COC table (be familiar with the footnotes)
- POCs: interactions with enzyme-inducing drugs, POCs and surgery,

changing from COC, after childbirth, action to be taken if one or more pills are missed, action to be taken in case of diarrhoea and vomiting, note the cautions and contraindications (such as arterial disease), POCs and breast cancer, **guidance on the use of medroxyprogesterone**, parenteral preparations and intra-uterine preparation of POCs available, preparations of intra-uterine devices available (associated risk of infection and any action required)

- Emergency contraception: time window for effectiveness of different preparations, patient counselling, interactions, contraindications and cautions
- Drugs for urinary retention: acute vs. chronic retention, alpha blockers (hypotension, concomitant blood pressure management, caution in cataract surgery, **driving, first-dose effect**)
- Drugs for urinary frequency, enuresis, and incontinence: duloxetine vs. antimuscarinic drugs, antimuscarinic cautions, contraindications and side effects, **duloxetine and withdrawal symptoms**, **maximum dose of fesoterodine** with concomitant interacting drugs, the management options for nocturnal enuresis in children
- Drugs for erectile dysfunction: **the Selected List Scheme prescribing criteria for PDE-5 inhibitors**, contraindications to PDE-5 inhibitors

8: Malignant Disease and Immunosuppression

- Common side effects of cytotoxic drugs, including their management (particularly oral mucositis, tumour lysis syndrome/hyperuricaemia, nausea and vomiting, bone marrow suppression)
- The use of folinic acid for the prevention of methotrexate-induced adverse effects vs. the treatment of suspected methotrexate overdose
- The use of mesna for the prevention of haemorrhagic cystitis associated with cyclophosphamide and ifosfamide
- Anthracyclines and cardiac effects (**concomitant use with trastuzumab**)
- **Vinca alkaloids: the NPSA alert on the route of administration (never intrathecal), neurotoxicity**
- Bevacizumab and sunitinib: **MHRA/CHM advice on osteonecrosis of the jaw, no intrathecal administration for bortezomib**
- **MHRA/CHM advice on keratitis and ulcerative keratitis associated with the use of epidermal growth factor receptor inhibitors**
- Platinum compounds and renal function/nephrotoxicity

- Protein kinase inhibitors: QT interval prolongation, **dasatinib and pulmonary arterial hypertension**
- **Trastuzumab and cardiotoxicity**
- Antiproliferative immunosuppressants: **bone marrow suppression,** mycophenolate and 'brand specificity'
- **Ciclosporin: nephrotic syndrome, interactions, 'brand specificity'**
- **Tacrolimus: driving, cardiomyopathy, 'brand specificity'**
- Rituximab and severe cytokine release syndrome
- **Lenalidomide: thromboembolism, neutropenia and thrombocytopenia, second primary malignancy, contraception**
- **Thalidomide: thromboembolism, peripheral neuropathy, contraception**
- **Tamoxifen: endometrial changes, risk of thromboembolism**
- **Cyproterone: hepatotoxicity, driving**

9: Nutrition and Blood

- Iron-deficiency anaemias: **iron content of different iron salts (know how to convert between different preparations),** side effects and how they can be managed, patient counselling, indications for parenteral iron and **risk of anaphylaxis with some preparations**
- Drugs used in megaloblastic anaemias: hydroxocobalamin vs. cyanocobalamin, the use of folic acid for the prevention of **neural tube defects (what dose should be taken by women in different risk groups)**
- **Erythropoietins: MHRA/CHM advice on erythropoietins and haemoglobin concentration, MHRA/CHM advice on erythropoietins and tumour progression and survival in patients with cancer, erythropoietins and red cell aplasia, NICE guidance on the use of epoetin alfa, beta and darbepoetin alfa for cancer treatment-induced anaemia,** routes of administration for different preparations
- Sickle-cell disease: principles of pharmaceutical management
- Iron overload: indications for use of desferrioxamine, deferasirox and deferiprone, **deferiprone and blood disorders**
- **G6PD deficiency: the tables of drugs with definite and with possible risk of haemolysis**
- Drugs used in neutropenia: indications for granulocyte-colony stimulating factors, acute respiratory distress syndrome

- **Fluids and electrolytes: be able to find the tables of electrolyte concentrations in IV fluids and electrolyte content in gastrointestinal secretions (use them when calculating the total daily electrolyte requirement for a patient)**
- Potassium: groups of patients in whom the loss of potassium may be associated with particular risks (e.g. patients on digoxin therapy), the management of hyperkalaemia
- Oral vs. IV sodium bicarbonate (indications, doses and rate of administration/frequency of administration)
- Sodium chloride vs. balanced solutions (e.g. Hartmann's solution), risk of hyperchloraemic acidosis
- Parenteral preparations for fluid and electrolyte imbalance: familiarise yourself with different preparations available to be able to prescribe appropriate amounts of each fluid in order to meet the daily fluid/ electrolyte requirements for a specific patient
- Plasma and plasma substitutes: 'colloids' vs. 'crystalloids'
- Calcium and magnesium: indications for calcium supplementation, treatment of severe acute hypocalcaemia or hypocalcaemic tetany, treatment of severe hypercalcaemia and hyperparathyroidism (**note NICE guidance on cinacalcet**), treatment of (symptomatic) hypomagnesaemia, the use of magnesium sulphate in the presence of arrhythmias, myocardial infarction and eclampsia/pre-eclampsia, **know the equivalence of grams (of magnesium sulphate) to millimoles of magnesium ions**
- Phosphorus: the indications of oral vs. parenteral phosphate, know the preparations of phosphate-binding agents available, sevelamer and bowel obstruction
- Vitamin A: the use in pregnancy/breastfeeding
- Vitamin B group: **MHRA/CHM advice on thiamine and serious allergic adverse reactions**, know the regimens of Pabrinex® used in the prophylaxis and treatment of Wernicke's encephalopathy, **pyridoxine and neuropathy with doses of 200 mg or more a day**
- Vitamin D: treatment of simple vitamin D deficiency, treatment of vitamin D deficiency caused by intestinal malabsorption or chronic liver disease, treatment of hypothyroidism-associated hypocalcaemia, the use of alfacalcidol and calcitriol in patients with severe renal impairment (note the use of nanograms as dose units)

- Vitamin K: the use of water-soluble vitamin K (menadiol) in patients with biliary obstruction or hepatic disease, the use of vitamin K to prevent bleeding in neonates
- Multivitamin preparations: Ketovite® tablets vs. liquid, the standard dose of Dalivit® oral drops
- Acute porphyrias: the use of haem arginate in acute porphyria crises, **the tables of drugs that are unsafe for use in acute porphyrias**

10: Musculoskeletal and Joint Diseases

- The principles of pharmaceutical management of osteoarthritis (in conjunction with relevant NICE guidance)
- The principles of pharmaceutical management of rheumatoid arthritis (in conjunction with relevant NICE guidance)
- Non-steroidal anti-inflammatory drugs (NSAIDs): non-selective NSAIDs vs. selective COX-2 inhibitors, side effects, cautions and contraindications (particularly renal impairment, **asthma, NSAIDs and cardiovascular events, NSAIDs and gastrointestinal events**), NSAIDs and pregnancy/breastfeeding, interactions, **CHMP advice on piroxicam, CSM advice on tiaprofenic acid**
- Corticosteroids: the use of corticosteroids in the treatment of rheutmatoid arthritis, polymyalgia rheumatica, systemic lupus erythematosus and ankylosing spondylitis, intra-articular injections
- DMARDs: the onset of response to treatment (2–6 months), first-line drugs, management of juvenile idiopathic arthritis, **sodium aurothiomalate and patient counselling (blood disorders, pulmonary effects, hepatotoxicity), penicillamine (blood counts and urine tests, patient counselling), hydroxychloroquine (epilepsy, G6PD deficiency, acute porphyria, myasthenia gravis, screening for ocular toxicity, calculating the dose using ideal body weight), ciclosporin (additional cautions in rheumatoid arthritis), leflunomide (hepatotoxicity, washout procedure), methotrexate (as in other, earlier chapters, monitoring, interactions, patient counselling, methotrexate treatment booklets), sulfasalazine (blood disorders)**
- Cytokine modulators: **NICE guidance on the use of certolizumab, golimumab, adalimumab, etanercept, infliximab, rituximab, abatacept, anakinra, tocilizumab** (particularly that relating to the treatment of

rheumatoid arthritis), **tuberculosis and blood disorders with certain cytokine modulators, infliximab and hypersensitivity reactions**

- Gout and cytotoxic-induced hyperuricaemia: treatment of acute attacks of gout (no allopurinol, febuxostat or uricosurics), colchicine vs. NSAIDs, long-term control of gout (time window following an acute attack), **NICE guidance on febuxostat**, uricosuric drugs and crystallisation of urate, **allopurinol (rash and hypersensitivity reactions**, renal function, adequate fluid intake), **febuxostat and MHRA/CHM advice on serious hypersensitivity reactions**, indications of allopurinol and rasburicase when used for hyperuricaemia associated with cytotoxic drugs, dosing of rasburicase
- Anticholinesterases: indications, neostigmine and pyridostigmine (asthma, increased salivation, signs of overdose), the **use of atropine to counteract severe cholinergic reactions associated with edrophonium**
- Immunosuppressant treatment in generalised myasthenia gravis (corticosteroids, azathioprine, ciclosporin, mycophenolate)
- Skeletal muscle relaxants: **baclofen (withdrawal, drowsiness, cautions)**, cannabis extract (**Schedule 1 vs. Schedule 2 Controlled Drug**, specific indications, **driving** and other cautions), diazepam (**IM vs. PO vs. IV routes – see the note about IM diazepam injections in the BNF**), **tizanidine (withdrawal and driving)**
- Nocturnal leg cramps and quinine
- Management of extravasation
- Topical NSAIDs and photosensitivity

11: Eye

- Application of eye drops and eye ointments (counselling points, interval between applications)
- Antibacterials: be familiar with a range of antibacterial eye drops available and their clinical indications, the use of antibacterials with corticosteroids for the treatment of undiagnosed 'red eye', the frequency of application for eye drops and eye ointments
- Corticosteroids: 'red eye', 'steroid glaucoma', 'steroid cataract', **NICE guidance on dexamethasone intravitreal implant**, xylometazoline (Otrivine-Antistin®) and angle-closure glaucoma
- Mydriatrics and driving
- Phenylephrine and cardiovascular risk

- Treatment of glaucoma: primary open-angle vs. primary angle-closure glaucoma, stepwise approach to management, **beta blockers (systemic absorption may occur** – note cautions, contraindications and side effects, particularly the use in asthma or COPD), prostaglandin analogues (monitoring for change in eye colour, effects on eye lashes), **sympathomimetics (driving,** cardiovascular disease), carbonic anhydrase inhibitors (monitoring of electrolytes, sulphonamide hypersensitivity)
- Miotics: indications, cautions, driving
- Tear deficiency, ocular lubricants, and astringents: a range of eye drops available, preservative-free vs. non-preservative-free, ensure the strength of hypromellose is stated on the prescription
- **NICE guidance on ranibizumab and pegaptanib**
- **Contact lenses and drug treatment:** the use of unpreserved drops, contact lenses and eye ointment/oily eye drops, systemic drugs (oral contraceptives, drugs that reduce blink rate, drugs that increase or reduce lacrimation, isotretinoin, aspirin, rifampicin and sulfasalazine)

12: Ear, Nose and Oropharynx

- Treatment of otitis externa vs. otitis media and preparations available (indications for systemic antibacterials in otitis media)
- Treatment of acute vs. chronic otitis media
- Caution in patients with perforated tympanic membrane (risk of ototoxicity with topical aminoglycosides)
- The use of sodium chloride 0.9% solution (as a douche or 'sniff') following endonasal surgery
- The treatment of nasal allergies/allergic rhinitis
- Nasal corticosteroids: cautions and side effects (e.g. risk of systemic absorption following prolonged treatment)
- Nasal staphylococci: eradication regimens (the use of chlorhexidine (Naseptin® and nut allergy), neomycin, mupirocin), maximum duration for MRSA eradication regimen with mupirocin
- Drugs acting on oropharynx: unlicensed use of beclomethasone inhaler and betamethasone soluble tablets to treat oral ulceration, the use of doxycycline dispersible tablets for the treatment of recurrent aphthous ulceration
- Oropharyngeal anti-infective drugs: treatment of oral thrush/oropharyngeal candidiasis, duration of treatment

- Chlorhexidine: risk of brown staining of teeth, tongue discolouration, compatibility with toothpastes
- Treatment of dry mouth: drugs that may be causing it (e.g. antispasmodics, tricyclic antidepressants, some antipsychotics, diuretics, radiation therapy), treatment options available, **pilocarpine and driving**

13: Skin

- Creams vs. ointments vs. gels vs. lotions (e.g. gels are particularly suitable for applications to face and scalp)
- **The table of suitable quantities of dermatological preparations to be prescribed for specific areas of the body**
- **The table of excipients that are associated with sensitisation**
- Application of emollients (the risk of folliculitis, sensitisation)
- Treatment of nappy rash
- Topical corticosteroids: choice of formulation (based on clinical presentation), cautions (psoriasis and rebound relapse, prolonged use), contraindications and side effects, **know how to minimise the side effects**, define the 'fingertip unit', **the table of suitable quantities of corticosteroid preparations to be prescribed for specific areas of the body, be familiar with the table of topical corticosteroid preparation potencies**
- Preparations for eczema: treatment options available, **alitretinoin (NICE guidance on alitretinoin for the treatment of severe chronic hand eczema in adults, pregnancy prevention**, contraindications)
- Preparations for psoriasis: treatment options available, **acitretin (pregnancy prevention, hyperlipidaemia)**
- **Drugs affecting the immune response: NICE guidance on tacrolimus, pimecrolimus, adalimumab, etanercept, efalizumab, infliximab and ustekinumab, ciclosporin and additional cautions in atopic dermatitis and psoriasis, ustekinumab and tuberculosis**
- Acne and rosacea: treatments of mild to moderate, moderate to severe and severe acne, treatment of rosacea, cautions with topical retinoids, **co-cyprindiol and venous thromboembolism, isotretinoin (pregnancy prevention, counselling, monitoring, side effects)**
- Sunscreen preparations: definition of sun protection factor, UVA vs. UVB protection, options available, guidance on optimum photoprotection and use of sunscreens, photodamage

- Finasteride and minoxidil for androgenetic alopecia
- The principles of treatment of fungal skin and nail infections
- The topical treatment of labial herpes simplex infections (cold sores)
- The treatment of scabies and head lice (**special attention to be paid to the table of suitable quantities of parasiticidal preparations**)
- **The use of povidone-iodine on large open wounds (risk of systemic adverse effects)**

14: Immunological Products and Vaccines

- **Different types of vaccines (live attenuated, inactivated, detoxified exotoxins and extracts of a microorganism)**
- **The table of excipients that have been implicated in hypersensitivity reactions**
- Other contraindications to vaccines (e.g. live vaccines and immunosuppression
- Side effects of vaccines
- **Post-immunisation pyrexia in infants**
- **Predisposition to neurological problems and vaccines**
- **Be able to navigate the immunisation schedule** (including vaccination of preterm babies)
- Vaccines that are recommended for asplenic patients
- Be aware of the chapter focused on relevant vaccines (e.g. diphtheria vaccines) and preparations available (e.g. Pediacel®)
- The clinical indications of human normal immunoglobulin
- Know which disease-specific immunoglobulins are available
- **Immunisation and international travel: able to identify the vaccines required for patients travelling to a certain part of the world**

15: Anaesthesia

- Surgery and long-term medication: corticosteroid requirements, drugs that are not to be discontinued prior to surgery, drugs that are to be withheld prior to surgery (time frame before and after surgery), risks associated with these drugs if they are not withheld, prophylaxis of acid aspiration
- **Halothane and hepatotoxicity**
- The use of nitrous oxide for analgesia (note the cautions)
- Overdosage with midazolam used for conscious sedation

Appendix 1: Interactions

- Pharmacodynamic vs. pharmacokinetic interactions
- **Information about cytochrome P450 interactions reported in the BNF**
- Be able to navigate the interactions table to find the relevant interaction(s)

Appendix 3: Cautionary and Advisory Labels

- Know how to find the cautionary/advisory labels for different medicines (may be required for patient counselling purposes)

Appendix 4: Intravenous Additives

- Common incompatibilities (factors that may be implicated, e.g. pH changes, beta-lactams, blood products, IV fat emulsions)
- Method of administration (using ready-prepared infusions, 'layering' effect with potassium chloride, the use of intermittent infusions, addition via the drip tubing)
- **Be able to find the information about the infusion of a relevant medicine in the table**

Other

- **Cardiovascular Risk Prediction Charts**: which patient groups are excluded from these charts, when should these charts not be used to determine the need for an anti-hypertensive or a lipid-lowering medication, the definition of 'current smoker', how to calculate total cholesterol/HDL-C level when the HDL-C value is not available, the additional cardiovascular risks for patients from ethnic minorities and those with a family history of premature cardiovascular disease, differences from **the NICE clinical guideline 67, be able to use the charts to determine an individual's risk of cardiovascular disease**
- Medical emergencies in the community: **be able to find the relevant emergency treatment pathway**
- Approximate conversions and units, and prescribing for children
- **The table of E numbers**

Reference

1. British Medical Association; Royal Pharmaceutical Society. *British National Formulary 65*. London: Pharmaceutical Press; 2013.

CPD with Radcliffe

You can now use a selection of our books to achieve CPD (Continuing Professional Development) points through directed reading.

We provide a free online form and downloadable certificate for your appraisal portfolio. Look for the CPD logo and register with us at: www.radcliffehealth.com/cpd

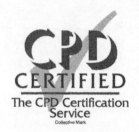